1998
YEAR BOOK OF
FAMILY PRACTICE®

Statement of Purpose

The YEAR BOOK Service

The YEAR BOOK series was devised in 1901 by practicing health professionals who observed that the literature of medicine and related disciplines had become so voluminous that no one individual could read and place in perspective every potential advance in a major specialty. In the final decade of the 20th century, this recognition is more acutely true than it was in 1901.

More than merely a series of books, YEAR BOOK volumes are the tangible results of a unique service designed to accomplish the following:

- to *survey* a wide range of journals of proven value
- to *select* from those journals papers representing significant advances and statements of important clinical principles
- to provide *abstracts* of those articles that are readable, convenient summaries of their key points
- to provide *commentary* about those articles to place them in perspective

These publications grow out of a unique process that calls on the talents of outstanding authorities in clinical and fundamental disciplines, trained literature specialists, and professional writers, all supported by the resources of Mosby, the world's preeminent publisher for the health professions.

The Literature Base

Mosby and its editors survey more than 1,000 journals published worldwide, covering the full range of the health professions. On an annual basis, the publisher examines usage patterns and polls its expert authorities to add new journals to the literature base and to delete journals that are no longer useful as potential YEAR BOOK sources.

The Literature Survey

The publisher's team of literature specialists, all of whom are trained and experienced health professionals, examines every original, peer-reviewed article in each journal issue. More than 250,000 articles per year are scanned systematically, including title, text, illustrations, tables, and references. Each scan is compared, article by article, to the search strategies that the publisher has developed in consultation with the 270 outside experts who form the pool of YEAR BOOK editors. A given article may be reviewed by any number of editors, from one to a dozen or more, regardless of the discipline for which the paper was originally published. In turn, each editor who receives the article reviews it to determine whether the article should be included in the YEAR BOOK. This decision is based on the article's inherent quality, its probable usefulness to readers of that YEAR BOOK, and the editor's goal to represent a balanced picture of a given field in each volume of the YEAR BOOK. In addition, the editor indicates when to include figures and tables from the article to help the YEAR BOOK reader better understand the information.

Of the quarter million articles scanned each year, only 5% are selected for detailed analysis within the YEAR BOOK series, thereby assuring readers of the high value of every selection.

The Abstract

The publisher's abstracting staff is headed by a seasoned medical professional and includes individuals with training in the life sciences, medicine, and other areas, plus extensive experience in writing for the health professions and related industries. Each selected article is assigned to a specific writer on this abstracting staff. The abstracter, guided in many cases by notations supplied by the expert editor, writes a structured, condensed summary designed so that the reader can rapidly acquire the essential information contained in the article.

The Commentary

The YEAR BOOK editorial boards, sometimes assisted by guest commentators, write comments that place each article in perspective for the reader. This provides the reader with the equivalent of a personal consultation with a leading international authority—an opportunity to better understand the value of the article and to benefit from the authority's thought processes in assessing the article.

Additional Editorial Features

The editorial boards of each YEAR BOOK organize the abstracts and comments to provide a logical and satisfying sequence of information. To enhance the organization, editors also provide introductions to sections or individual chapters, comments linking a number of abstracts, citations to additional literature, and other features.

The published YEAR BOOK contains enhanced bibliographic citations for each selected article, including extended listings of multiple authors and identification of author affiliations. Each YEAR BOOK contains a Table of Contents specific to that year's volume. From year to year, the Table of Contents for a given YEAR BOOK will vary depending on developments within the field.

Every YEAR BOOK contains a list of the journals from which papers have been selected. This list represents a subset of the more than 1,000 journals surveyed by the publisher and occasionally reflects a particularly pertinent article from a journal that is not surveyed on a routine basis.

Finally, each volume contains a comprehensive subject index and an index to authors of each selected paper.

The 1998 Year Book Series

Year Book of Allergy, Asthma, and Clinical Immunology: Drs. Rosenwasser, Borish, Gelfand, Leung, Nelson, and Szefler

Year Book of Anesthesiology and Pain Management®: Drs. Tinker, Abram, Chestnut, Roizen, Rothenberg, and Wood

Year Book of Cardiology®: Drs. Schlant, Collins, Gersh, Graham, Kaplan, and Waldo

Year Book of Chiropractic®: Dr. Lawrence

Year Book of Critical Care Medicine®: Drs. Parrillo, Balk, Calvin, Franklin, and Shapiro

Year Book of Dentistry®: Drs. Meskin, Berry, Jeffcoat, Leinfelder, Roser, Summitt, and Zakariasen

Year Book of Dermatologic Surgery®: Drs. Greenway, Papadopoulos, Whitaker, and Barrett

Year Book of Dermatology®: Dr. Thiers

Year Book of Diagnostic Radiology®: Drs. Osborn, Groskin, Dalinka, Maynard, Pentecost, Rebner, Ros, Smirniotopoulos, and Young

Year Book of Drug Therapy®: Drs. Lasagna and Weintraub

Year Book of Emergency Medicine®: Drs. Wagner, Dronen, Davidson, King, Niemann, and Roberts

Year Book of Endocrinology®: Drs. Bagdade, Braverman, Horton, Kannan, Landsberg, Molitch, Morley, Nathan, Odell, Poehlman, Rogol, and Ryan

Year Book of Family Practice®: Drs. Berg, Bowman, Davidson, Dexter, and Scherger

Year Book of Gastroenterology®: Drs. Aliperti and Fleshman

Year Book of Geriatrics and Gerontology®: Drs. Beck, Burton, Ostwald, Rabins, Reuben, Roth, Shapiro, and Whitehouse

Year Book of Hand Surgery®: Drs. Amadio and Hentz

Year Book of Hematology®: Drs. Spivak, Bell, Ness, Quesenberry, Wiernik, and Horowitz

Year Book of Infectious Diseases: Drs. Keusch, Barza, Bennish, Poutsiaka, Skolnik, and Snydman

Year Book of Medicine®: Drs. Klahr, Cline, McCallum, Frishman, Utiger, Malawista, Mandell, and Jett

Year Book of Neonatal and Perinatal Medicine®: Drs. Fanaroff, Maisels, and Stevenson

Year Book of Nephrology, Hypertension, and Mineral Metabolism: Drs. Schwab, Bennett, Emmett, Hostetter, Kumar, and Toto

Year Book of Neurology and Neurosurgery®: Drs. Bradley and Gibbs

Year Book of Nuclear Medicine®: Drs. Gottschalk, Blaufox, Neumann, Strauss, and Zubal

Year Book of Obstetrics, Gynecology, and Women's Health: Drs. Mishell, Herbst, and Kirschbaum

Year Book of Occupational and Environmental Medicine®: Drs. Emmett, Frank, Gochfeld, and Hessl

Year Book of Oncology®: Drs. Ozols, Eisenberg, Glatstein, Loehrer, Tallman, and Wiersma

Year Book of Ophthalmology®: Drs. Wilson, Augsburger, Cohen, Eagle, Grossman, Laibson, Maguire, Nelson, Penne, Rapuano, Sergott, Spaeth, Tipperman, Ms. Gosfield, and Ms. Salmon

Year Book of Orthopedics®: Drs. Morrey, Beauchamp, Currier, Tolo, Trigg, Swiontkowski

Year Book of Otolaryngology–Head and Neck Surgery®: Drs. Paparella and Holt

Year Book of Pathology and Laboratory Medicine®: Drs. Raab, Cohen, Olson, Sirgi, and Stanley

Year Book of Pediatrics®: Dr. Stockman

Year Book of Plastic, Reconstructive, and Aesthetic Surgery®: Drs. Miller, Bartlett, Garner, McKinney, Ruberg, Salisbury, and Smith

Year Book of Psychiatry and Applied Mental Health®: Drs. Talbott, Ballanger, Frances, Lydiard, Meltzer, Schowalter, and Tasman

Year Book of Pulmonary Disease®: Drs. Jett, Maurer, Ryu, Strollo, and Wenzel

Year Book of Rheumatology®: Drs. Panush, Hadler, LeRoy, Liang, Reichlin, Simon, and Weinblatt

Year Book of Sports Medicine®: Drs. Shephard, Drinkwater, Eichner, Torg, Alexander, and Mr. George

Year Book of Surgery®: Drs. Copeland, Bland, Deitch, Eberlein, Howard, Luce, Seeger, Souba, and Sugarbaker

Year Book of Thoracic and Cardiovascular Surgery®: Drs. Ginsberg, Wechsler, and Williams

Year Book of Urology®: Drs. Andriole and Coplen

Year Book of Vascular Surgery®: Dr. Porter

1998

The Year Book of FAMILY PRACTICE®

Editor
Alfred O. Berg, M.D., M.P.H.

Associate Editors
Marjorie A. Bowman, M.D., M.P.A.
Robert C. Davidson, M.D., M.P.H.
William W. Dexter, M.D.
Joseph E. Scherger, M.D., M.P.H.

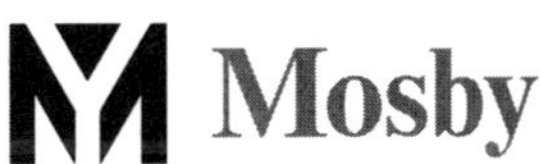 **Mosby**

St. Louis Baltimore Boston Carlsbad Naples New York Philadelphia Portland London
Madrid Mexico City Singapore Sydney Tokyo Toronto Wiesbaden

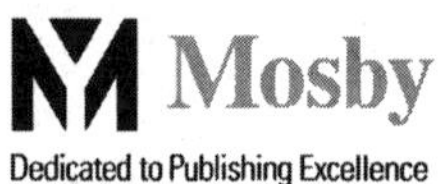 Mosby

Dedicated to Publishing Excellence

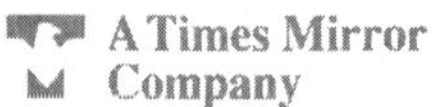 A Times Mirror
Company

Associate Publisher: Gretchen C. Murphy
Developmental Editor: Jaime Chatman
Manuscript Editor: Pat Costigan
Project Supervisor, Production: Joy Moore
Production Assistant: Karie House
Manager, Literature Services: Idelle L. Winer
Illustrations and Permissions Coordinator: Chidi C. Ukabam

1998 EDITION

Printed in the United States of America
Composition by Reed Technology and Information Services, Inc.
Printing/binding by Maple–Vail

Editorial Office:
Mosby, Inc.
11830 Westline Industrial Drive
St. Louis, MO 63146
Customer Service: customer.support@mosby.com
          www.mosby.com/Mosby/CustomerSupport/index.html

International Standard Serial Number: 0147–1996
International Standard Book Number: 0–8151–9629–6

Editorial Board

Editor
Alfred O. Berg, M.D., M.P.H.
Professor and Associate Chair, Director, Affiliated Residency Network, Department of Family Medicine, University of Washington, Seattle, Washington

Associate Editors
Marjorie A. Bowman, M.D., M.P.A.
Professor and Chair, Department of Family Practice and Community Medicine, University of Pennsylvania Health Systems, Philadelphia, Pennsylvania

Robert C. Davidson, M.D., M.P.H.
Associate Professor, Department of Family and Community Medicine; Director, Family Medicine Center, University of California, Davis, California

William W. Dexter, M.D.
Director, Sports Medicine; Assistant Director, Family Practice Residency, Maine Medical Center, Portland, Maine

Joseph E. Scherger, M.D., M.P.H.
Professor and Chair, Department of Family Medicine; Associate Dean for Clinical Affairs, University of California, Irvine, California

Table of Contents

Journals Represented

Mosby and its editors survey more than 1,000 journals for its abstract and commentary publications. From these journals, the editors select the articles to be abstracted. Journals represented in this YEAR BOOK are listed below.

Academic Emergency Medicine
Acta Dermato-Venereologica
Acta Neurologica Scandinavica
Acta Obstetricia et Gynecologica Scandinavica
Acta Ophthalmologica Scandinavica
Acta Paediatrica
Age and Ageing
American Family Physician
American Journal of Cardiology
American Journal of Clinical Nutrition
American Journal of Emergency Medicine
American Journal of Epidemiology
American Journal of Gastroenterology
American Journal of Kidney Diseases
American Journal of Medicine
American Journal of Obstetrics and Gynecology
American Journal of Preventive Medicine
American Journal of Psychiatry
American Journal of Public Health
Annals of Allergy, Asthma, & Immunology
Annals of Emergency Medicine
Annals of Internal Medicine
Annals of Surgery
Archives of Dermatology
Archives of Disease in Childhood
Archives of Family Medicine
Archives of General Psychiatry
Archives of Internal Medicine
Archives of Neurology
Archives of Otolaryngology-Head and Neck Surgery
Archives of Pediatrics and Adolescent Medicine
Archives of Surgery
Arthritis and Rheumatism
British Journal of Cancer
British Journal of General Practice
British Journal of Obstetrics and Gynaecology
British Journal of Psychiatry
British Journal of Sports Medicine
British Journal of Urology
British Medical Journal
Canadian Family Physician
Canadian Journal of Surgery
Canadian Medical Association Journal
Chest
Circulation
Clinical Infectious Diseases
Clinical Pediatrics

Clinical Pharmacology and Therapeutics
Contact Dermatitis
Contraception
Dermatology
Diabetes
Diabetes Care
Diabetic Medicine
European Heart Journal
European Journal of Cancer
Family Medicine
Fertility and Sterility
Gastroenterology
Gerontologist
Gut
Hypertension
International Journal of Cancer
International Journal of Dermatology
International Journal of Epidemiology
International Journal of Obesity
Investigative Ophthalmology and Visual Science
Israel Journal of Medical Sciences
Journal of Adolescent Health
Journal of Allergy and Clinical Immunology
Journal of Bone and Joint Surgery (British Volume)
Journal of Clinical Endocrinology and Metabolism
Journal of Clinical Microbiology
Journal of Family Practice
Journal of General Internal Medicine
Journal of Hypertension
Journal of Infectious Diseases
Journal of Marriage and the Family
Journal of Nervous and Mental Disease
Journal of Otolaryngology
Journal of Pain and Symptom Management
Journal of Pediatrics
Journal of Reproductive Medicine
Journal of Sports Sciences
Journal of Urology
Journal of the American Board of Family Practice
Journal of the American College of Cardiology
Journal of the American Geriatrics Society
Journal of the American Medical Association
Journal of the National Cancer Institute
Journal of the Neurological Sciences
Kidney International
Lancet
Maturitas
Mayo Clinic Proceedings
Medical Care
Medical Economics
Medical Journal of Australia
Neurology

New England Journal of Medicine
New Zealand Medical Journal
ORL (Journal for Oto-Rhino-Laryngology)
Obstetrics and Gynecology
Occupational and Environmental Medicine
Optometry and Vision Science
Orthopedics
Otolaryngology — Head and Neck Surgery
PACE — Pacing and Clinical Electrophysiology
Pediatric Infectious Disease Journal
Pediatrics
Pharmacotherapy
Psychiatric Services
Psychosomatic Medicine
Public Health Reports
Research Quarterly for Exercise and Sport
S.A.M.J./S.A.M.T. — South African Medical Journal
Southern Medical Journal
Sports Medicine
Stroke
Urology

STANDARD ABBREVIATIONS

The following terms are abbreviated in this edition: acquired immunodeficiency syndrome (AIDS), cardiopulmonary resuscitation (CPR), central nervous system (CNS), cerebrospinal fluid (CSF), computed tomography (CT), deoxyribonucleic acid (DNA), electrocardiography (ECG), health maintenance organization (HMO), human immunodeficiency virus (HIV), intensive care unit (ICU), intramuscular (IM), intravenous (IV), magnetic resonance (MR) imaging (MRI), and ribonucleic acid (RNA).

NOTE

The YEAR BOOK OF FAMILY PRACTICE is a literature survey service providing abstracts of articles published in the professional literature. Every effort is made to assure the accuracy of the information presented in these pages. Neither the editors nor the publisher of the YEAR BOOK OF FAMILY PRACTICE can be responsible for errors in the original materials. The editors' comments are their own opinions. Mention of specific products within this publication does not constitute endorsement.

To facilitate the use of the YEAR BOOK OF FAMILY PRACTICE as a reference tool, all illustrations and tables included in this publication are now identified as they appear in the original article. This change is meant to help the reader recognize that any illustration or table appearing in the YEAR BOOK OF FAMILY PRACTICE may be only one of many in the original article. For this reason, figure and table numbers will often appear to be out of sequence within the YEAR BOOK OF FAMILY PRACTICE.

Foreword

The 1998 YEAR BOOK OF FAMILY PRACTICE turns 21 this year, coming of age during a time of rapid change for just about everything family physicians do. In recent years, the editors have expanded the scope of the YEAR BOOK OF FAMILY PRACTICE to incorporate new fields of medical practice and areas of activity such as HIV infection, clinical practice policies, health economics, and cost containment.

This year the editors are responding to new interest in making clinical practice "evidence-based." Family physicians have always used evidence, of course, but standards and definitions are changing. Increasingly, "evidence-based" practice means paying attention to intervention studies that are of the highest scientific quality, usually interpreted to mean well-constructed and meticulously conducted randomized controlled trials (RCTs).

This year the editors made a special effort to collect RCTs that have the potential for making a real clinical difference. At the conclusion of each chapter introduction, the abstract numbers in that chapter reporting RCTs are listed. The commentaries point out strengths and weaknesses of the studies that are abstracted.

Readers will note that RCTs are a small minority of the articles presented. Many important clinical topics will never be subjected to an RCT. The 1998 YEAR BOOK OF FAMILY PRACTICE also presents the best descriptive studies we could find, along with provocative case series, case reports, rigorous reviews, and thoughtful editorials.

The process the editors used in selecting and presenting the articles in this volume from among the 10,000 articles in nearly 1,000 journals that we reviewed has not changed. We have grouped articles in chapters and sections and have cross-referenced other articles of interest. The introductions for each chapter give a quick overview of the topics that follow. Full text copies of articles can be obtained through your local medical library.

In the aggregate, the editors have selected the best and most interesting medical literature that we came across and attempted a new focus on high-quality RCTs. We hope that readers find useful and thought-provoking material here and will share the editors' enthusiam for this distinctive publishing enterprise.

Alfred O. Berg, M.D., M.P.H.

1 Cardiovascular Diseases

Introduction

The editors comment on many provocative articles in this section, opening with studies linking hypertension to birthweight and sodium intake, and the effects of sour milk on blood pressure control.

The section on coronary artery disease risk covers secular trends and such unconventional risk factors as serum iron, plasma homocysteine, and anger, in addition to the more conventional ones such as physical activity, alcohol, and diet.

The following 5 articles address angina and myocardial infarction, followed by a selection of 4 articles on secondary prevention (i.e., after a primary event): lipid-lowering agents, aspirin, digoxin, and β-blockers.

The final 2 sections cover other vascular diseases (claudication, DVT, and abdominal aortic aneurysm) and miscellaneous articles on defining normal sinus rhythm, treating atrial fibrillation in the elderly, and (mostly) reassuring advice about pacemakers and cellular telephones.

Randomized controlled trials: Abstracts 1–3, 1–4, 1–7, 1–8, 1–18, 1–26, 1–27, 1–28, and 1–31.

Alfred O. Berg, M.D., M.P.H.

Hypertension

Is Blood Pressure Inversely Related to Birth Weight? The Strength of Evidence From a Systematic Review of the Literature

Law CM, Shiell AW (Univ of Southampton, England)
J Hypertens 14:935–941, 1996
1–1

Purpose.—It has been suggested that adult cardiovascular disease may be linked to undernutrition during fetal and infant life. However, this theory is controversial. Blood pressure is the most widely studied of the various cardiovascular risk factors. The possible link between blood pressure and birth weight was examined in a retrospective literature review.

Methods.—The review included 34 studies, published since 1956, examining the relationship between blood pressure and birth weight. The studies included more than 66,000 individuals, ranging in age from 0 to 71 years. Fifteen studies used multiple regression analyses, with adjustment for current size; 12 used other quantitative analyses; and 5 used repeated measures.

Results.—Most studies found that blood pressure declined as birth weight increased, independent of current size. This was so for both children and adults, although the findings for adolescents were inconsistent. Newborns showed a positive association between blood pressure and birth weight. The few studies with repeated measures supported the link between blood pressure and birth weight as the research subjects aged from childhood to adolescence—none of these studies included adults. The relationship held across methods of analysis, academic research groups, and countries.

Conclusions.—The available evidence suggests an inverse relationship between birth weight and blood pressure in children and adults. This relationship holds in newborns but is inconsistent in adolescents, perhaps because of the unusual growth dynamics seen during these phases of growth. The authors call for research into the mechanisms underlying the link between birth weight and blood pressure.

▶ I have read with interest several articles on the relationship between birth weight and subsequent blood pressure. I selected this article because it is the most thorough that I have seen. It is a retrospective literature review combining 34 studies with over 66,000 study subjects.

This exhaustive review of the world's literature regarding this issue finds a very strong inverse relationship between birth weight and subsequent blood pressure readings. Unfortunately, the authors could find no plausible explanation from this review of the world's literature on why blood pressure fell with increasing birth weight.

In practical terms, there is very little practicing physicians can do with this information. Low birth weight infants are at higher risk for elevated blood pressure and subsequent hypertension. There is no information that any innovations might alter the course of this. In theory, if we more closely follow up individuals with low birth weight, we might advise them more strongly than usual to monitor their blood pressure and use known preventive measures for hypertension. However, there's no evidence that this will change the blood pressure of these individuals in later life.

R.C. Davidson, M.D., M.P.H.

Heritability of Salt Sensitivity in Black Americans
Svetkey LP, McKeown SP, Wilson AF (Duke Univ, Durham, NC; Louisiana State Univ, New Orleans, NIH, Baltimore, Md)
Hypertension 28:854–858, 1996   1–2

Introduction.—A change in blood pressure in response to changes in salt and water homeostasis is the definition of salt sensitivity. Generally considered a hallmark of hypertension in blacks, salt sensitivity is found in 73% of hypertensive and 36% of normotensive blacks. There is a suggestion of a genetic influence on salt sensitivity if the higher prevalence of salt sensitivity in blacks than in whites is taken into account. The extent to which salt sensitivity is correlated in black families was determined and its heritability was estimated.

Methods.—Twenty black families, comprising 30 parent-offspring pairs and 115 adult sibling pairs, participated in the study. The mean age was 36 years, and 66% of the participants were women. Using an IV sodium-loading, furosemide volume-depletion protocol, hypertensive and normotensive adults were phenotyped according to their salt sensitivity. The difference between sodium-loaded and volume-depleted blood pressure was the definition of salt sensitivity.

Results.—Overall average systolic pressure was 118 ± 15 mm Hg, average diastolic pressure was 79 ± 12 mm Hg, and mean arterial pressure was 92 ± 12 mm Hg. From the sodium-loaded state, systolic pressure decreased by an average of 8.6% ± 8%, diastolic pressure decreased by 0.9% ± 9%, and mean arterial pressure decreased by 4% ± 9%. An age adjustment was made to calculate the correlation coefficient because of the known relation between salt sensitivity and age. An underlying genetic heterogeneity of salt sensitivity may be reflected by the higher correlations in equal weight to pedigrees than to pairs. There were 3-fold correlations for mean arterial pressure and systolic blood pressure responses in some families, which suggested high heritability for these traits.

Conclusions.—There is a heritable component of salt sensitivity. A foundation is laid by these data for a comprehensive search for hypertensive genes in the black population.

▶ Numerous studies have found a high correlation between black Americans, hypertension, and salt sensitivity. Because this high correlation between salt sensitivity and hypertension carries through all socioeconomic classes of black Americans, we have assumed that it is transmitted on a heritable basis.

This was a unique study of 20 black American families. Both hypertensive and normotensive adults were studied with a standard protocol to determine salt sensitivity. The findings strongly suggest a heritable component of salt sensitivity. When this direct evidence is combined with the known epidemiologic data, I think it is safe to conclude that salt sensitivity in blacks is transmitted on a heritable basis.

The importance of this study to me is the reminder to work with my black hypertensive patients to try to modify and reduce risk factors for hypertension in their children. Low-salt diets, weight maintenance, and avoidance of smoking are more important than ever in these children because of the increased risk they have inherited from their hypertensive parents.

R.C. Davidson, M.D., M.P.H.

Comparison of Single Versus Multiple Lifestyle Interventions: Are the Antihypertensive Effects of Exercise Training and Diet-induced Weight Loss Additive?

Gordon NF, Scott CB, Levine BD (Presbyterian Hosp of Dallas; Univ of Texas, Dallas; Candler Hosp, Savannah, Ga)
Am J Cardiol 79:763–767, 1997   1–3

Background.—Lifestyle modifications are widely used as definitive or adjunctive therapy for high blood pressure. Separately, aerobic exercise training and diet-induced weight loss have been shown to reduce blood pressure. However, the possible additive effect of their combined use is unknown. This issue was addressed in a 3-way randomized trial.

Methods.—Fifty-five sedentary, overweight adults with high-normal blood pressure or stage 1 or 2 hypertension participated in the study. The patients were assigned into 3 intervention groups, each intervention to last 12 weeks. One group was assigned aerobic exercise only; they exercised for 30 to 45 minutes 3 to 5 days a week at 60% to 85% of maximal heart rate. Another group was assigned to dietary modification only, with reduction of energy intake and dietary fat for the purpose of weight loss. The third group was assigned to both exercise training and dietary modification. Outcome measures included blood pressure, body weight, and maximal graded treadmill testing.

Results.—Seven patients dropped out of the study for various reasons, leaving 48 patients for analysis. The mean reduction in body weight was 7 kg with exercise plus diet, compared with 6 kg with diet only and 1 kg with exercise only. Patients assigned to both diet and exercise also had a greater improvement in maximal oxygen uptake: 4.3 mL/kg/min, compared with 1.9 mL/kg/min with diet only and 2.5 mL/kg/min with exercise only. However, there was no significant difference between groups in the mean blood pressure reduction achieved: 12.5/8 mm Hg with exercise plus diet, 11/7.5 mm Hg with diet only, and 10/6 mm Hg with exercise only.

Conclusion.—Although each is effective in reducing hypertension, aerobic exercise training and diet-induced weight loss do not have additive effects on blood pressure. In terms of blood pressure only, no greater effect is to be expected when both diet and exercise are prescribed for patients with high-normal blood pressure or stage 1 or 2 hypertension. However, both interventions have important benefits aside from their antihypertensive effect.

▶ How many hundreds of times have I given my talk to patients with hypertension regarding nonpharmacologic ways that they can reduce their elevated blood pressure. Exercise and diet are always 2 of the most important. I would include alcohol and smoking as 2 other high priority items.

This study compared the efficacy of diet alone, exercise alone, and a combination of the 2 on blood pressure reduction. The authors found that each intervention resulted in a lowering of both systolic and diastolic blood pressure. However, they found no additive effect when the 2 were combined.

Unfortunately, the number of study subjects in this protocol was quite low, each arm of the research protocol having between 14 and 19 subjects. There was also no way to measure the sustainability of blood pressure reduction in this population. These were some secondary effects in the exercise group which appeared very significant to me. These included a significant increase in maximal oxygen uptake. I think we should continue to vigorously counsel our patients with hypertension on the positive aspects of both appropriate exercise and weight reduction and not be dissuaded by whether or not they are additive.

R.C. Davidson, M.D., M.P.H.

A Placebo-controlled Study of the Effect of Sour Milk on Blood Pressure in Hypertensive Subjects
Hata Y, Yamamoto M, Ohni M, et al (Kyorin Univ, Tokyo; Calpis Food Industry Co Ltd, Kanagawa, Japan)
Am J Clin Nutr 64:767–771, 1996   1–4

Background.—Dietary treatments have an important role to play in the control of blood pressure in patients with hypertension. Previous experiments suggest that sour milk—skim milk fermented with a starter culture containing *Lactobacillus helveticus* and *Saccharomyces cerevisae*—has antihypertensive activity in rats. The effects of sour milk on blood pressure were studied in elderly research subjects with hypertension.

Methods.—The randomized, placebo-controlled study included 30 elderly patients with hypertension, most of whom were receiving antihypertensive medication. They were assigned to 1 of 2 treatment groups: 1 group received the sour milk product, 95 mL/day, for 8 weeks, whereas the other group received the same amount of artificially acidified milk. Blood pressure and serum biochemical values were measured before, during, and after treatment.

Results.—Systolic blood pressure decreased significantly in the research subjects drinking sour milk, by 9 mm Hg at 4 weeks and 14 mm Hg at 8 weeks. Diastolic blood pressure decreased by 7 mm Hg at 8 weeks. In contrast, the research subjects drinking placebo milk showed no significant declines in blood pressure. Patients in the sour milk group tended to have greater reductions in systolic and diastolic pressure. Neither group showed any significant changes in pulse rate, body weight, blood serum values, or other variables.

Conclusions.—Dietary supplementation with sour milk appears to aid blood pressure control for elderly patients with hypertension. The mechanism of action likely involves 2 kinds of tripeptides that act as angiotensin-converting enzyme (ACE) inhibitors. No side effects are noted, even in patients who are already taking ACE inhibitors.

▶ The editors of this YEAR BOOK review hundreds of articles to select the 65 or so that each of us include. This article on the relationship between intake of sour milk and blood pressure caught my interest because of its incongruity with my understanding of hypertension. I thought it might also interest you, the reader.

This research project from Japan studied a small group of 30 elderly patients with hypertension. They were able to use a sour milk placebo to study the effect of sour milk on systolic and diastolic blood pressure. They found a significant reduction in both systolic and diastolic blood pressure because of ingestion of sour milk. The daily dose was 100 mL of sour milk.

There are some major problems with this study. The first is that it does not look at any of the potential side effects of adding 100 mL of sour milk to an individual's diet, 1 of which could be changes in the serum cholesterol level. This study was also supported by a Japanese food industry company that I presume markets sour milk. I chuckle when I envision the look on my patients' faces when I suggest that they add sour milk to their regimen but eliminate all other lipids. Oh well, perhaps my cynicism is just all sour milk.

R.C. Davidson, M.D., M.P.H.

Higher Incidence of Discontinuation of Angiotensin Converting Enzyme Inhibitors Due to Cough in Black Subjects

Elliott WJ (Rush-Presbyterian-St Luke's Med Ctr, Chicago)
Clin Pharmacol Ther 60:582–588, 1996

1–5

Background.—Researchers have recently suggested that race or ethnicity may play a role in the differential rates of angioedema with angiotensin converting enzyme (ACE) inhibitors, the risk being higher among black patients. The prevalences of ACE inhibitor–associated cough in different racial and ethnic groups were investigated.

Methods.—Eight hundred ninety-two patients receiving their first dose of ACE inhibitor were studied. Surveillance for cough was begun in 1986 and included a routine trial of sinusitis therapy, followed by withdrawal and rechallenge before drug discontinuation.

Findings.—The prevalence of cough necessitating ACE inhibitor discontinuation was 9.6 per 100 among black patients and 2.4 per 100 among nonblacks. The discontinuation rates of the 3 most commonly used ACE inhibitors—captopril, enalapril, and lisinopril—did not differ significantly. Women more frequently had cough. After adjustment for baseline differences, black patients had a relative risk of 2.58 of ACE inhibitor discontinuation because of cough.

Conclusion.—There appear to be racial or ethnic differences in the prevalence of cough caused by ACE inhibitor therapy. Although a race-related difference in ACE gene polymorphism has been proposed, further research is needed to determine the biological reason for and pathophysiology of these differences.

▶ I included this article because it quantifies an observation that I have made in my own practice. It seemed to me that my black patients had more trouble with cough related to ACE inhibitors. This author studied a registry of patients in a tertiary hypertension clinic. Nearly 10% of the black patients discontinued their use of ACE inhibitors because of cough. Only 2% of white patients had similar problems.

There are some problems with the methodology in this study. There is a very skewed patient population in a tertiary hypertension clinic. There was also a retrospective analysis of charts, and there was no randomization or other characteristics that would make the findings more statistically valid. However, the fourfold increase in incidence among the black population is hard to explain by any reason other than ethnicity.

Because many black hypertensive patients have high renin levels, one would expect that ACE inhibitors might be a good choice for many of these patients. However, the increased incidence of cough may be a limiting factor in our ability to use this medication.

R.C. Davidson, M.D., M.P.H.

Safety and Feasibility of Dobutamine-Atropine Stress Testing in Hypertensive Patients
Elhendy A, van Domburg RT, Roelandt JRTC, et al (Erasmus Univ, Rotterdam, The Netherlands)
Hypertension 29:1232–1239, 1997   1–6

Objective.—Although dobutamine-atropine stress echocardiography (DSE) is being more commonly used to diagnose and evaluate function in coronary artery disease, its effect in hypertensive patients has not been investigated. The safety and feasibility of DSE for evaluation of myocardial ischemia in hypertensive patients unable to perform exercise stress testing was compared with results of normotensive patients.

Methods.—Dobutamine-atropine stress echocardiography was performed in 446 hypertensive (group 1) and 718 normotensive patients (group 2) for evaluation of myocardial ischemia. The test was considered feasible if the patient could reach 85% of the maximal heart rate for the patient's age or an ischemic endpoint was reached. Lesions were quantified by coronary angiography 3 months after DSE. A stenosis diameter exceeding 50% was defined as significant coronary artery disease. Results from the 2 groups were compared statistically.

Results.—Compared with baseline values, DSE significantly increased heart rate (72 compared with 134 beats/min) and systolic pressure (133 compared with 137 mm Hg) in both groups. Diastolic pressure decreased significantly from 76 to 72 mm Hg. Rate pressure product at peak stress was similar for both groups, as were heart rates before and after administration of atropine. Group 1 had higher resting and peak stress blood pressures. Group 2 had a significant increase in systolic pressure at peak stress. A total of 305 patients experienced angina. Side effects included nausea, flushing, dizziness, anxiety, headache, and chills. Eighty percent of patients achieved their target heart rate. Baseline systolic pressure exceeding 140 mm Hg, older age, and medication with calcium-channel blockers were significant predictors of hypotension according to multivariate analysis. Hypotension occurred significantly more frequently in group 1. The prevalence of arrhythmias was similar for both groups. Wall-motion scores increased significantly during DSE in both groups. Compared with coronary angiography, DSE as a diagnostic tool for detecting significant coronary artery stenosis in hypertensive patients had a sensitivity of 77%, specificity of 85%, and accuracy of 80%. For patients without hypertension, the respective values were 71%, 86%, and 77%.

Conclusion.—Dobutamine-atropine stress echocardiography is a safe, feasible method for evaluating coronary artery disease in hypertensive patients. The sensitivity, specificity, and accuracy of the technique are similar for hypertensive and nonhypertensive patients.

▶ The evaluation of coronary artery disease is complicated in patients with hypertension. Standard treadmill exercise electrophysiology is reduced in its predictive value, and many of these patients cannot comply with the exercise requirements of a valid test. Dobutamine-atropine stress echocardiography can evaluate ventricular wall motion under simulated exercise conditions. This study looked at the safety of this test in more than 1,000 patients. They found no significant difference in complication rates between patients with hypertension and those who were normotensive. It seems that DSE is safe for patients with hypertension, and its predictive value for coronary artery disease is valid.

R.C. Davidson, M.D., M.P.H.

Effect of Diuretic-based Antihypertensive Treatment on Cardiovascular Disease Risk in Older Diabetic Patients With Isolated Systolic Hypertension

Curb JD, for the Systolic Hypertension in the Elderly Program Cooperative Research Group (John A Burns School of Medicine, Honolulu, Hawaii)
JAMA 276:1886–1892, 1996   1–7

Introduction.—Oral diuretics given to control elevated blood pressure reduce cardiovascular morbidity and mortality, but adverse effects have also been noted. Among the undesirable effects of diuretic treatment are increases in blood glucose, total cholesterol, and levels of low-density lipoprotein cholesterol. A multicenter, randomized trial assessed the effect of low-dose, diuretic-based antihypertensive treatment on cardiovascular disease (CVD) risk in older, non–insulin-treated diabetic patients with isolated systolic hypertension (ISH).

Methods.—The double-blind trial—the Systolic Hypertension in the Elderly Program (SHEP)—enrolled men and women aged 60 years and older who had ISH at baseline. The study group included 583 patients with non–insulin-dependent diabetes and 4,149 who were nondiabetic. Those randomly assigned to active treatment received a low dose of chlorthalidone (12.5–25.0 mg/day) with a step-up to atenolol (25–50 mg/day) or reserpine (0.05–0.10 mg/day) if needed. Patients in the placebo group took placebo and any active antihypertensive drugs prescribed by the patient's private physician for persistently high blood pressure. The primary end point in SHEP was nonfatal plus fatal stroke. Also recorded were 5-year rates of major CVD events, nonfatal myocardial infarction, fatal coronary heart disease, major coronary heart disease events, and all-cause mortality.

Results.—The 4 patient subgroups (active treatment, placebo, diabetic, and nondiabetic) were generally comparable in baseline characteristics and adherence to the study regimen. Both diabetic and nondiabetic patients had their blood pressure lowered with the SHEP antihypertensive drug regimen, and all outcome rates were lower for the active treatment group than for the placebo group. The 5-year major CVD rate was 34% for active treatment compared with placebo, and this effect was seen in both diabetic and nondiabetic patients. Reflecting the higher CVD risk of diabetic patients, the absolute risk reduction with active treatment was twice as great for diabetic patients as for nondiabetic patients. No adverse effects were associated with the antihypertensive regimen.

Discussion.—The SHEP low-dose antihypertensive treatment, with chlorthalidone as the step 1 drug, substantially reduced the 5-year relative risk and absolute risk of nonfatal and fatal CVD events in older, diabetic and nondiabetic men and women with ISH. These positive effects were not negated by any adverse effects of treatment, a finding that contrasts with a recent report suggesting an excess mortality rate among diabetic patients who receive diuretic therapy for hypertension.

▶ Current guidelines for the treatment of uncomplicated ISH recommend low-dose diuretics as the treatment of choice. Those of us who have been practicing for more than 15 years understand that this is a return to a previous step-therapy set of recommendations in which diuretics were the first step of a pyramid approach.

Because many of the diuretics—particularly the thiazide diuretics—do alter glucose metabolism, their efficacy in older patients with ISH and diabetes has been questioned. This large study of almost 5,000 men and women aged 60 years and older with ISH shows that low-dose thiazide diuretics are a safe and appropriate first step toward reducing the effects of this disease. Of course, we will need to monitor their diabetes more closely. However, considering the known side effects of many of the other antihypertensive medications, I concur with the authors that utilizing a low-dose diuretic as a first step is appropriate.

R.C. Davidson, M.D., M.P.H.

Effects of Losartan on Insulin Sensitivity in Hypertensive Subjects

Laakso M, Karjalainen L, Lempiäinen-Kuosa P (Kuopio Univ, Finland)
Hypertension 28:392–396, 1996
1–8

Introduction.—In most populations, it is generally believed that insulin resistance has an important role in the pathogenesis of essential hypertension. Insulin sensitivity has been shown to worsen with thiazide diuretics and β-blocking agents, but to remain neutral with calcium-channel blockers, angiotensin-converting enzyme inhibitors, α_1-receptor antagonists. However, these studies have not differentiated between insulin-resistant and insulin-sensitive patients with hypertension. The first specific and orally available angiotensin II receptor antagonist is losartan, a potent antihypertensive drug with low toxicity and few side effects in human studies. The effects of losartan and metoprolol on insulin sensitivity were compared in hyperinsulinemic, or insulin-resistant, patients with hypertension.

Methods.—In 20 hyperinsulinemic patients with essential hypertension, the effects of losartan (50 mg daily) were compared with the effects of metoprolol (95 mg daily) on insulin sensitivity, insulin secretion, glucose tolerance, and lipid and lipoprotein levels.

Results.—The use of losartan resulted in a greater fall in blood pressure than did the use of metoprolol. After 12 weeks of treatment, insulin sensitivity did not change in either group, as evaluated by the euglycemic clamp technique. During the last 30 minutes of the 3-hour euglycemic clamp, glucose oxidation and non-oxidation remained unchanged. With losartan, glucose oxidation was 17 ± 0.9 versus 16.9 ± 1 µmol/kg/min, and with metoprolol, it was 17.9 ± 1.3 versus 16.8 ± 1.6 µmol/kg/min. With losartan, non-oxidation was 22.3 ± 4 versus 23.5 ± 3.4 µmol/kg/min, and with metoprolol, it was 23.3 ± 4 versus 25.6 ± 4.7 µmol/kg/min. There were no significant adverse effects on lipoproteins or lipid levels, glucose tolerance, or insulin secretion with metoprolol or losartan.

Conclusions.—There are no significant adverse effects on glucose or lipid metabolism with losartan, which is metabolically neutral. This new class of antihypertensive drugs, Ang II receptor antagonists, may offer a good alternative in treating patients with hypertension.

▶ The angiotensin II receptor antagonists, a relatively new class of antihypertensive drugs, are gaining increasing popularity. They have been proven to be potent antihypertensive drugs with an apparently low incidence of side effects. This study looked at the drugs' effects on insulin sensitivity. Many physicians are reluctant to use thiazide-type diuretics in patients with hypertension who concurrently have insulin-resistant type II diabetes. This study found no effect on insulin sensitivity with this new class of antihypertensive drugs. Therefore, for our patients with both hypertension and type II diabetes, when we are having trouble controlling them on the standard first-line drugs, then this new class of angiotensin II receptor antagonists appears to be a good alternative.

I suspect that we will see several other brand-name drugs from this same class come on the market in the next several years. We always must take caution that the first blush of enthusiasm we often have for a new drug sometimes wanes as we find unsuspected negative attributes with increasing use. However, this is a promising new class of antihypertensive drugs that seems to be neutral in its effect on type II diabetes.

R.C. Davidson, M.D., M.P.H.

Coronary Artery Disease Risk

The Recent Decline in Mortality From Coronary Heart Disease, 1980–1990: The Effect of Secular Trends in Risk Factors and Treatment
Hunink MGM, Goldman L, Tosteson ANA, et al (Harvard Med School, Boston; Univ of Groningen, The Netherlands; Univ of California, San Francisco; et al)
JAMA 277:535–542, 1997   1–9

Background.—Coronary heart disease is still the major cause of morbidity and mortality in the United States, even though the incidence of and death rate from coronary disease have been decreasing in recent decades. Possible explanations for this are the effect of risk factor reductions in decreasing the incidence of coronary disease and event rates in patients with existing coronary heart disease, and improved treatment of current patients with coronary disease. It is unclear to what extent each of these factors have affected mortality rates. A computer simulation model was designed by the coronary heart disease policy model research group to replicate *Vital Statistics of the United States 1980*, and has been updated for 1986. The model was used to determine whether secular trends in risk factors and treatment can account for the decrease in mortality from coronary disease between 1980 and 1990.

Methods.—Data from the medical literature, health surveys, clinical trials, and United States statistics were collected. A computer simulation state-transition model of individuals between ages 35 and 84 years was developed to predict the death rate from coronary heart disease.

Results.—In 1990, the actual death rate from coronary heart disease in the United States was 34% lower than would have been predicted if risk factor levels, case-fatality rates, and event rates in individuals with and without coronary disease were the same as in 1980. After secular changes in these factors were included in the model, the predicted death rate from coronary disease for 1990 was within 3% of the actual death rate, and 92% of the decrease was accounted for. Primary prevention accounted for 25% of the decrease, secondary reduction of risk factors in patients with coronary heart disease accounted for 29% of the decrease, and other improvements in treatment of patients with coronary disease accounted for 43% of the decrease.

Discussion.—Primary and secondary reductions in risk factors account for 50% of the decrease in mortality from coronary heart disease in the United States between 1980 and 1990. More than 70% of the overall decline in the death rate has been in current patients with coronary heart disease.

▶ This is a very interesting article, although I must admit I do not understand the methodology used in the prediction model. By review of the literature and the use of U.S. statistics, the authors computed a 34% decline in coronary mortality between 1980 and 1990. They then used a complicated computer model to assign portions of this mortality decline to various preventive and treatment modalities.

The authors conclude that roughly 25% of the morbidity reduction is related to primary prevention with well patients, with most of this related to better control of lipoprotein levels. Reduction of risk factors in patients with known coronary artery disease added another 30% to risk factor reduction benefit. This means that slightly more than half of the overall mortality reduction is related to risk factor reduction. The other half, the authors conclude, is related to improved treatment modalities, including more aggressive medical and surgical treatment of coronary artery disease and acute myocardial infarction.

Although I cannot put too much validity on the accuracy of the authors' actual percentages, I think this is an interesting research study attempting to get at the "why" question of the well-demonstrated reduction in coronary heart disease mortality over this decade. Because most family physicians will deal predominantly with the risk factor reduction, it is important to understand that this at least equals the benefit of the interventional cardiologists and surgeons.

R.C. Davidson, M.D., M.P.H.

Serum Iron Level, Coronary Artery Disease, and All-cause Mortality in Older Men and Women
Corti M-C, Guralnik JM, Salive ME, et al (NIH, Bethesda, Md; Ospedale I Fraticini, Florence, Italy; Catholic Univ, Rome; et al)
Am J Cardiol 79:120–127, 1997   1–10

Background.—Studies of the possible association between iron levels and coronary artery disease (CAD) mortality have yielded conflicting findings. The association between serum iron and CAD, cardiovascular disease, and all-cause mortality was assessed in 1 large cohort.

Methods.—The cohort included 3,936 patients aged 71 years and older. All participants were interviewed, underwent serum iron determination, and survived at least 1 year after baseline determinations. The median follow-up was 4.4 years. Relative risks (RRs) were calculated, adjusting for age, race, education, creatinine, serum albumin, serum lipids, use of iron supplementation, smoking, use of alcohol, blood pressure, body mass index, and presence of chronic conditions.

Findings.—As serum iron levels increased, the RRs of CAD, cardiovascular disease, and all-cause mortality declined gradually. Men in the highest quartile of iron levels were one fifth as likely to die of CAD as men in the lowest quartile. Women in the highest quartile were at half the risk of women in the lowest quartile. Compared with the risk in the lowest quartile, the risk of all-cause mortality was reduced by 38% in men in the highest iron quartile and by 28% in women in the highest quartile. Similar

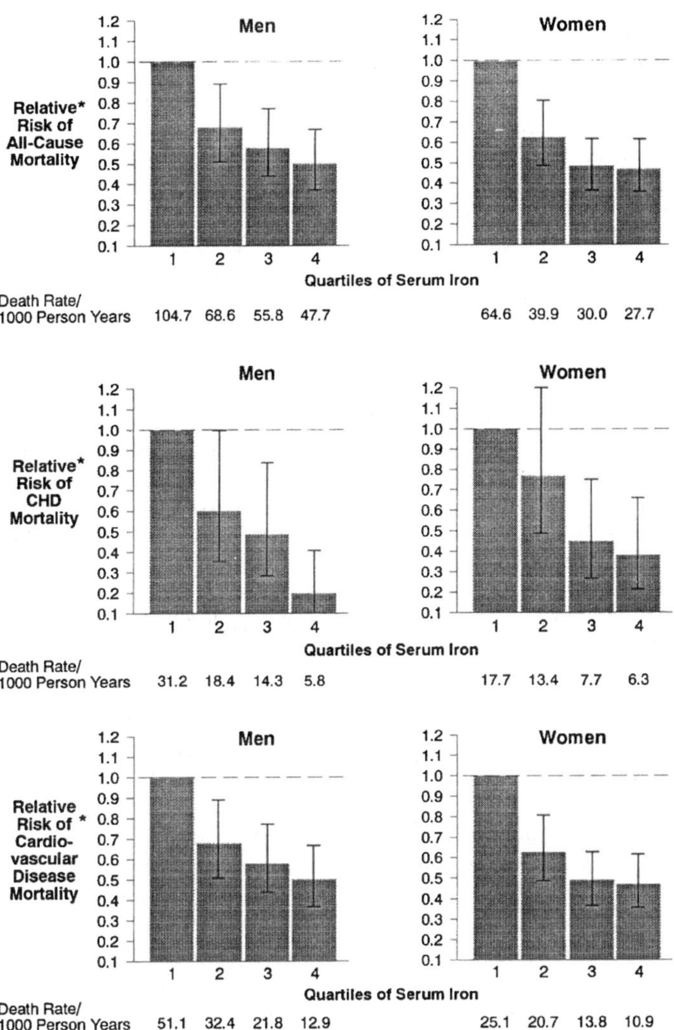

FIGURE 2.—Age-adjusted relative risks of death according to serum iron level quartiles in men and women, with 95% confidence intervals (*vertical lines*), Death rates are per 1000/person-years. All events during the first year were excluded. *Asterisk* indicates that relative risks and 95% confidence intervals were calculated from community-stratified proportional-hazards regression models, adjusted for age. *Abbreviation: CHD*, coronary heart disease. (Reprinted by permission of the publisher from Corti M-C, Guralnik JM, Salive ME, et al: Serum iron level, coronary artery disease, and all-cause mortality in older men and women. *American Journal of Cardiology* 79:120–127, copyright 1997 by Excerpta Medica, Inc.)

findings were obtained for cardiovascular disease mortality and in analyses excluding the first 3 years of follow-up (Fig 2).

Conclusion.—In this cohort, consistent evidence showed that the risk of mortality increases at lower serum iron levels. Lower levels were associated with an increased risk of CAD, cardiovascular disease, and all-cause mortality.

▶ I found this a disturbing but important and well-designed study. The authors studied a cohort of nearly 4,000 patients for a mean follow-up time of 4.4 years. These patients completed an interview and had a serum iron determination. In both men and women, an inverse association between serum iron levels and risk of mortality was found.

Unfortunately, the authors were not able to investigate whether attempting to raise the iron levels of older men and women will, in any way, reduce their mortality. Until we know that, there seems to be little value in routinely measuring serum iron levels in older patients, unless there is a concurrent anemia. In fact, much of the affect found in this study may well be related to an underlying anemia or malnutrition.

I included this study because it does raise an important issue. However, we will need to await further studies before we change our screening and treatment criteria for older patients in relation to their serum iron level.

R.C. Davidson, M.D., M.P.H.

Plasma Homocysteine as a Risk Factor for Vascular Disease: The European Concerted Action Project

Graham IM, Daly LE, Refsum HM, et al (Trinity College, Dublin, Ireland; Royal College of Surgeons in Ireland, Dublin; Univ College, Dublin, Ireland; et al)
JAMA 277:1775–1781, 1997   1–11

Background.—Increased plasma homocysteine is known to be a risk factor for atherosclerotic vascular disease. However, the strength of the association and interaction of plasma homocysteine with other risk factors are unclear.

Methods.—Seven hundred fifty men and women with atherosclerotic vascular disease and 800 control subjects seen at 19 centers in 9 European countries were enrolled in the case-control study. All subjects were younger than 60 years. Plasma total homocysteine was measured while subjects were fasting and after a standardized methionine-loading test. Other parameters were also measured.

Findings.—Compared to the bottom four fifths of the control fasting total homocysteine distribution, the top fifth had a relative risk of 2.2 for vascular disease. Methionine loading identified another 27% of patients at risk. There was a dose-response effect between total homocysteine level and risk. Although the risk was similar to and independent of that of other risk factors, interactive effects were evident between homocysteine and these risk factors. When both sexes were analyzed together, increased fasting homocysteine levels showed a more than multiplicative effect on risk in smokers and hypertensive individuals. Total homocysteine levels were inversely associated with red blood cell folate, cobalamin, and pyridoxal phosphate, all modulators of homocysteine metabolism. The small number of subjects taking vitamin supplements appeared to have a markedly lower risk of vascular disease compared to nonusers, a proportion of which was attributable to lower plasma homocysteine levels.

Conclusions.—Increased plasma total homocysteine levels confer an independent risk of vascular disease, comparable to that of smoking and hyperlipidemia, strongly increasing the risk associated with smoking and hypertension. Randomized controlled trials of the effects of vitamins that decrease plasma homocysteine levels on the risk of vascular disease are now needed.

▶ Diagnosis and treatment seemed so simple when we were focused on cholesterol and its high-density and low-density components. Now we worry about apo-lipoprotein fractions, antioxidant levels, and also homocysteine levels.

These authors studied 750 patients with known atherosclerotic vascular disease and 800 controls. They found a significant relationship between elevated fasting homocysteine levels and risk of cardiovascular event. These were compounded with other known risk factors such as elevated cholesterol, smoking, and hypertension.

It is very clear that the interactive set of risk factors for atherosclerotic disease and coronary artery disease in particular is a complex interaction. Attempting to deal with only one risk factor may help, but does not address the interaction of the multiple factors. Homocysteine appears to be one of those risk factors. Whether it is genetic or diet-induced, elevated fasting homocysteine appears to be a risk factor for cardiovascular events. Whether this proves out in additional studies to warrant preventive testing and prophylactic treatment or both is yet unknown.

R.C. Davidson, M.D., M.P.H.

A Prospective Study of Anger and Coronary Heart Disease: The Normative Aging Study

Kawachi I, Sparrow D, Spiro A III, et al (Harvard Med School, Boston; Brigham and Women's Hosp, Boston; Beth Israel Hosp, Boston)
Circulation 94:2090–2095, 1996   1–12

Introduction.—Earlier findings indicate that anger and hostility are related to the incidence of coronary heart disease (CHD). The relationship between anger and overall CHD risk was prospectively evaluated in the Veterans Administration Normative Aging Study, on ongoing cohort of older community-dwelling men.

Methods.—Mean participant age was 61 years. The revised Minnesota Multiphasic Personality Inventory (MMPI-2) was administered to 1,305

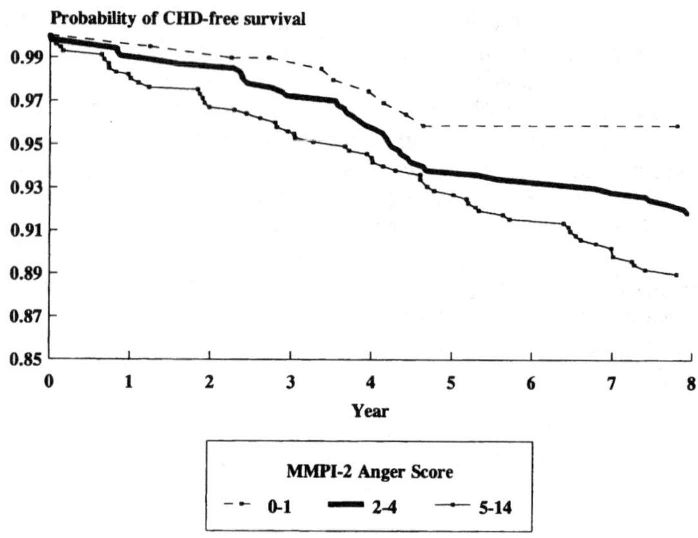

FIGURE 2.—CHD-free survival according to MMPI-2 Anger Content scale score. (Courtesy of Kawachi I, Sparrow D, Spiro A III, et al: A prospective study of anger and coronary artery disease: The Normative Aging Study. *Circulation* 94:2090–2095, 1996. Reproduced with permission of *Circulation*. Copyright 1996 American Heart Association.)

men with no diagnosis of CHD. Research subjects were categorized according to their responses to the MMPI-2 Anger content scale. All participants underwent physical examination, medical history update, measurement of a variety of biochemical values, and were assessed for morbidity and mortality. Average follow-up was 7 years.

Results.—Research subjects who scored high on anger were younger, heavier, more likely to be current smokers, and somewhat more likely to drink at least 2 alcoholic drinks daily. During follow-up, 110 new coronary events occurred in 1,305 men: 30 nonfatal myocardial infarction (MI), 20 fatal CHD, and 60 angina pectoris. Men with higher levels of anger experienced increased risks of CHD. Men who scored in the highest category of anger had about a 60% excess risk of nonfatal MI and increased risk of incident angina pectoris. Men with higher levels of anger had shorter periods of CHD-free survival. (Fig 2) A dose-response association was observed between level of anger and overall CHD risk.

Conclusion.—Anger was associated with a twofold to threefold increased risk of total CHD and angina pectoris in older men. These findings need to be explored in other populations before anger management programs can be suggested as a means to help reduce the risk of CHD events.

▶ As I read this interesting study, the lyrics from some Caribbean song whose title I have forgotten kept ringing in my ears, "Don't worry—be happy." These authors identified a subset of 1,300 men who were high anger responders to a MMPI-2. They then followed the entire cohort during a 7-year follow-up period. Those men who scored high on the anger scale were 3 times more likely to have a significant coronary event.

This intuitively makes sense to me. The problem is what do we do about it? I have enough trouble trying to get my patients to deal with weight control and exercise. I personally feel helpless in trying to change an anger response in my patients. In fact, if I tell them they are 3 times more likely to have a coronary artery event, this may make them more angry and push them into a higher risk.

R.C. Davidson, M.D., M.P.H.

Leisure-time Physical Activity But Not Work-related Physical Activity Is Associated With Decreased Plasma Viscosity: Results From a Large Population Sample
Koenig W, Sund M, Döring A, et al (Ulm Univ, Germany; MEDIS Inst; Inst of Epidemiology, Neuherberg, Germany; et al)
Circulation 95:335–341, 1997   1–13

Background.—Regular leisure-time physical activity (LTPA) has been found to be related inversely to coronary heart disease (CHD), mainly because of its effect on traditional CHD risk factors. Recently, regular LTPA was also found to lower fibrinogen, which largely determines plasma viscosity. To date, no one has studied the effect of work activity (WA) on plasma viscosity.

Methods and Findings.—Data were obtained on LTPA, WA, plasma viscosity, and other CHD risk factors in 3,522 men and women 25–64 years of age. In both sexes, LTPA and plasma viscosity were inversely associated. In men, the unadjusted mean differences in plasma viscosity between no activity and the highest activity levels were 0.024 mPa·sec in winter and 0.024 mPa·sec in summer. After adjusting for age, cholesterol, smoking status, blood pressure, body mass index, and years of education, the mean differences declined but were still significant. Findings in women were comparable. After controlling for covariates, WA was not appreciably associated with plasma viscosity.

Conclusion.—Regular LTPA was found to be inversely associated with plasma viscosity independent of other risk factors, whereas WA was not. Reduced plasma viscosity may represent 1 mechanism through which LTPA reduces the risk of CHD.

▶ I included this article because of its very interesting finding that physical activity and its effect on the body are quite different when it is LTPA rather than WA. The authors studied plasma viscosity, which is predominantly related to the fibrinogen level. A major study in 1987,[1] found a reduction in risk of CHD and death with increased LTPA. This study of plasma viscosity showed a reduction with LTPA, which may well help to explain the morbidity and mortality reduction. Surprising to me, however, was that the authors did not find the same plasma viscosity reduction related to WA. The obvious

TABLE 7.—Estimated Incidence Rates and Attributable Risks Per 10^6 Woman-Years Associated With Current OC Use by Age and Smoking Status Among European Women

	Incidence per 10^6 woman-years		Attributable risk
	Non-users of OCs	Users of OCs	
Women <35 years			
Non-smokers	0.83	3.56	2.73
Smokers	7.78	42.7	34.9
Women ≥35 years			
Non-smokers	9.45	40.4	31.0
Smokers	88.4	484.6	396.2

(Courtesy of Poulter NR, and the WHO Collaborative Study of Cardiovascular Disease and Steroid Hormone Contraception: Acute myocardial infarction and combined oral contraceptives: Results of an international multicentre case-control study. *Lancet* 349:1202–1209, 1997. Copyright by the *Lancet* Ltd., 1997.)

Hysterectomy, Oophorectomy, and Heart Disease Risk Factors in Older Women

Kritz-Silverstein D, Barrett-Conner E, Wingard DL (Univ of California, San Diego)
Am J Public Health 87:676–680, 1997

1–16

Background.—Several studies have reported an increased risk of heart disease and atherosclerosis after bilateral oophorectomy. Heart disease has been associated less consistently with hysterectomy and conservation of at least 1 ovary. The relationship of hysterectomy and oophorectomy to heart disease risk factors was examined.

Methods and Findings.—Data on 1,150 women, age 50 to 89 years, were analyzed. Hysterectomy with bilateral oophorectomy had been performed in 21.8%, and hysterectomy with ovarian conservation in 22.1%. Compared with women who had not had hysterectomy, oophorectomized women had increased lipids, lipoproteins, glucose, and insulin. This was especially true in women 20 years or more passed menopause. Current estrogen users had increased blood pressures. Women who underwent hysterectomies with ovarian conservation had comparable or more favorable risk factors than women who had not had hysterectomy.

Conclusions.—The association of bilateral oophorectomy with more unfavorable heart disease risk factors many years after surgery, not completely alleviated by estrogen replacement, has important implications. Physicians should reconsider the use of routine bilateral oophorectomy to prevent cancer. Additional research is needed.

Estrogen Replacement Therapy and Prognosis After First Myocardial Infarction
Newton KM, LaCroix AZ, McKnight B, et al (Group Health Cooperative of Puget Sound, Seattle; Univ of Washington, Seattle; Fred Hutchinson Cancer Research Ctr, Seattle)
Am J Epidemiol 145:269–277, 1997   1–17

Background.—The effects of estrogen replacement on prognosis in women with coronary disease has not been definitively established. The effects of such therapy on reinfarction and survival of a first myocardial infarction were studied.

Methods.—A cohort of 726 women, with a mean age of 66.2 years, was included in the retrospective study. These women had survived to hospital discharge after a first myocardial infarction between 1980 and 1991. A total of 122 women were receiving estrogen replacement therapy. Of these participants, 135 had reinfarctions, and 183 deaths occurred through 1993.

Findings.—The relative risk (RR) for reinfarction associated with current estrogen replacement treatment after myocardial infarction was 0.64, after adjustment for age and time since infarction. The RR for past estrogen replacement therapy was 0.90. That for all-cause mortality associated with current estrogen replacement therapy was 0.50 and was 0.79 for past estrogen replacement therapy. Estrogen users were less likely than nonusers to have a history of diabetes or congestive heart failure. However, adjustment for these and other prognostic factors did not greatly change the risk estimated. Estrogen replacement therapy after first myocardial infarction was unrelated to an increased risk of reinfarction or mortality (Fig 1).

Conclusions.—Estrogen replacement therapy appears to be safe after myocardial infarction. Such therapy after a first myocardial infarction was unassociated with an increased risk of reinfarction or all-cause mortality in postmenopausal women.

▶ I combined these 3 interesting studies (Abstract 1–15 to 1–17) because they have a common theme. Each studies the relationship of estrogen, either natural or supplemented, to the risk of myocardial infarction and other heart diseases.

The first of these is an international multicenter case-controlled study of the use of oral contraceptives and the risk of acute myocardial infarction. The good news here is that the authors found a very low incidence of myocardial infarction in all women. There was a particularly low incidence among nonsmokers and younger women. The authors concluded that only in women older than 35 years who regularly smoked cigarettes was there a significant risk increase for myocardial infarction. The data in Table 7 show a slight increased risk for myocardial infarction with the use of oral contraceptives. Remember, however, that these incidence rates are per 10 million women-years. It also does not factor in the increased risks of not using oral

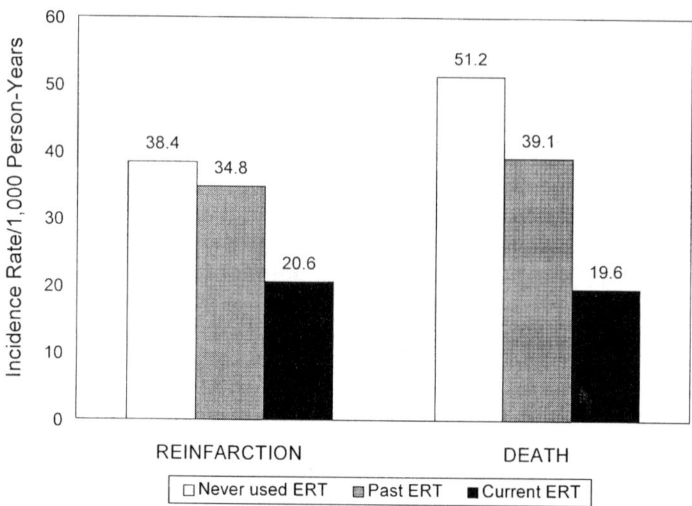

FIGURE 1.—Age-standardized rates of reinfarction and death (standardized to age distribution of the cohort) in relation to postmenopausal estrogen replacement therapy (ERT) among postmenopausal women less than 80 years old who survived first myocardial infarction to hospital discharge, Group Health Cooperative of Puget Sound, 1980–1991. (Courtesy of Newton KM, LaCroix AZ, McKnight B, et al: Estrogen replacement therapy and prognosis after first myocardial infarction. *Am J Epidemiol* 145:269–277, 1997.)

contraceptives such as unwanted pregnancies and the risks associated with these.

My analysis of this study is to reassure my younger women patients that the risk of their using oral contraceptives in relationship to myocardial infarction and coronary artery disease is very low, as long as they don't smoke cigarettes.

The second study looked at older women who had either hysterectomy or hysterectomy and bilateral oophorectomy and their heart disease risk factors. The authors studied 11,050 women as part of an ongoing community-based heart disease risk factor study. They found that women who had their ovaries removed showed evidence of long-term negative consequences for heart disease risk factors. These factors were reduced but not removed by estrogen replacement. The authors conclude that there is something cardio-protective in maintaining ovarian use as long as possible and that this is probably something beyond just the estrogen production by the ovaries.

The decision to have hysterectomy is a difficult one. Two decades ago, hysterectomy was the most frequent surgical procedure on older women. A number of studies questioned the necessity for these and the incidence in an era of cost-conscious managed care has plummeted. When the decision to have hysterectomy is made, however, there is a second major decision regarding sparing the ovaries. Most surgeons in this community recommend taking the ovaries out at the time of surgery and using estrogen replace-ment. They cite the difficulty of detecting ovarian cancer as the reason to remove the ovaries. This study, however, would give an additional reason to not remove the ovaries as they seem to be cardioprotective. This is obviously a woman's choice and both the surgeon and primary care physician need to give complete information so that they can make their decision with as much information as possible.

The third study looked at estrogen replacement therapy following first myocardial infarction. This was a retrospective cohort study of 726 women mean aged 66.2 years that had been diagnosed as first myocardial infarction. It was good news that the authors found that estrogen replacement therapy was not associated with increased risk for reinfarction or mortality. I think we can reassure our women patients who have had myocardial infarction that the use of estrogen replacement therapy does not increase their risk for repeat infarction.

R.C. Davidson, M.D., M.P.H.

Effects of Low-Fat, High-Carbohydrate Diets on Risk Factors for Ischemic Heart Disease in Postmenopausal Women
Jeppesen J, Schaaf P, Jones C, et al (Stanford Univ, Calif; Shaman Pharmaceuticals Inc, South San Francisco, Calif)
Am J Clin Nutr 65:1027–1033, 1997   1–18

Objective.—Although current dietary information for postmenopausal women advises them to replace saturated fat with carbohydrate, the approach decreases low-density lipoprotein and high-density lipoprotein cholesterol and increases fasting triglyceride levels. There is speculation that the more insulin-resistant the individual, the greater the undesirable effect of a low-fat, high-carbohydrate diet on glucose, insulin, and lipoprotein metabolism. Results of a study of the effects of a low-fat, high-carbohydrate diet on risk factors for ischemic heart disease in healthy postmenopausal women not taking hormone replacement therapy were presented.

Methods.—Insulin resistance was determined in 10 nondiabetic postmenopausal women (average age, 66 years) who were then randomly assigned to a diet of either 15% protein, 45% fat, and 40% carbohydrate, or 15% protein, 25% fat, and 60% carbohydrate. After 3 weeks on 1 diet, each woman was crossed over to the other diet for 3 weeks. After each arm, the metabolic effects of each diet were assessed. Data were compared statistically.

Results.—Plasma insulin and triacylglycerol levels were significantly higher in women consuming the 60% carbohydrate diet. Daylong plasma triacylglycerol concentrations were significantly higher in women consuming the 60% carbohydrate diet. Steady-state plasma glucose (SSPG) concentrations were significantly correlated with increases in daylong ambient glucose ($r = 0.68$), insulin concentrations ($r = 0.82$), postprandial triacylglycerol ($r = 0.72$ to 0.77), postprandial retinyl palmitate concentrations ($r = 0.68$) and for S_f greater than 400 triacylglycerol ($r = 0.77$), S_f 20 to 400 triacylglycerol ($r = 0.72$), and S_f greater than 400 retinal palmitate (r = 0.75) lipoprotein fractions. Body mass index and waist-to-hip ratios did not change significantly with diet.

Conclusion.—Low-fat, high-carbohydrate diets increase the risk of ischemic heart disease in postmenopausal women.

▶ Women often can lose weight and have lower total cholesterol values on a low fat diet; however, their ratios of high-density lipoprotein (HDL) cholesterol to low-density lipoprotein cholesterol, their triglycerides, and their total HDL cholesterol appear to get worse. This study verifies the fact that the provision of the same total calories but more unsaturated fat, rather than carbohydrates, results in a better lipid profile. The authors extrapolate this to better long-term cardiac outcomes, but I am not as convinced that we know that. These women were all postmenopausal and, on average, were slightly overweight; none were taking hormones.

From my reading of much literature on cholesterol and diet, I believe the authors are correct that the lipid profile is best when women lower total calories but continue fats at a reasonable level (here it was 45% of calories), with most of the fat monounsaturated or polyunsaturated. Unfortunately, I find this diet more difficult to describe than the "count your fat grams" approach. The American Heart Association Step I diet listing the sources of good and bad fat remains a terrific source of information for this type of diet.

M.A. Bowman, M.D., M.P.A.

Intra-abdominal Adipose Tissue, Physical Activity and Cardiovascular Risk in Pre- and Post-Menopausal Women
Hunter GR, Kekes-Szabo T, Treuth MS, et al (Univ of Alabama at Birmingham)
Int J Obes 20:860–865, 1996   1–19

Background.—Although the association of cardiovascular disease (CVD) with physical activity (PA) and with fat distribution is well established, little is known about the interrelationships among these 3 variables. These interrelationships were investigated to determine whether the beneficial effect of PA on CVD risk is mediated through the effects of activity on intra-abdominal adipose fat (IAF).

Methods and Findings.—Two hundred twenty Caucasian women, aged 17 to 77 years, were enrolled in the cross-sectional study. Intra-abdominal adipose fat, subcutaneous abdominal adipose fat (SAF), percent fat, age, menopausal status, and 4 indices of PA were consistently associated with CVD risk. After adjustment for age, menopausal status, SAF, and percent fat, IAF was negatively correlated with PA, which indicates that more active women had relatively small IAF compared with other fat deposits. After adjustment for IAF, menopausal status, and age, none of the PA indices were correlated with any of the CVD risk factors except, for the cholesterol/high-density lipoprotein ratio. After adjustment for PA, menopausal status, and age, however, IAF was correlated with all CVD risk factors except cholesterol.

Conclusion.—These data support the hypothesis that the relationship between PA and CVD risk is mediated mainly through changes in IAF. Physically active women have lower absolute and relative IAF, and, thus, their risk of CVD, as measured by blood lipid profile and blood pressure, is reduced.

▶ I can use these data to reassure some of my patients and, hopefully, to keep them exercising. Intra-abdominal adipose fat appears to be the key factor influencing cholesterol and blood pressure. This IAF decreased with exercise, regardless of changes in total body fat, SAF, or weight. Thus, even when patients cannot see the difference ("My stomach does not seem smaller"; "My weight is not lower"), they are probably still benefiting. The results also seem to suggest why maximum oxygen uptake (VO_2) improvement exercise is not required to lower cardiac risk factors.

M.A. Bowman, M.D., M.P.A.

Serious Cardiovascular Side Effects of Large Doses of Anabolic Steroids in Weight Lifters

Nieminen MS, Rämö P, Viitasalo M, et al (Helsinki Univ; Central Military Hosp, Helsinki)
Eur Heart J 17:1576–1583, 1996
1–20

Introduction.—Anabolic steroids have been shown to increase ventricular wall thickness, end-diastolic volume, and left ventricular mass and to significantly prolong isovolumetric relaxation time in weight lifters. Anabolic steroids are considered atherogenic and have been linked to arterial occlusion in several reports. The pathologic cardiovascular manifestations in 4 young men who used high doses of anabolic steroids for several years in combination with weight training were studied.

Methods.—Patients were referred for evaluation because of a long history of massive anabolic steroid use (patient 1); ventricular fibrillation during exercise (patient 2); clinically manifest heart failure (patient 3); and arterial thrombus in the lower left leg (patient 4). Ages ranged from 27 to 33 years. All patients underwent history-taking, physical examination, and cardiovascular evaluation.

Results.—All 4 patients had abnormal cardiac hypertrophy. Two patients who underwent endomyocardial biopsy had diffuse myocardial fibrosis. Patients 3 and 4 had signs of heart failure, patient 2 had impairment of coronary flow, and patient 3 had impairment of perfusion. A large lobular intraventricular thrombus was observed in both the left and right ventricles of patient 4 during echocardiography. Two patients had improved left ventricular function after cessation of anabolic steroids. Despite warnings, both patients restarted use of anabolic steroids.

Conclusion.—Two of the 4 weight lifters using anabolic steroids had potentially lethal side effects: malignant ventricular arrhythmia in 1 and massive intracardiac thrombosis in the other. All men had cardiac hypertrophy. All physicians and athletes should be warned about the serious risks involved in continuous use of large doses of anabolic steroids.

▶ The fact that large doses of anabolic steroids are a health risk is not news to primary care physicians. I chose this article because of its documentation of serious cardiovascular side effects of the use of this elicit substance. Even though fear is generally not a good motivator for behavioral change, the more data we can supply to our patients who are asking for or utilizing anabolic steroids, the better chance we have of getting them to change their high-risk behavior.

This study describes the serious cardiovascular effects in 4 patients. All 4 of the patients had cardiac hypertrophy. All of them showed significant cardiac changes and were at increased risk for myocardial infarction and/or sudden death.

I'm sure that when we know a patient is taking large doses of anabolic steroids as a body-building or performance-enhancing drug, we counsel them against it. However, we need to remember to ask the question when we see muscular weight lifters in our practice.

R.C. Davidson, M.D., M.P.H.

Coronary Artery Disease and Myocardial Infarction

Relation Between Severity of Magnesium Deficiency and Frequency of Anginal Attacks in Men With Variant Angina

Satake K, Lee J-D, Shimizu H, et al (Fukui Med School, Japan)
J Am Coll Cardiol 28:897–902, 1996

1–21

Purpose.—Death from ischemic heart disease is inversely correlated with magnesium intake. The relationship between magnesium deficiency and the severity of variant angina remains unclear, however. Men with variant angina were studied to determine the relationship between the severity of magnesium deficiency and the frequency of anginal attacks.

Methods.—The study included 18 men with variant angina. Seven men had 4 or more attacks of angina per week (group 1), and 11 had less than 4 attacks per week (group 2). Body magnesium status was assessed in all patients, including measurement of magnesium concentrations in serum, urine, mononuclear cells, and erythrocytes. The 24-hour magnesium retention rate was studied as well. Correlations were sought between the severity of magnesium deficiency and the activity of variant angina.

Results.—The mean 24-hour magnesium retention rate was 7.6% in men with more frequent anginal attacks vs. 24.9% in those with less frequent anginal attacks. The intracellular concentration of magnesium in mononuclear cells was 156.3 fg per cell in group 1 vs. 212.1 fg per cell in group 2. The concentration in erythrocytes was 3.5 fg per cell for group 1 vs. 5.2 fg per cell for group 2. Thus, the men with more frequent anginal attacks had magnesium deficiency. For the overall group, the frequency of attacks was significantly correlated with the 24-hour magnesium retention rate and with the intracellular concentrations of magnesium in mononuclear cells and erythrocytes.

Conclusions.—In men with variant angina, the frequency of anginal attacks is significantly correlated with magnesium status. This connection may arise because of magnesium's role in modulating calcium's action on the vascular smooth muscle. Further studies will tell whether correcting the magnesium deficiency can reduce the frequency of attacks.

▶ What a wonderfully complex organism the human body is. We continually find new biochemical correlations with known disease patterns. However, their clinical significance is often not recognized, or it is impractical to do anything about them.

This is an interesting study from Japan looking at the relationship between intracellular magnesium levels and the frequency of angina. This is a small, controlled study of only 18 patients. It also used a method of measuring intracellular magnesium that is not available outside of very sophisticated research laboratories. Therefore, its practicality to physicians is limited, especially because the authors found no relationship between serum magnesium levels and anginal frequency. There was a very high correlation between intracellular magnesium levels and anginal attacks. As the authors state, there's no way to know whether this is causative or is an effect of the angina.

I included this article because of the increasing interest in a variety of common ions in relationship to coronary artery disease. We thought we understood calcium metabolism and its relationship to angina. However, more recent studies have called into question the efficacy of the calcium channel blockers. These authors studied a related ion by measuring intracellular magnesium levels. I suspect that we will hear more regarding magnesium and probably will read an article in the near future regarding a research project for supplemental magnesium in patients with angina. Until then, stay tuned.

R.C. Davidson, M.D., M.P.H.

Effects of Mental Stress on Myocardial Ischemia During Daily Life
Gullette ECD, Blumenthal JA, Babyak M, et al (Duke Univ, Durham, NC; Ohio State Univ, Columbus; Uniformed Services Univ, Bethesda, Md)
JAMA 277:1521–1526, 1997   1–22

Objective.—Myocardial ischemia, an important indicator of future cardiac events in patients with coronary artery disease (CAD), can be triggered by stress. A prospective case-crossover investigation was conducted to determine the effect of generalized vs. specific emotional stress on initiation of ischemia.

Methods.—Ambulatory ECG monioring was performed during a 48-hour period on 132 patients with CAD and recent evidence of exercise-induced ischemia. Patients received no antiischemic medication and kept a diary of major activities during the monitoring period. Information about emotional arousal, time of day, and physical activity level were correlated with ST-segment episodes.

Results.—Two of the 58 patients experiencing myocardial ischemia during the monitoring period were excluded from the study. No physical activity was recorded for 2,311 of the 2,760 hours during the monitoring period. Although most patients did not report high levels of negative emotions, the percentage of ischemic hours was highest during high levels of negative emotions that included 101 hours of tension levels >2, 98 hours of high frustration, and 28 hours of sadness. The percentage of ischemic hours was lower during the high levels of positive emotions. Unadjusted relative risk for high levels of negative emotions was 3.0 for tension, 2.9 for sadness, and 2.6 for frustration. When adjusted for time and day and level of activity, the relative risk diminished to 2.2 for all 3 emotions.

Conclusion.—These findings indicate that everyday mental stress can trigger myocardial ischemia. Stress management techniques are recommended and should be evaluated for use in patients with CAD.

▶ This was an interesting small study of 132 patients with known CAD and recent evidence of exercise-induced ischemia. During a 48-hour ambulatory EKG monitoring period, the effects of mental stress on their ischemic changes was measured. The authors found that these patients were 3 times more likely to have evidence of myocardial ischemia during periods of high levels of negative emotion described as tension, sadness, and frustration.

This is an important message to get across to our patients. In addition to risk factor reversal, they must understand the relationship between stress and myocardial ischemia and pursue ways of stress reduction. This study offers objective evidence that stress may cause myocardial ischemia.

R.C. Davidson, M.D., M.P.H.

A Comparison of Thrombolytic Therapy With Primary Coronary Angioplasty for Acute Myocardial Infarction
Every NR, for the Myocardial Infarction Triage and Intervention Investigators (Seattle Veterans Affairs Med Ctr, Wash)
N Engl J Med 335:1253–1260, 1996   1–23

Background.—Various studies have shown that the short-term outcome of primary coronary angioplasty is better than the outcome of thrombolytic treatment in patients with acute myocardial infarction. Because these studies have used small populations, the benefit of primary angioplasty beyond 30 days cannot be determined. There is little information on the long-term use of resources associated with these 2 treatments. It is unclear whether the results of these smaller studies can be duplicated in larger studies. The short-term and long-term outcomes of primary angioplasty and thrombolytic therapy in patients with acute myocardial infarction were compared.

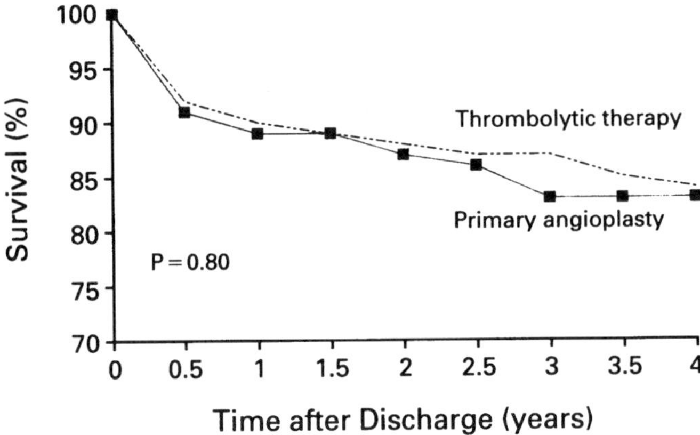

FIGURE 3.—Cumulative survival among 1,050 patients in the primary angioplasty group and 2,095 patients in the thrombolytic therapy group. (Reprinted by permission of the *New England Journal of Medicine*, courtesy of Every NR, for the Myocardial Infarction Triage and Intervention Investigators: A comparison of thrombolytic therapy with primary coronary angioplasty for acute myocardial infarction. *N Engl J Med* 335:1253–1260, Copyright 1996, Massachusetts Medical Society. All rights reserved.)

Methods.—Short-term and long-term mortality and the use of resources were compared for 1,050 patients treated with primary angioplasty and 2,095 patients treated with thrombolysis for acute myocardial infarction. Patients were chosen from the Myocardial Infarction Triage and Intervention Project Registry. Analyses were also performed on several subgroups to compensate for selection bias.

Results.—There were no significant differences in short-term mortality or long-term follow-up between patients who had primary angioplasty or thrombolytic therapy (Fig 3) No differences were seen in mortality rates between subgroups of patients at high risk selected from the 2 treatment groups. Patients who had thrombolytic therapy underwent fewer procedures and had lower costs at hospital discharge and at 3 years.

Conclusion.—There were no differences in mortality in patients treated with primary angioplasty or thrombolysis for acute myocardial infarction. Costs and rates of subsequent procedures were higher in patients treated with primary angioplasty. If the savings from patients given thrombolytic therapy were applied to the patients eligible for thrombolysis, there could be considerable savings nationwide.

▶ The debate continues regarding the "best" therapeutic options for patients with acute myocardial infarction. This interesting study investigated a population of over 12,000 patients admitted with acute myocardial infarction between 1988 and 1994. They found no difference in the 4-year survival rate between patients who had received primary angioplasty and those who had received thrombolytic therapy as the initial treatment modality. Hospital costs, however, were significantly reduced in patients who had received thrombolytic therapy.

Prevalence of Unrecognized Silent Myocardial Ischemia and Its Association With Atherosclerotic Risk Factors in Noninsulin-Dependent Diabetes Mellitus

Faglia E, and the Milan Study on Atherosclerosis and Diabetes (MiSAD) Group (Ospedale Niguarda, Milan, Italy)
Am J Cardiol 79:134–139, 1997

1–25

Background.—Unrecognized silent coronary artery disease (CAD) in diabetic patients has a reported prevalence ranging from 9% to 48%. This wide variability may be a result of different patient selection criteria and diagnostic approaches. The prevalence of unrecognized silent myocardial ischemia was further investigated.

Methods.—Nine hundred non–insulin-dependent diabetic outpatients aged 40 to 65 years were included in the study. All were free from symptoms, known CAD, advanced diabetic retinopathy, nephropathy, severe hypertension, and poor prognosis disease. The patients underwent exercise ECG and, if results were abnormal, exercise thallium scintigraphy.

Findings.—Exercise ECG test results were abnormal in 12.1% of the patients. Six percent had perfusion defects on thallium scintigraphy. When more restrictive criteria were used, the prevalence of silent CAD was 6.4%. In a multivariate analysis, associated independent risk factors in the whole population and in the men included age, total cholesterol, proteinuria, and ST-T abnormalities on ECG at rest. This last factor had the highest odds ratio and was the only one that was also a risk factor in women.

Conclusion.—The relevance of ST-T abnormalities on ECG at rest as a predicting factor for silent CAD underscores the importance of periodic ECG at rest in non–insulin-dependent diabetic patients. In addition, it suggests an indication for performance of further investigations in the presence of these abnormalities.

▶ This study by Italian investigators measured the incidence of myocardial ischemia in a population of 925 non–insulin-dependent diabetic patients free from known CAD. The study excluded patients with advanced diabetes and screened the remainder with exercise ECG tests. The authors found that 12% of these patients had myocardial ischemia and that 6% of the screened population had perfusion defects by thallium scan.

To me, the take-home message from this study is that we need to maintain a high level of suspicion for CAD in our adult non–insulin-dependent diabetic population. Even when patients have normal lipid levels and no symptoms, this study would suggest a more aggressive screening with exercise ECGs.

R.C. Davidson, M.D., M.P.H.

Secondary Prevention of Coronary Artery Disease

The Effect of Pravastatin on Coronary Events After Myocardial Infarction in Patients With Average Cholesterol Levels
Sacks FM, for the Cholesterol and Recurrent Events Trial Investigators (Harvard Med School, Boston)
N Engl J Med 335:1001–1009, 1996   1–26

Background.—Lowering cholesterol levels in patients with high levels is known to decrease the risk of coronary events. However, the effect of lowering cholesterol levels in the majority of patients with coronary disease, whose cholesterol levels are average, is unclear.

Methods.—A 5-year, double-blind study included 3,583 men and 576 women with myocardial infarction who had plasma total cholesterol levels of less than 240 mg/dL and low-density lipoprotein (LDL) cholesterol levels of 115 to 174 mg/dL. The patients were given either 40 mg of pravastatin per day or placebo. A fatal coronary event and nonfatal myocardial infarction were the primary end points.

Findings.—Primary end points occurred in 10.2% of pravastatin recipients and in 13.2% of placebo recipients—a 24% decrease in risk with pravastatin. Ten percent of the patients in the placebo group and 7.5% in the pravastatin group needed coronary bypass surgery (a 26% reduction in risk). Coronary angioplasty was required in 8.3% of the pravastatin recipients and in 10.5% of the placebo recipients (a 23% reduction) (Fig 1) Pravastatin reduced the frequency of stroke by 31%. Overall rates of mortality and mortality from noncardiovascular causes did not differ significantly between groups. Pravastatin decreased the rate of coronary events more among women than among men. Also, the decrease in coronary events was greater in patients with higher pretreatment levels of LDL cholesterol.

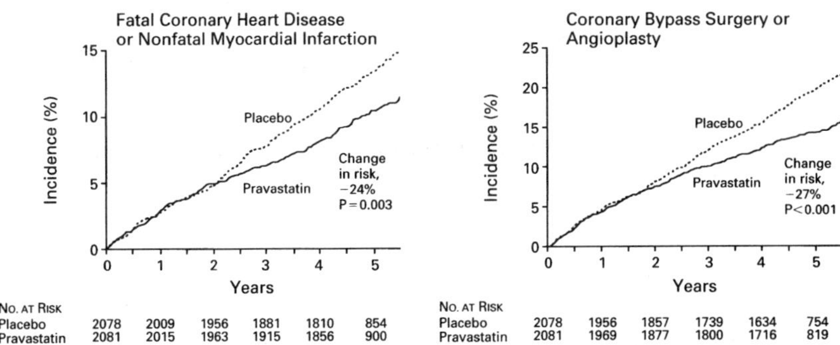

Figure 1.—Kaplan-Meier estimates of the incidence of coronary events in the pravastatin and placebo groups. **Left panel** shows data for the primary end point: fatal coronary heart disease or nonfatal myocardial infarction. **Right panel** shows data for coronary bypass surgery or angioplasty. Changes in risk are those attributable to prevastatin. *P* values and changes in risk are based on Cox proportional hazards analysis. (Reprinted by permission of the *New England Journal of Medicine*, courtesy of Sacks FM, for the Cholesterol and Recurrent Events Trial Investigators: The effect of pravastatin on coronary events after myocardial infarction in patients with average cholesterol levels. *N Engl J Med* 335:1001–1009, copyright 1996, Massachusetts Medical Society. All rights reserved.)

Conclusion.—Cholesterol-lowering treatment is of value for most patients with coronary disease and average cholesterol levels. The majority of myocardial infarction survivors appear to benefit.

▶ A number of research studies proved the reduction in risk for myocardial infarction by reducing LDL cholesterol. Although several classes of drugs can be used to reduce LDL cholesterol, hepatic hydroxymethylglutaryl coenzyme A (HMG-CoA) reductase inhibitor drugs have become the most commonly prescribed for this condition. Their safety profile so far appears very good, and their ease of administration and low incidence of side effects make them the first choice of most patients and physicians.

Previous studies addressed patients with elevated total and LDL serum cholesterols. This very interesting study found a significant reduction in risk for repeat cardiac events in patients who had had previous myocardial infarction but maintained total cholesterol and LDL cholesterol levels in areas previously thought to be "normal." Our current guideline of a total cholesterol level of 200 mg/dL is, of course, an arbitrary number. Other studies have shown that a total cholesterol value below 200 mg/dL further reduces the risk of myocardial infarction.

This study investigated a population of people who had had previous myocardial infarction but who maintained total and LDL cholesterol levels in a range believed to be low risk. Using a randomized, double-blind protocol, the authors showed a significant reduction in risk for repeat infarction by using 40 mg of pravastatin, an HMG-CoA reductase inhibitor.

Each year we seem to find out more and more about the risk factors related to serum cholesterol and coronary artery disease. It makes sense to me that patients who are known to be at very high risk for myocardial infarction could be assisted by further reducing their LDL cholesterol. Certainly a population of patients who have had a previous myocardial infarction would constitute a high-risk group. It seems that, along with aspirin and β-blockade, we should now be giving our post–myocardial infarction patients cholesterol-lowering drugs.

R.C. Davidson, M.D., M.P.H.

Effect of Aspirin on Mortality in Women With Symptomatic or Silent Myocardial Ischemia
Harpaz D, for the Israeli BIP Study Group (Chaim Sheba Med Ctr, Tel-Hashomer, Israel)
Am J Cardiol 78:1215–1219, 1996　　　　　　　　　　　　　　　　1–27

Introduction.—The benefit of aspirin therapy among women with coronary artery disease is not well established. There were 15,502 men and women, aged 45 to 74 years, with coronary artery disease who were screened for a 21-month clinical trial, the Bezafibrate Infarction Prevention study. In a large cohort of women with coronary artery disease who participated in this trial, the effect of aspirin therapy on intermediate-term cardiovascular and total mortality was assessed.

Methods.—An analysis was conducted on data from 2,418 screened women from this trial, and 45% of these reported taking aspirin therapy. These women were not randomly assigned to receive either Bezafibrate or placebo, but had their vital status ascertained. The women were divided into 2 groups, 45% receiving aspirin and 55% not receiving aspirin. During the screening period, the dosage of aspirin these women were administered was 100 to 500 mg/day. Multivariate analysis of independent predictors of mortality was performed.

Results.—At 3.1 ± 0.9 years of follow-up, the cardiovascular mortality rate was 2.7% in the aspirin group, compared to 5.1% in the no-aspirin group. In the aspirin group, the all-cause mortality rate was 5.1%, and in the no-aspirin group, it was 9.1%. An independent predictor of reduced cardiovascular and all-cause mortality was treatment with aspirin. This was adjusted for possible confounders such as history of myocardial infarction, age, diabetes mellitus, systemic hypertension, current smoking, peripheral vascular disease, and concomitant treatment with digitalis. The older, diabetic, symptomatic women who had a previous myocardial infarction benefited the most from aspirin therapy. The 4-year actuarial survival rate of women treated with aspirin was higher than that of women not treated with aspirin (Fig 1).

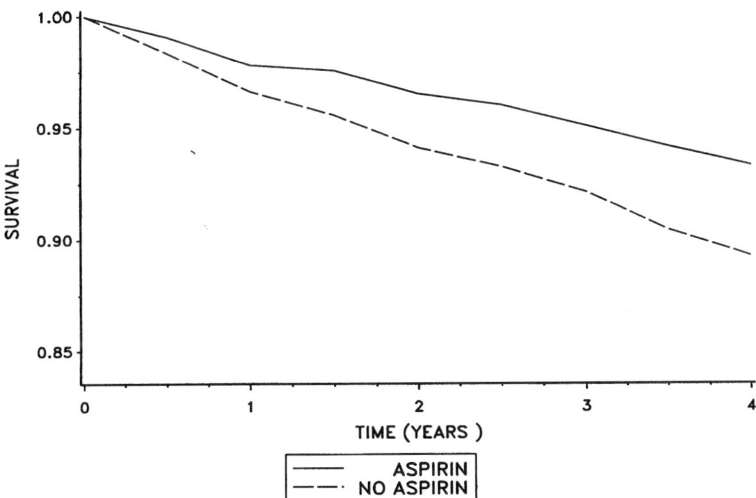

FIGURE 1.—Four-year actuarial survival curves for women with coronary artery disease treated with and without aspirin. (Courtesy of Harpaz D, for the Israeli BIP Study Group: Effect of aspirin on mortality in women with symptomatic or silent myocardial ischemia. *Am J Cardiol* 78:1215–1219, 1996. Reprinted by permission of the publisher. Copyright 1996 by Excerpta Medica, Inc.)

Conclusion.—Unless specific contraindications exist, women with coronary artery disase should be treated with aspirin.

▶ I selected this study for 2 reasons. The first is to remind all of us of the cardio-protective value of using low-dose aspirin in patients with known coronary artery disease. The second is to report on these authors' findings that previous studies showing a reduction of risk for myocardial infarction in men is replicated in a population of women with similar coronary artery disease risks. This was a large study of more than 2,400 women with coronary artery disease. Although all the women seemed to benefit from the use of aspirin, the women who benefited the most were older, diabetic, symptomatic, or had a previous myocardial infarction.

We all know that coronary artery disease is not limited to men. Studies like this continue to show that women have the same risks, although they are somewhat protected by their estrogen and can be helped by postmenopausal estrogen replacement. For women who are at risk for coronary artery disease, aspirin appears to be just as valuable as it is in men.

R.C. Davidson, M.D., M.P.H.

The Effect of Digoxin on Mortality and Morbidity in Patients With Heart Failure

Gorlin R, and the Digitalis Investigation Group (Mount Sinai Med Ctr, New York)
N Engl J Med 336:525–533, 1997

1–28

Background.—Digoxin is a common drug used to treat heart failure, but its long-term safety and efficacy are unclear. Recent studies have shown that discontinuing digoxin in patients with heart failure can worsen functional status, exercise capacity, and left ventricular ejection fraction. The effects of digoxin on hospitalization and mortality rates in patients with heart failure were assessed in a randomized, double-blind, placebo-controlled trial.

Methods.—Patients with heart failure and a left ventricular ejection fraction of 0.45 or less were treated with digoxin or placebo, plus angiotensin-converting enzyme inhibitors and diuretics. The median dose of digoxin was 0.25 mg/day. The average follow-up was 37 months. In a substudy of patients with a left ventricular ejection fraction of 0.45 or more, 492 patients were treated with digoxin and 496 were given placebo.

Results.—In the main study, mortality was similar in both groups of patients. In patients treated with digoxin, there was a trend toward a lower risk of death from worsening heart failure. Also in patients treated with digoxin, the hospitalization rate was 6% less than in patients given placebo, and fewer patients were admitted for worsening heart failure. In the substudy, the mortality and hospitalization rates from worsening heart failure were consistent with the rates in the main study.

Discussion.—In these patients, digoxin did not affect overall mortality in patients also receiving angiotensin-converting enzyme inhibitors and diuretics, but it lowered the death and hospitalization rates from worsening heart failure. In clinical practice, it is unlikely that digoxin would affect survival rates.

▶ Although the use of digitalis in patients with heart failure is one of the oldest known medical interventions, it remains a controversial issue in modern medicine. All of us remember our lectures on the use of the foxglove plant in patients with "dropsy." However, more recent studies have raised questions of its overall efficacy.

This landmark study was designed to address this exact question. It is a random study of almost 7,000 patients divided between those receiving digoxin and those receiving placebo in addition to appropriate diuretics and angiotensin-converting enzyme inhibitors.

There seems to be good news and bad news. The authors found that digoxin did not reduce overall mortality but did reduce the rate of hospitalization, both overall and for worsening heart failure. The authors conclude that the use of digoxin in patients with heart failure is indicated and should continue to be a part of the medical regimen for treatment of heart failure.

R.C. Davidson, M.D., M.P.H.

Adverse Outcomes of Underuse of β-Blockers in Elderly Survivors of Acute Myocardial Infarction

Soumerai SB, McLaughlin TJ, Spiegelman D, et al (Harvard Med School, Boston; Harvard School of Public Health, Boston; Brigham and Women's Hosp, Boston)
JAMA 277:115–121, 1997   1–29

Purpose.—β-Blocker treatment is highly effective in reducing cardiovascular mortality and reinfarction after acute myocardial infarction. Few data are available, however, on how many and which patients receive β-blockers, especially among elderly patients living in the community. Levels, determinants, and outcomes of β-blocker treatment among elderly survivors of acute myocardial infarction were studied.

Methods.—The retrospective study used Medicare and drug-claims data covering the years 1987–1992. It included a cohort of 5,332 elderly patients who survived for 30 days after acute myocardial infarction. Of these, 3,737 met eligibility requirements for β-blocker treatment. The analysis looked at the use of β-blockers and calcium channel blockers in the first 90 days after hospital discharge. Mortality and cardiac hospital readmission rates were evaluated for the 2 years after discharge, with adjustment for sociodemographic and baseline risk variables. Factors associated with underuse of β-blockers, and the consequences of that underuse, were assessed. The relative risks (RRs) for survival in patients

TABLE 5.—Four-Year Probability of Intermittent Claudication for Persons Aged 45–84 Years, Framingham Heart Study

Risk Factor	Risk Factor Points								Line Score
	0	+1	+2	+3	+4	+5	+6	+7	
Age, y	45-49	50-54	55-59	60-64	65-69	70-74	75-79	80-84	
Sex	Female			Male					
Cholesterol, mg/dL	<170	170-209	210-249	250-289	>289				
Blood pressure	Normal	High normal	Stage 1		Stage 2+				
Cigarettes/d, n	0	1-5	6-10	11-20	>20				
Diabetes	No					Yes			
CHD	No					Yes			
								Point total	

Points	4-Year Probability
<10	<1%
10-12	1%
13-15	2%
16-17	3%
18	4%
19	5%
20	6%
21	7%
22	8%
23	10%
24	11%
25	13%
26	16%
27	18%
28	21%
29	24%
30	28%

Note: Stage 1 indicates stage 1 hypertension; stage 2+, greater than or equal to stage 2 hypertension.
Abbreviation: CHD, coronary heart disease.
(Reproduced with permission from Murabito JM, D'Agostino RB, Silvershatz H, et al: Intermittent claudication: A risk profile from the Framingham Heart Study. *Circulation* 96:44–49, 1996. Copyright 1997, American Heart Association.)

simple probability risk table, however, may be useful in helping a patient with known risk factors to understand his or her risk for IC. This just might provide the added emphasis to help patients institute the lifestyle changes necessary to reduce their risk.

R.C. Davidson, M.D., M.P.H.

Randomised Trial of Effect of Compression Stockings in Patients With Symptomatic Proximal-Vein Thrombosis

Brandjes DPM, Büller HR, Heijboer H, et al (Academic Med Ctr, Amsterdam)
Lancet 349:759–762, 1997   1–31

Background.—The manifestations of postthrombotic syndrome range from mild edema to incapacitating swelling with pain and ulceration. The rate of postthrombotic syndrome after a first episode of deep-vein thrombosis was studied, and the preventive effect of direct applications of a sized-to-fit graded compression stocking evaluated.

Methods.—By random assignment, 194 patients were given compression stockings or no stockings. The made-to-measure, graded compression elastic stockings were worn for at least 2 years. Assessments were made every 3 months for 2 years and every 6 months thereafter for 5 years or longer. Median follow-up time was 76 months.

Findings.—Twenty percent of the patients in the stocking group and 47% in the control group had mild-to-moderate postthrombotic syndrome. Severe postthrombotic syndrome developed in 11% of the patients wearing stockings and in 23% of those not wearing stockings. The syndrome developed within 24 months of the acute thrombotic event in most patients in both groups (Fig 2).

Conclusions.—Postthrombotic syndrome develops in about 60% of patients with a first episode of proximal deep-vein thrombosis. The use of a sized-to-fit compression stocking decreases this rate by about half.

▶ This is an interesting study from The Netherlands looking at the efficacy of the use of compression stockings following a first-event proximal deep-vein thrombosis. The study is a prospective randomly assigned study protocol. Investigators obviously could not use a blinded protocol because it is hard to mask compression stockings with some type of placebo. Although the study size was small (194 patients), they did find a significant difference in symptomatology between the 2 study groups. Patients who used compression stockings had a reduction in postthrombotic symptomatology, both in incidence and intensity.

These findings make common sense. Part of the problem with deep-vein thrombosis is the inadequacy of the valves in the veins. If we compensate for this with compression stockings, we should be able to improve blood flow and therefore reduce symptoms. Patients who are symptomatic following a thrombotic event should be advised to use compression stockings.

R.C. Davidson, M.D., M.P.H.

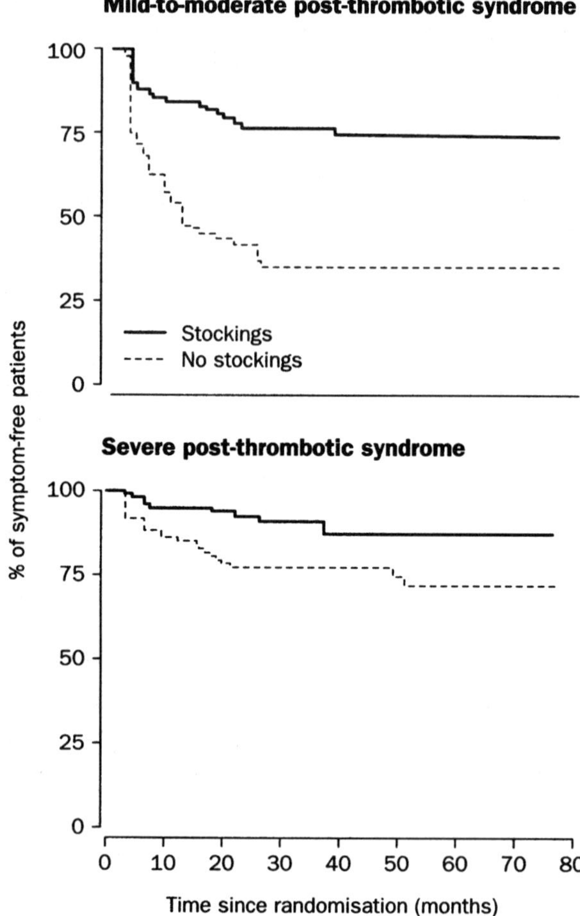

FIGURE 2.—Proportions of patients without symptoms of mild-to-moderate or severe postthrombotic syndrome. (Courtesy of Brandjes DPM, Buller HR, Heijboer H, et al: Randomised trial of effect of comparison stockings in patients with symptomatic proximal-vein thrombosis. *Lancet* 349:759–762, 1997. Copyright by the *Lancet* Ltd., 1997.)

Prevalence and Associations of Abdominal Aortic Aneurysm Detected Through Screening

Lederle FA, for the Aneurysm Detection and Management (ADAM) Veterans Affairs Cooperative Study Group (Veterans Affairs Med Ctr, Minneapolis)
Ann Intern Med 126:441–449, 1997   1–32

Objective.—Although abdominal aortic aneurysm (AAA) is an important cause of death, key questions remain about its cause and epidemiology. Most epidemiologic data on this condition have come from screening studies. There have been no multivariate analyses in large populations of patients to determine the independent risk factors for AAA. Risk factors for AAA and the prevalence of previously unrecognized AAA were studied as part of a large cross-sectional screening study.

Methods.—The study included 73,451 subjects undergoing ultrasonographic screening at 15 VA medical centers. The veterans, aged 50 to 79 years at the time of the screening, had no history of AAA (Table 1). The screening findings, together with the responses to a prescreening questionnaire, were used to determine the prevalence of AAA in various demographic and risk groups. Factors independently associated with AAA were evaluated as well.

Results.—The prevalence of previously unrecognized AAA was 1.4%. The main risk factor was smoking; the odds ratio (OR) for an AAA measuring 4 cm or larger was 5.57, compared with normal aortas with an infrarenal aortic diameter of less than 3.0 cm. The greater the number of years smoked, the greater the risk of AAA. This risk decreased progressively as the number of years since quitting smoking increased. Smoking-related risk explained 78% of all AAAs measuring 4 cm or larger. Factors negatively associated with AAA were female sex (OR, 0.22), African-American race (OR, 0.49), and diabetes (OR, 0.54). Subjects with a family history of AAA were at double the risk (OR, 1.95); however, just 5% of the veterans studied reported such a history. Age, height, coronary artery

TABLE 1.—Characteristics of Veterans Screened for Abdominal
Aortic Aneurysm

Characteristic	Value
Mean age ± SD, *y*	66.2 ± 7.1
Male, %	97.2
Race, %	
White	87.0
Black	8.2
Other	4.9
Mean height ± SD, *cm*	176.4 ± 7.2
Mean weight ± SD, *kg*	84.8 ± 15.7
Mean waist circumference ± SD, *cm*	96.4 ± 11.3
Family history of abdominal aortic aneurysm, %	5.1
Ever smoked regularly, %*	75.5
Mean duration of smoking history ± SD, *y*	30.1 ± 14.6
Current smoker, %	18.7
Hypertension, %	55.1
High cholesterol levels, %	52.3
Coronary artery disease, %	39.0
Claudication, %	6.7
Cerebral vascular disease, %	11.5
Any atherosclerosis, %	46.0
Deep venous thrombosis, %	7.4
Diabetes mellitus, %	18.1
Chronic obstructive pulmonary disease, %	14.4
Cancer at site other than skin, %	12.4
Abdominal imaging in past 5 years, %	19.5

Note: Values represent percentages of patients unless otherwise noted.
*More than 100 cigarettes over lifetime.
(Courtesy of Lederle FA, for the Aneurysm Detection and Management (ADAM) Veterans Affairs Cooperative Study Group. *Ann Intern Med* 126:441–449, 1997.)

disease, atherosclerosis, high cholesterol, and high blood pressure were also independently associated with AAA.

Conclusion.—Many different factors are related to risk of AAA. However, smoking is the major risk factor and may account for most clinically significant instances of previously undiagnosed AAA. The prevalence of previously undiagnosed AAA in this large screening population was about 1%.

▶ Surprise! Surprise! Smoking is bad for us. This was a very large study of over 73,000 predominantly older white male veterans who were screened for AAA through Department of Veterans Affairs medical centers. The authors defined a normal abdominal aorta as one of less than 3.0 cm in diameter and one with an aneurysm as having a greater than 4.0–cm diameter. The risk for AAA was increased by 5½ times if the veteran smoked. The excess prevalence with smoking accounted for 78% of all AAAs in the study sample.

Interestingly, the incidence for black veterans was half that for white veterans. Unfortunately, only 8% of the sample was black. However, because the study population was so large this was statistically significant.

With an overall incidence of previously unrecognized AAA of 1.4% in the screened population, it probably does not make sense to use routine ultrasound for screening for AAA. However, with a greater than fivefold increase in risk in patients who smoke, we must carefully consider whether we would screen for AAA in the smoking population.

R.C. Davidson, M.D., M.P.H.

Miscellaneous

Normal Sinus Heart Rate: Appropriate Rate Thresholds for Sinus Tachyardia and Bradycardia

Spodick DH (Univ of Massachusetts, Worcester)
South Med J 89:666–667, 1996   1–33

Purpose.—In a patient at rest, the accepted range of normal sinus rhythm is 60/min to 100/min. Faster and slower rates prompt a search for a cause of tachycardia and bradycardia, respectively. However, these rate limits were established by consensus and have never been formally studied. Clinical experience suggests that both the high and low limits are too high. Five hundred normal subjects were studied to investigate the value of conventional thresholds for tachycardia and bradycardia.

Methods.—The patients all underwent ECG recording of resting heart rate. All examinations were performed in the afternoon, which is the time of day most nonemergency patients are seen.

Results.—Across age groups, the mean heart rate was approximately 70/min, with only small differences between the sexes. The results were very similar to those reported in larger cohorts—the 5,000-subject cohort of the Framingham study and the nearly 20,000 cohort of the EPICORE Center group. Extreme values corresponding to standard deviations for normal resting sinus rate were 46/min to 93/min for men and 51/min to 95/min for women. These figures were rounded to 50/min and 90/min.

Conclusions.—Based on measurements in normal subjects, the authors propose that 50/min to 90/min be considered the appropriate range for normal sinus heart rate. Using these thresholds for bradycardia and tachycardia, respectively, should increase the specificity of bradycardia detection and the sensitivity of tachycardia detection.

▶ The concept of what is "normal" has always interested me. We set arbitrary standards for blood pressure, pulse, and other parameters such as weight. This interesting study looked at the parameters for what is considered a normal sinus heart rate. Traditionally, these parameters have been 100 beats per minute as a threshold for tachycardia and 60 beats per minute as the threshold for bradycardia. The authors studied 500 normal individuals and compared these with the 5,000-subject cohort of the Framingham study and 18,000-subject cohort of the EPICORE study. Their conclusion is that the appropriate rate range for normal sinus rhythm should be lowered by 10 beats per minute for both upper and lower limits. They therefore recommend a definition of bradycardia as below 50 beats per minute and tachycardia above 90 beats per minute. They suggest that this will improve the sensitivity of diagnosing tachycardia and reduce unnecessary evaluations of patients with pulse rates between 50 and 60 beats per minute.

R.C. Davidson, M.D., M.P.H.

Cardioversion of Atrial Fibrillation in the Elderly
Carlsson J, for the ALKK-Study Group (Klinikum Lippe-Detmold, Germany)
Am J Cardiol 78:1380–1384, 1996   1–34

Introduction.—There is a strong relation between increasing age and the prevalence of atrial fibrillation. About 70% of patients with atrial fibrillation are between 65 and 85 years old, and this group has a higher stroke rate than younger patients, creating therapeutic problems. Because physicians are reluctant to prescribe anticoagulants for older patients, they may turn to cardioversion for long-term maintenance of sinus rhythm. However, there is still some controversy over whether age is correlated with the success rate of cardioversion or the maintenance of sinus rhythm. Complication and success rates of elective cardioversion in elderly patients with atrial fibrillation were presented.

Methods.—From 61 cardiology clinics, 1,152 patients were enrolled in this prospective study. They were divided into 2 groups: 570 were younger than 65 years and 582 were 65 years or older. Demographic, procedural, and outcome data on patients who underwent cardioversion of atrial fibrillation were recorded.

Results.—In the group younger than 65, the overall success rate of cardioversion was 76.1%, and in the group aged 65 or older, it was 72.7%. Predictors of success were left atrial size and New York Heart

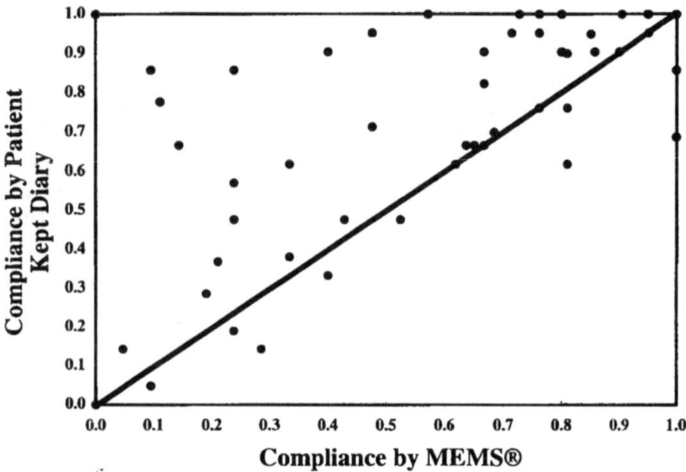

FIGURE 2.—The concordance between the compliance rates recorded by the MEMS vials and those recorded in the patient-kept diaries. Each data point represents the compliance values for a single patient, and the solid line depicts the line of identity. (Courtesy of Straka RJ, Fish JT, Benson SR, et al: Patient self-reporting of compliance does not correspond with electronic monitoring: An evaluation using isosorbide dinitrate as a model drug. *Pharmacotherapy* 17:126–132, 1997).

in a Medication-Event Monitoring System (MEMS-4) monitor fitted as a bottle cap and designed to record each time the bottle is opened. The study was divided into a contiguous 2-week run-in phase, 4-week monitoring phase, and 3-week self-assessment phase. Data collected by the monitor were compared with diary entries.

Results.—Of the 55 patients (20 men, average patient age, 67 years) who completed the study, 3 did not complete all days during the assessment phase. Patients had received isosorbide for an average of 2.1 years and were taking an additional 4.1 oral medications on average. Level 3 compliance for diaries and MEMS vials was significantly different (71% compared with 55%) (Fig 2). Compared with MEMS data, diaries underestimated compliance by 16%, overestimated compliance by 67%, and were the same in 16% of cases. The average number of errors between diaries and the MEMS system was 18.4. When MEMS data were used, the compliance rate during the monitoring phase was 46%; and during the self-assessment phase, the compliance rate was 55%.

Conclusion.—Although keeping a patient diary increased compliance, the diaries tend to overestimate compliance by as much as 29%. Because of findings of poor compliance overall in this study, results suggest a reevaluation of the effectiveness of 3-times-daily dosing of isosorbide dinitrate.

▶ The findings from this study are not new. I included it to remind us of the relatively poor compliance of patients whose recommended drug regimens involve taking medicine more than once per day. These pharmacy researchers evaluated an oral nitrate recommended to be taken 3 times per day. As shown in the concordant graph (Fig 2), there was very poor correlation between the patient-completed medication diary and the more accurate electronic monitoring drug-dispensing unit.

Although it is not always feasible, comparison of alternate therapies must factor in the noncompliance with regimens involving taking medicine several times per day drug. If we ask our patients to take drugs more than twice a day, their compliance begins to drop dramatically.

R.C. Davidson, M.D., M.P.H.

2 Metabolism

Introduction

The section on adult nutrition opens with studies of 11,000 vegetarians, vitamin status and health, and nutrition labeling. The pediatric section focuses on breast feeding, but adds 2 articles on growth under age 3 and fat intake, and use of fortified cereals in schoolchildren. The 3 articles in the obesity section avoid the drug treatment controversy of the last year, instead presenting studies on morbidity in adolescents, body size perception, and an interesting article about use of refeeding diets in highly controlled circumstances.

Randomized controlled trials: Abstracts 2–4 and 2–11.

Alfred O. Berg, M.D., M.P.H.

Adult Nutrition

Dietary Habits and Mortality in 11000 Vegetarians and Health Conscious People: Results of a 17 Year Follow Up
Key TJA, Thorogood M, Appleby PN, et al (Radcliffe Infirmary, Oxford, England; London School of Hygiene & Tropical Medicine; Univ of Wales, Cardiff)
BMJ 313:775–779, 1996   2–1

Introduction.—Between 1973 and 1979, the relationship between dietary habits and mortality was assessed in a cohort of 11,000 British males and females. Follow-up of this cohort until 1980–1985 revealed that habitual consumption of wholemeal bread was not significantly correlated with mortality, but that a vegetarian diet was associated with a significant decrease in mortality from ischemic heart disease. Follow-up through 1995 was reported.

Methods.—The mortality ratios for vegetarianism and for daily vs. less-than-daily consumption of wholemeal bread, bran cereals, nuts or dried fruits, fresh fruit, and raw salad were assessed to determine any correlations between dietary habits and all causes of mortality, and mortality from ischemic heart disease, cerebrovascular disease, all malignant neoplasms, lung cancer, colorectal cancer, and breast cancer. A total of 4,336 males and 6,435 females were recruited through health food shops, vegetarian societies, and magazines.

Results.—Research subjects were followed for a mean of 16.8 years. Of 10,771 participants, 2,064 (19%) smoked, 4,627 (43%) were vegetarian, 6,699 (62%) ate wholemeal bread daily, 4,091 (38%) ate nuts or dried fruit daily, 2,948 (27%) ate bran cereals daily, 8,304 (77%) ate fresh fruit daily, and 4,105 (38%) ate raw salad daily. There were 1,343 deaths before 80 years of age at the 1995 follow-up. The cohort of health-conscious individuals had an overall mortality rate of about half that of the general population. Daily consumption of fresh fruit in the cohort was correlated with significantly lower mortality from ischemic heart disease, cerebral vascular disease, and for all causes combined. Limitations to the study include: the design of the survey instrument, which did not include a comprehensive food survey or questions about related health factors such as exercise of socioeconomic status; and that dietary habits of those in the cohort changed over time.

Conclusions.—After adjusting for smoking, the daily consumption of fruit in vegetarians and health-conscious research subjects was associated with a 24% reduction in mortality from ischemic heart disease, a 32% decrease in mortality from cerebrovascular disease, and a 21% reduction in all causes of mortality.

▶ This study certainly fits in well with the accumulating evidence of the benefits of eating low on the food chain. Don't bank on the conclusions, though. Read the limitations carefully. They range from an incomplete initial questionnaire to lack of follow-up, and potential confounders were not evaluated. I included this study as a reminder that, despite the hype and my acceptance of the basic validity of the concept, the evidence is not always as solid as it is portrayed.

W.W. Dexter, M.D.

Do Nutrition Label Readers Eat Healthier Diets? Behavioral Correlates of Adults' Use of Food Labels

Kreuter MW, Brennan LK, Scharff DP, et al (Saint Louis Univ)
Am J Prev Med 13:277–283, 1997   2–2

Introduction.—The first step in making personal dietary changes is knowledge of the relative nutritional value of different foods. Little is known about consumer use of nutrition labels and what effects label reading has on dietary behaviors. A self-administered survey was used to determine characteristics of adult primary care patients who do and do not read nutrition labels, to describe patterns of label use and perception of label understandability among individuals who read nutrition labels, and to identify behavioral and health status correlates of nutrition label reading.

Methods.—Research subjects were adult patients from 4 community-based family medicine clinics from 3 towns in southeastern Missouri. A self-administered questionnaire was completed by participants while in the waiting area of their doctor's office. Of 915 questionnaires completed in a 2-week period, 885 were able to be used for data collection.

Results.—Nutrition labels were significantly more likely to be read by patients who were female rather than male; had more years of education; ate diets lower in fat; ate diets higher in fruits, vegetables, and fiber; had accurate perceptions of their own dietary fat consumption; and had been told by their doctors within the last 6 months to eat less fat. Patients with a diagnosis of high blood pressure were 63% more likely than patients with normal or low blood pressure to read labels for sodium content, but not other information. Patients with high cholesterol levels were more likely to read nutrition labels for cholesterol and saturated fat content, but not other information. Ease in reading nutrition labels increased with educational level.

Conclusions.—Rates of nutrition label reading were lower in males, patients with less than a high school education, and those with no specific medical condition requiring dietary modification. The role of nutrition labels could be expanded from current practices using educational programs emphasizing their importance in disease prevention. New strategies are needed for encouraging males and individuals with less education to use nutrition labels.

▶ When working with patients ready for change in their dietary habits, we often discuss paying close attention to food choices. Label reading can be a critical step in making informed choices. The conclusion here comes as no surprise. But be careful; while the association is clear, whether label reading leads to improved dietary practices is not. In fact, less than half the respondents felt that reading labels influenced their choices. What's to make of this? Label reading behavior may only identify individuals who have already made changes, but it also might help facilitate positive change. It is, at least, a useful skill and I encourage my patients to develop this shopping habit.

W.W. Dexter, M.D.

Intake of Vitamins E, C, and A and Risk of Lung Cancer: The NHANES I Epidemiologic Followup Study
Yong L-C, Brown CC, Schatzkin A, et al (Natl Cancer Inst, Bethesda, Md; Natl Center for Health Statistics, Hyattsville, Md)
Am J Epidemiol 146:231–243, 1997   2–3

Introduction.—It has been suggested that vitamins E and C and the carotenoids, with their antioxidant properties, and vitamin A, which functions in cell differentiation, may have protective effects against cancer. Several reports have found an inverse correlation between the risk of lung cancer and frequency of consumption of fruits and vegetables, which are major food sources of these nutrients. The relation of intakes of dietary and supplemental vitamins E, C, and A, and fruits and vegetables to subsequent risk of lung cancer was examined. Also, the role of cigarette

(always hard to change) don't easily meet or exceed RDA's, supplementation also makes sense.

W.W. Dexter, M.D.

Vitamin A Status, Other Risk Factors and Acute Respiratory Infection Morbidity in Children

Dudley L, Hussey G, Huskissen J, et al (Univ of Cape Town, South Africa)
S Afr Med J 87:65–69, 1997   2–5

Background.—The effects of vitamin A supplementation on mortality rate and the occurrence of infectious diseases (acute respiratory tract infection [ARI] and gastroenteritis) among children are currently under investigation worldwide. However, no one has studied the relationship between vitamin A status and illness severity. The relationship between vitamin A status and ARI-associated morbidity was reported.

Methods.—Thirty-five hospitalized children with severe ARI and 32 treated as outpatients for mild ARI were included. Fifty-four children with noninfectious diseases seen as outpatients comprised the control group. The groups were matched by age and area of residence.

Findings.—Mean vitamin A levels were 22.09 µg/dl for the control group, 20.27 µg/dl for the mild ARI group, and 13.79 µg/dl for the severe ARI group. All pairwise comparisons were significant. After vitamin A levels were dichomotized, odds ratios were 2.1 for severe versus mild ARI, 2.9 for mild versus no ARI, and 6.0 for severe versus no ARI. Risk factors correlated with disease status were a history of hospitalization in the preceding 6 months, no clinic card, poor housing, and lack of electricity for indoor fuel use. Poor vitamin A status was associated with low weight for age, previous diarrheal disease, and poor housing conditions. Vitamin A status and disease status were associated independently in a logistic regression model.

Conclusions.—Vitamin A status is strongly associated with infection severity, with an apparent dose-response effect. Thus, these data support vitamin A supplementation for groups considered at risk, though its role in a broader health initiative needs to be better defined.

Marginal Vitamin and Mineral Intakes of Young Adults: The Bogalusa Heart Study

Zive MM, Nicklas TA, Busch EC, et al (Univ of California, San Diego; Tulane Ctr for Cardiovascular Health, New Orleans, La)
J Adolesc Health 19:39–47, 1996   2–6

Background.—A knowledge of the dietary intakes and eating patterns of young adults is important, because this is the age of childbearing and the formation of lifestyles that affect later health. The vitamin and mineral intakes, vitamin supplement use, and food consumption patterns of young adults were reported.

Methods.—Between 1988 and 1991, 24-hour dietary recall histories were obtained from a cross-sectional sample of 504 young adults, 19 to 28. Fifty-eight percent were female, and 70% were white.

Findings.—According to recommended dietary allowances (RDAs), these subjects had inadequate intakes of vitamins A, B_6, E, D, and C; folacin; magnesium; iron; zinc; and calcium. More women than men reported nutrient intakes less than two thirds of the RDA. About 10% reported taking a vitamin and mineral supplement during the 24-hour survey period. Additional food source data showed that the main contributors of the vitamins and minerals consumed were breads and grains, milk, vegetables, soups, fruits, and beef.

Conclusions.—Young adults need to be educated on practical strategies for making wise food choices with adequate nutrient content relative to energy value. More objective measures now need to be applied to examine the extent to which RDAs are useful in identifying deficiency or marginal nutritional status, as well as optimal nutrition.

▶ As noted in Abstracts 2–5 and 2–6, evidence is accumulating to support a rationale for dietary supplementation with vitamins. Having been a young adult once, I can attest to the paucity of vitamin and mineral–laden foods in the diet of this age group. About half the young adults in this study did not even approach the RDA for many vitamins and minerals. Older adults do not fare much better. Am I simply taking the easy way out in suggesting that we use supplements? Is meeting or exceeding the RDAs a nutritional goal with supplements worth the potential downside? Does recommending a supplement imply tacit acceptance of poor nutritional habits? Perhaps. Clearly, we need to develop strategies to help folks change their eating patterns to at least meet the minimum RDA standards. Ten percent of the population studied were already taking supplements. I do not necessarily see this as the default option—proper diet is still the best way to go—but I am becoming increasingly convinced that supplements, although not always needed, can play a role in health maintenance.

W.W. Dexter, M.D.

Pediatric Nutrition

Maternal Employment and Breast-feeding: Findings From the 1988 National Maternal and Infant Health Survey
Visness CM, Kennedy KI (Univ of Denver)
Am J Public Health 87:945–950, 1997   2–7

Objective.—The low rate of breast-feeding in the U.S. is commonly blamed on the increasing number of women in the workforce. Whether breast-feeding and working outside the home are mutually exclusive activities was examined by exploring the factors associated with initiation and duration of breast-feeding using data from the 1988 National Maternal and Infant Health Survey (NMIHS).

Methods.—The 9,087 eligible NMIHS respondents were asked if and how they had breast-fed their babies. The women were stratified by socio-economic and demographic factors.

Results.—A total of 53.4% of respondents breast-fed. The median duration of breast-feeding was less than 1 week among all respondents, including bottle-feeders. Only 25% of women breast-fed for more than 9 weeks. Those who initiated breast-feeding averaged 13 weeks. Twenty-five percent breast-fed for 6 weeks or less. Women employed before giving birth were more likely to breast-feed than women who were not employed. Only 24% of black women breast-fed whereas more than 50% of white, Hispanic, and "other" women breast-fed. Older, higher income, more educated, and married women were more likely to breast-feed. Normal weight infants were more likely to be breast-fed than were low birthweight infants. Nonparticipants in the Special Supplemental Food Program were 62% more likely to breast-feed than were participants. Professional women were most likely and manufacturing women were least likely to breast-feed. Approximately half of nonworking women breast-fed.

Conclusion.—Low rates of breast-feeding are not ascribable to working women, although returning to work is associated with earlier weaning.

▶ Overcoming the barriers to breast-feeding can be troublesome. Lack of support at the work site is a problem encountered all too frequently, even within health care settings. Let's get the problems with this study out of the way: old data (1988) and possible selection bias. I was surprised and disappointed that, as the authors point out, this is the most current source of information available on this topic. I agree that postpartum employment is not solely responsible for the low rates of breast-feeding, but it is clearly a barrier to maintaining breast-feeding, and, in my experience, to initiation. We should strive to support our patients in the choice to breast-feed. Begin this process early in the pregnancy, establish a relationship with a lactation consultant, and work with your patients' employers to facilitate this choice.

W.W. Dexter, M.D.

Breastfeeding and Catch-up Growth in Infants Born Small for Gestational Age

Lucas A, Fewtrell MS, Davies PSW, et al (Inst of Child Health, London; MRC Dunn Nutrition Unit, Cambridge, England; Addenbrookes Hosp, Cambridge, England)
Acta Paediatr 86:564–569, 1997   2–8

Objective.—The risks of growth failure and other problems are elevated among infants born small for gestational age (SGA). There are few data on how postnatal nutrition affects growth in SGA infants. The influence of breast-feeding versus formula feeding on growth in SGA infants was assessed.

Methods.—The prospective study included 54 term infants who were SGA at birth. Half were fed breast milk and half were fed a standard term infant formula; feeding was not randomly assigned. Postnatal growth was measured at intervals until 1 year.

Results.—Infants who were breast-fed had a 0.36 standard deviation (SD) increase in weight at 2 weeks and a 0.64 SD increase at 3 months. This gain persisted beyond the breast-feeding period, with a continued 0.64 SD increase at 1 year. Catch-up growth in head circumference and

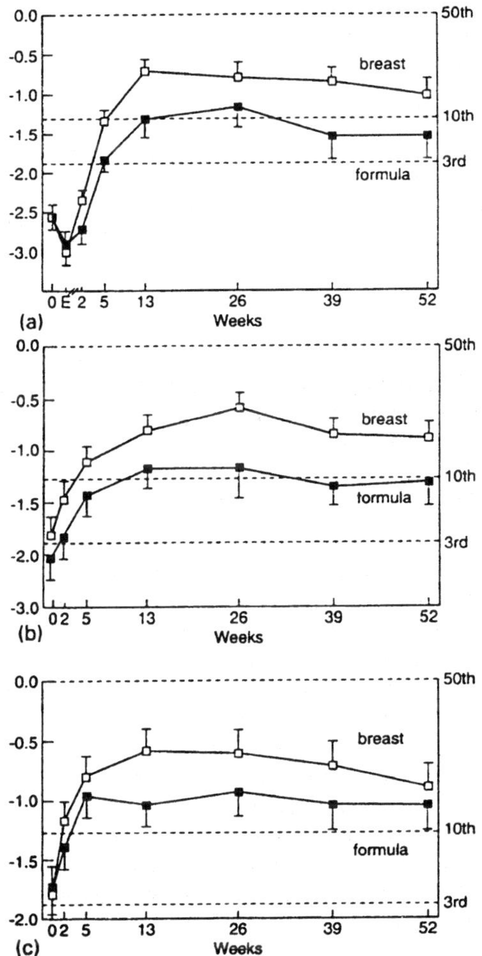

FIGURE 1.—A, Body weight; B, length; and C, head circumference SDs at different ages from birth to 12 months in term growth-retarded infants, according to diet. Values are mean. The third, tenth, and fiftieth percentiles are marked for reference. Error bars represent SE. *0*, Birth; *E*, time of enrollment in the study. (Courtesy of Lucas A, Fewtrell MS, Davies PSW, et al: Breastfeeding and catch-up growth in infants born small for gestational age. *Acta Paediatr* 86:564–569, 1997.)

body length were also greater in the breast-fed group (Fig 1). The improved growth in breast-fed infants was independent of potential obstetric, social, and demographic confounders.

Results.—For term SGA infants, breast-feeding may be associated with faster growth than formula feeding. More research is needed to see whether the risks of adverse outcomes associated with being SGA are affected by postnatal nutrition.

▶ I am not surprised by the outcome here. The results confirm earlier observations regarding the benefit of breast-feeding in SGA infants. The study design was reasonably tight, though not randomized, which certainly may have introduced significant bias. The analysis of the data, however, was quite detailed, lending weight to the findings. Another solid reason to encourage breast-feeding, particularly in this population.

I must admit to some puzzlement, though. Why must we (medical science) strive to prove that breast-feeding is better than formula? It should be the other way around. It seems to me that a certain human arrogance is at work when our baseline assumption is that we can create in a laboratory a better source of nutrition for infants. Nevertheless, this seems to be a pervasive attitude, and I am delighted to read and share studies that support breast-feeding.

W.W. Dexter, M.D.

The Influence of Medroxyprogesterone on the Duration of Breast-feeding in Mothers in an Urban Community

Hannon PR, Duggan AK, Serwint JR, et al (Johns Hopkins Univ, Baltimore, Md)
Arch Pediatr Adolesc Med 151:490–496, 1997   2–9

Background.—Many new mothers feel they have to choose between breast-feeding their infants and using a hormonal method of contraception (which may have negative effects on lactation). The effects on lactation of medroxyprogesterone acetate (a long-acting progesterone that is a highly effective contraceptive) given immediately postpartum were evaluated.

Methods.—Ninety-five women were enrolled in the study, of which 43 chose to use medroxyprogesterone acetate and 52 chose to use a nonhormonal method of contraception. Inclusion criteria included delivery of a healthy term neonate, breast-feeding at discharge, and the intention to breast-feed at home. Telephone interviews at postpartum weeks 1–8, 12, and 16 assessed the duration and frequency of breast-feeding, when formula was introduced, why breast-feeding was stopped, and the current means of contraception.

Findings.—The 2 groups showed no significant differences in lactation parameters at enrollment (including planned duration of lactation, prior experience with lactation, and start of formula use). Follow-up data on 90 women (96% of sample) showed that the groups had similar rates in the frequency of lactation, the duration of lactation, and the timing of the introduction of formula.

Conclusions.—Medroxyprogesterone acetate given immediately postpartum had no detrimental effect on the duration of breast-feeding, the frequency of feedings, or the introduction of formula for the first 16 weeks postpartum.

▶ The desire for a chemical contraceptive method postpartum raises questions and sometimes interferes with the choice of breast-feeding. Data on the safety and effectiveness of breast-feeding during the use of contraceptive methods will reassure patients and promote more widespread use of breast-feeding. This study confirms that women may receive injectable medroxyprogesterone acetate immediately postpartum and go on to breast-feed their infants.

J.E. Scherger, M.D., M.P.H.

Does Early Supplementation Affect Long-term Breastfeeding?
Hill PD, Humenick SS, Brennan ML, et al (Univ of Illinois, Chicago; Univ of Wyoming, Laramie)
Clin Pediatr 36:345–350, 1997   2–10

Purpose.—Most previous studies have suggested that supplemental formula feeding reduces the duration of breast-feeding, particularly for infants who start supplementation in the early postpartum period. Other studies—including data disseminated by a formula manufacturer—suggest the opposite relationship. Data from a previous longitudinal study were analyzed to determine the effect of early formula supplementation on the duration of breast-feeding.

Methods.—The analysis included 2 convenience samples of breast-feeding mothers: 120 mothers in 1 group and 223 in the other. They were prospectively followed up through the twentieth postpartum week or until weaning occurred. Breast-feeding duration was compared for women who fed their infants only breast milk versus those who supplemented with formula.

Results.—In the first sample, the breast-feeding rate at 20 weeks was 63% for mothers who breast-fed exclusively during the second postpartum week versus 28% for those who supplemented with formula during the first 2 weeks. In the second sample, these figures were 60% and 24%, respectively (Fig 1). The mothers who did and did not continue breast-feeding were similar with respect to intended duration of breast-feeding.

Conclusions.—Early supplementation with formula is associated with a reduced duration of breast-feeding by the mothers of term infants. Health care professionals should be aware of the importance of exclusive breast-feeding and the negative effects of early supplementation when offering advice to breast-feeding mothers. Other factors affecting the mother's

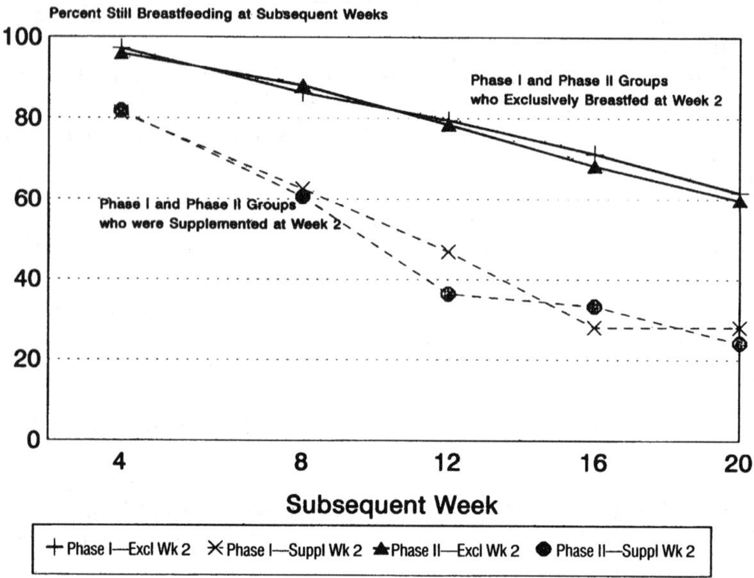

FIGURE 1.—Breastfeeding rates at weeks 4 through 20 subsequent to feeding pattern at week 2. (Courtesy of Hill PD, Humenick SS, Brennan ML, et al: Does early supplementation affect long-term breastfeeding? *Clin Pediatr* 36:345–350, 1997.)

decision to supplement with formula, especially during the first few postpartum weeks, should be examined as well.

▶ My wife Cindy, a lactation consultant, has preached this for years. Early supplementation, despite the patient's stated intentions, reduces duration of breast-feeding. I would like to see this study repeated with more stringent controls and a larger, more representative sample. Nevertheless, the findings support her contention. A good case is made for working toward reducing, if not eliminating, early supplementation in healthy term infants. This is not as easy as it would appear on the surface. Supplementation is a behavior that is well ingrained in our thoughts, behaviors, and birthing unit policies, both stated and unstated. It is also promulgated and fostered by formula companies, for obvious reasons. Having recently concluded a successful campaign to achieve recognition for her hospital (Alice Peck Day Hospital, Lebanon, N.H.), through the World Health Organization's Baby Friendly Initiative, Cindy can attest to the size of the task. Reaching a breast-feeding target of 80% (the Healthy People 2000 goal is 75%; currently, it is less than 60% in the United States), took the concerted effort of physicians, nurses, lactation consultants, administrators, and patients. Lend your support; in the office and at the birthing center, this is a laudable and attainable goal.

W.W. Dexter, M.D.

Growth Until 3 Years of Age in a Prospective, Randomized Trial of a Diet With Reduced Saturated Fat and Cholesterol
Niinikoski H, Lapinleimu H, Viikari J, et al (Univ of Turku, Finland; Social Insurance Institution, Turku, Finland)
Pediatrics 99:687–694, 1997   2–11

Purpose.—It has been suggested that modifying fat intake during childhood could reduce the risk of future atherosclerosis in children. However, too great a reduction in fat intake could lead to growth failure. The effects of a diet low in saturated fat on growth during the first 3 years of life were evaluated in a randomized trial.

Methods.—The study included 1,062 healthy 7-month-old infants. They were randomized into an atherosclerosis risk factor reduction group and a control group. The intervention group received individual dietary counseling geared toward reducing the babies' exposure to atherosclerosis risk factors. Both groups underwent regular assessments of growth and serum lipid levels. At intervals of 5–12 months, 3- to 4-day food records were completed to assess the children's nutrient intakes. The children were monitored until they reached 3 years of age.

Results.—Energy intake was slightly and consistently lower in the intervention group than it was in the control group. For both groups, mean fat intake was lower than expected, particularly in the first 2 years of life. For formula-fed children at 8 months of age, mean fat intake as a percentage of energy intake (E%) was about 29% in both groups. This figure was 26% in the intervention group and 28% in the control group at 13 months; 30% and 32% at 24 months; and 31% and 33%, respectively, at 36 months. From 13 to 36 months, children in the intervention group had a significantly lower baseline adjusted mean serum cholesterol concentration. For boys in the intervention group, the true mean of height during the study was at most 0.34 cm more or 0.57 cm less than for boys in the intervention group. The difference in weight was at most 0.19 kg more or 0.22 kg less. The pattern was similar for girls. The 2 groups were comparable in their proportions of slim children.

Conclusions.—For young children, following a diet low in saturated fat and low in cholesterol does not impair growth during the first 3 years of life. This is despite the fact that children following such a diet have consistently lower mean energy and fat intakes than control children. The findings of this study suggest that young children have a lower fat intake than is generally assumed.

▶ Eating habits are established early and are learned behaviors. Debate has raged over the advisability of restricting young children's consumption of fats, weighing the potential benefit of reduction in atherosclerotic disease vs. the perception that lower-fat diets may cause growth disturbances. I have always favored the former, and this study gives my bias some credence. I should note, however, that the study population was all-volunteer. It was a significant undertaking, not at all randomized and not particularly

well-controlled. It was instructive to note that the energy consumption in the intervention group was consistently lower. I remain concerned that, accepting these results as fact, without significant effort on our part and motivation on the part of our patients, appropriate nutrition to ensure proper growth and development might be problematic. This is not the final word, but with adequate counseling about nutrition, a diet for toddlers that is lower in fat than is customary would seem safe and appropriate.

W.W. Dexter, M.D.

Nutrient Intakes and Impact of Fortified Breakfast Cereals in School-children
McNulty H, Eaton-Evans J, Cran G, et al (Univ of Ulster, Coleraine, Northern Ireland; The Queen's Univ, Belfast, Northern Ireland; Inst of Clinical Science; et al)
Arch Dis Child 75:474–481, 1996   2–12

Objective.—Diet in childhood determines resistance to disease and lays down eating patterns. Adequate intake of micronutrients is a concern after recent surveys have confirmed that children's dietary habits are increasingly characterized by informal eating and frequent snacking. Micronutrient intakes in a random sample of Northern Ireland school children were determined to establish the extent to which eating a good breakfast contributes to overall nutrient intakes and achievement of current dietary recommendations.

Methods.—Body mass index, skinfold thicknesses, blood pressure, cardiorespiratory fitness, and estimates of total cholesterol were recorded for 1,015 school children, aged 12 and 15. Dietary data were collected and converted into energy and nutrient intakes. Median daily intakes were divided into centiles.

Results.—Thiamin, riboflavin, niacin, vitamin B-6, vitamin B-12, retinol, iron, zinc, and copper intakes were significantly higher in 15-year-old boys than in either 12-year-old boys or in girls. Folate and vitamin E levels were also significantly higher in 15-year-olds compared with 12-year-olds; the levels were higher in boys than in girls. Of those consuming fortified breakfast cereals, 95% and 92% were 12- and 15-year-old boys and 87% and 78% were 12- and 15-year-old girls. Folate intake was low for boys and girls and iron intake was low for girls. Children who did not eat fortified cereals had low intakes of riboflavin, niacin, folate, iron (for girls), and vitamin B-12.

Conclusion.—Mean micronutrient intake appears to be adequate (except for folate in boys and girls and iron in girls) in children in Northern Ireland who eat fortified breakfast cereals. Children who did not eat fortified breakfast cereals had low intakes of several vitamins and iron.

▶ Who reads cereal boxes over breakfast? We surely do in our house. And it is not just for breakfast anymore. Many of the cereal choices in our

supermarkets are fortified to one extent or another. It is gratifying, at least as a parent who probably too frequently defaults to the cereal option, to note that cereal really can be a nutritious choice. My one concern, given the mixed evidence on supplementation of vitamins, is whether fortification provides the same nutrient availability of the appropriate foods, or is equivalent to supplementation. I am not sure, but for now, I will feel better about our breakfast (and sometimes lunch and dinner) choices and continue to read the boxes.

W.W. Dexter, M.D.

Obesity

Relationship Between Morbidity and Extreme Values of Body Mass Index in Adolescents

Lusky A, Barell V, Lubin F, et al (Sheba Med School, Tel Hashomer, Israel; Israel Defense Force Med Corps)
Int J Epidemiol 25:829–834, 1996   2–13

Introduction.—Considerable evidence links being overweight with cardiovascular risk factors. However, few studies from industrialized countries have examined adolescent morbidity associated with underweight. A study of Israeli army recruits was performed to assess morbidity associated with body mass index (BMI) values at the extreme ends of the range.

Methods.—The study included approximately 110,000 Jewish Israeli boys, 17 years, who were required to undergo assessment for military service. This includes routine physical examination at an army induction center. Data from these examinations—including overall health profiles, specific physical and mental conditions, and height and weight—were analyzed to assess the relationship between BMI and morbidity. Any condition severe enough to preclude combat service was considered medically significant.

Results.—The prevalence of functional limitation was 149.5/1,000 among severely underweight recruits and 164.3/1,000 among severely overweight recruits, compared with 103.5/1,000 among recruits of normal weight. Hypertension occurred at a rate of 14.9/1,000 among severely overweight recruits. Other conditions associated with overweight included lower-extremity joint problems, particularly hip, ankle, and knee disorders. Asthma was present at a rate of 14.2/1,000 among mildly underweight recruits and 18.9/1,000 among severely underweight recruits. Other disorders associated with being underweight included scoliosis, intestinal conditions, and neurosis.

Conclusions.—Boys, 17 years, who are either overweight or underweight are apparently at increased risk for morbidity. Interventions to prevent or reduce morbidity should be directed toward adolescents and young adults. The study is the first to define the prevalence of pathology among adolescents along the entire spectrum of weight.

▶ Several things struck me about this study. First, the army has always been a fruitful area for research, because "volunteers" are plentiful. This is more true in Israel, where evaluation for military service is compulsory. It may be a stretch, though, to extrapolate these results to any other populations. Second, the prevalence of underweight among boys, 17 years, was about the same as that of overweight, which surprised me. I doubt that this is the case in the United States or other developed nations. The results otherwise are not striking—moderation wins the day. Finally, the investigators use BMI for their measurement, which might have underestimated overweight. I do agree with using BMI as a measure. BMI should be monitored in obese patients, because evaluation of weight alone may not provide adequate data to assess weight, particularly in growing children.[1]

W.W. Dexter, M.D.

Reference

1. Smith JC, Surey WH, Quebedeau D, et al. Use of body mass index to monitor treatment of obese adolescence. *J Adolesc Health* 20:466–469, 1997.

Black-White Differences in Body Size Perceptions and Weight Management Practices Among Adolescent Females
Neff LJ, Sargent RG, McKeown RE, et al (Univ of South Carolina, Columbia)
J Adolesc Health 20:459–465, 1997   2–14

Background.—Black women are twice as likely as white women to be overweight. This and other regional and ethnic differences suggest that sociocultural factors may play a role in the etiology of obesity. Adolescents may be the best target for interventions to reduce overweight and obesity. Black and white teenaged girls were compared with respect to body image perceptions, weight goals, and weight-management practices.

Methods.—The study included 1,824 black and 2,256 white female adolescents enrolled in South Carolina public high schools. The sample was selected to be representative of high school students statewide. The girls were asked to rate their body size as overweight, underweight, or about right. They were also asked about weight-management practices, such as dieting, exercise, and other measures, including use of diet pills and vomiting. Differences between the groups were assessed, including controlling for socioeconomic status.

Results.—The percentage of respondents perceiving themselves as overweight was 41% for white girls and 29% for black girls. Twenty-four percent of white girls and 13% of black girls reported dieting in the week before the questionnaire. Exercising to lose weight was reported by 34% of white girls versus 23% of black girls, whereas both dieting and exercising were reported by 45% of white girls and 16% of black girls. On logistic regression, white girls were twice as likely as black girls to think themselves overweight. Odds ratios suggested that white girls were 6 times more likely to use diet pills and vomiting, and nearly 4 times more likely to diet and exercise.

Conclusions.—Compared with black adolescent girls, white girls are more likely to think that they are overweight and more likely to use unhealthy weight-management practices. Black girls in this age group appear less motivated to be thin than are their white peers.

▶ The findings here support data on differences in obesity and eating disorders. I agree that most likely there are cultural differences at work here. This study points out some of these differences and suggests that we should at least be sensitive to them when dealing with these issues in the office. Broad generalizations such as these trouble me, though. These distinctions, although apparently real, are useful mainly as background, perhaps even in program design. It may not be appropriate to apply them broadly in the office to individual patients.

W.W. Dexter, M.D.

Inhibition of Regain in Body Weight and Fat With Addition of 3–Carbon Compounds to the Diet With Hyperenergetic Refeeding After Weight Reduction
Stanko RT, Arch JE (Montefiore Univ, Pittsburg, Pa; Univ of Pittsburgh, Pa)
Int J Obes 20:925–930, 1996   2–15

Introduction.—Animal and human investigations indicate that the use of 3–carbon compounds inhibits weight gain and body fat without deleterious effects on body protein. Numerous investigations have demonstrated that obese research subjects lose weight when they are partially or totally starved, but regain much of the weight when they resume eating. The efficacy of 3–carbon compounds in minimizing gain in body weight and fat with refeeding after weight reduction was evaluated in obese research subjects.

Methods.—Seventeen healthy obese research subjects were fed a regular diet during an initial 3-day period. For the next 21 days, the participants received a hypoenergetic diet consisting of fruits, vegetables, and eggs. The diet was supplemented with vitamins, minerals, and trace elements. The participants were asked to refrain from exercise throughout the study and were confined to bed except for trips to the bathroom or metabolic kitchen. At 3-week completion of the hypoenergetic diet, the participants were randomly assigned to receive a hyperenergetic refeeding diet and either the 3–carbon compounds pyruvate and dihydroxyacetone (PD) or placebo (PL). Body composition, resting energy expenditure, protein metabolism, and blood biochemical variables were measured at baseline and after refeeding and weight and fat gain.

Results.—The participants who received PD had significantly less weight gain when refed with a hyperenergetic diet, compared to those who received PL (1.8 versus 2.9 kg). Body fat regain was significantly less in the participants who received PD than in those who received PL (0.8 versus 1.8 kg). There were no between-group differences in body protein metabolism, as measured by nitrogen balance, serum protein concentrations, and fat-free mass.

Conclusion.—The substitution of 3–carbon compounds for carbohydrate in a hyperenergetic refeeding diet after weight reduction will decrease the regain of body weight and fat without preventing the regain of body protein.

▶ There are many claims that natural compounds and specific diets can prevent weight gain (just visit the local book or natural food store). This report shows that there may be some truth to this (i.e., at least pyruvate and dihydroxyacetone supplements inhibited fat and weight gain during refeeding). The setting was very well controlled. However, in creating this control, they also made the setting unnatural—these women were in bed except for short trips to the bathroom or kitchen for 45 days! It certainly would be nice if there were a natural, safe method for preventing obesity.

M.A. Bowman, M.D., M.P.A.

3 Endocrinology

Introduction

This chapter is dominated by reports on diabetes, appropriate given the dramatic increase in concern and visibility of the condition. The opening section includes an especially interesting article on diagnosis using glycosylated hemoglobin instead of blood sugar. The most immediately useful article in the section on Type I diabetes provides reassuring evidence about the safety of injecting insulin through layers of clothing. The 4 articles in the next section cover miscellaneous topics on Type II diabetes, including one on the beneficial effects of troglitazone, a drug under fire as of this writing. The section on diabetes complications includes an article recommending a relaxed schedule for eye exams in patients treated with diet alone, and data on electrical spinal cord stimulation for painful neuropathy.

A short selection of 3 articles on thyroid conditions concludes the chapter, covering a once-weekly treatment regimen, the effect of small changes in replacement, and a "tissue score" that might prove useful in evaluation.

Randomized controlled trials: Abstracts 3–13 and 3–18.

Alfred O. Berg, M.D., M.P.H.

Diabetes Risk and Diagnosis

Dietary Fiber, Glycemic Load, and Risk of Non–insulin-dependent Diabetes Mellitus in Women

Salmerón J, Manson JE, Stampfer MJ, et al (Harvard School of Public Health, Boston; Harvard Med School, Boston)
JAMA 277:472–477, 1997   3–1

Background.—Diets resulting in a high insulin demand may influence the risk of non–insulin-dependent diabetes mellitus. The relationship between specific dietary patterns and the risk of diabetes in 1 cohort was explored after controlling for the major known risk factors for diabetes.

Methods.—A cohort of 65,173 women 40 to 65 years of age completed a detailed dietary questionnaire in 1986. Usual intake of total and specific sources of dietary fiber, dietary glycemic index, and glycemic load were calculated. At the time of questionnaire completion, all subjects were free from cardiovascular disease, cancer, and diabetes.

Findings.—Nine hundred fifteen incident cases of diabetes were recorded during the 6-year follow-up. The dietary glycemic index was positively associated with the risk of diabetes after adjustment for age, body mass index, smoking, physical activity, family history of diabetes, alcohol and cereal fiber intake, and total energy intake. When the highest quintile was compared with the lowest, the relative risk of diabetes was 1.37. Glycemic load was positively correlated with diabetes, with a relative risk of 1.47. Comparing the extreme quintiles showed that cereal fiber intake was inversely associated with the risk of diabetes. The risk of diabetes was further increased by the combination of a high glycemic load and low cereal fiber intake, compared with a low glycemic load and high cereal fiber intake.

Conclusion.—These data support the hypothesis that diets with a high glycemic load and low cereal fiber content increase the risk of diabetes in women. Also, it appears that grains should be consumed in a minimally refined form to decrease the incidence of diabetes.

▶ An important distinction in this research report from the ongoing Nurses' Health Study was the fact that cereal fiber, but not fruit or vegetable fiber, was associated with a lower rate of development of diabetes. Foods low in glycemic index—i.e., those causing less rapid and less extreme increases in glucose and, thus, less demand for insulin—also were associated with less diabetes. All of these findings were, of course, controlled for body mass index, family history, physical activity, smoking, and alcohol consumption. The association of higher magnesium intakes with fewer incidences of diabetes could not be readily separated from the intake of a major source of magnesium, i.e., cereal fiber, but there are small studies suggesting that magnesium can improve diabetic control for some individuals.

Although this study was limited to women, I believe the same would be true for men. Overall, we can now provide better dietary information to patients, in the hopes of preventing diabetes. I would suggest targeting obese individuals, those with a family history of diabetes, and those gaining weight.

M.A. Bowman, M.D., M.P.A.

Effects of Smoking on the Incidence of Non–insulin-dependent Diabetes Mellitus: Replication and Extension in a Japanese Cohort of Male Employees

Kawakami N, Takatsuka N, Shimizu H, et al (Gifu Univ, Japan; Hitachi Gen Hosp, Ibaraki, Japan)
Am J Epidemiol 145:103–109, 1997   3–2

Introduction.—Three prospective epidemiologic investigations have indicated that smoking may be a risk factor for non–insulin-dependent diabetes mellitus (NIDDM). Data were analyzed from an 8-year follow-up of a Japanese cohort of 2,312 male employees of a large electric company to determine the effects of smoking, age at starting smoking, smoking cessation, and number of cigarettes smoked daily on the incidence of NIDDM.

Methods.—All employees were mailed a questionnaire regarding smoking habits and related information. The small number of female employees limited analysis to male employees only. Respondents were followed up for 8 years regarding smoking habits and incidence of NIDDM. Data were collected regarding age, education, occupation, shift work, obesity, leisure-time physical activity, alcohol drinking, and family history of diabetes. Respondents were evaluated for incidence of NIDDM by participation in a yearly screening program.

Results.—The overall crude incidence rate of NIDDM was 2.2 per 1,000 person-years. Men who currently were smoking 16 to 25 cigarettes daily were at 3.27 times greater risk for the development of NIDDM within the 8-year follow-up period, compared to nonsmokers. The risk of NIDDM did not increase when more than 25 cigarettes were smoked daily. There was a significant trend toward an increased risk of NIDDM and younger age at starting smoking.

Conclusions.—Findings of increased risk for NIDDM in heavy smokers are consistent with other reports. The risk for the development of NIDDM was 3.27 times higher for heavy smokers compared to nonsmokers. More investigation is needed to determine the association between smoking cessation and the incidence of NIDDM.

▶ Smoking multiplies the vascular damage of diabetes. Less well known is the fact that it also may encourage the development of diabetes. This study controls for known confounding factors well and was not dependent on individuals seeking medical care, but on annual diabetes screenings in a male employed cohort. The observation also is strengthened by the dose-response relation, and the fact that more diabetes was seen in individuals who started smoking earlier. This is yet one more reason to encourage patients to quit smoking.

M.A. Bowman, M.D., M.P.A.

A Clinical Approach for the Diagnosis of Diabetes Mellitus: An Analysis Using Glycosylated Hemoglobin Levels

Peters AL, for the Meta-analysis Research Group on the Diagnosis of Diabetes Using Glycated Hemoglobin Levels (Univ of California, Los Angeles)
JAMA 276:1246–1252, 1996   3–3

Background.—Diabetes is currently underdiagnosed. One reason for this is the difficulty encountered in adhering to diagnostic guidelines. The use of glycosylated hemoglobin levels may improve patient compliance with testing. A meta-analysis was performed to determine whether glycosylated hemoglobin levels can be used instead of an oral glucose tolerance test (OGTT) for diagnosing diabetes.

Methods.—Through an augmented MEDLINE search, all reports from 1966 through June 1994 that measured glycosylated hemoglobin concentrations concurrently with OGTT testing were identified. The authors were contacted for individual data on the patients tested. Eighteen were able to provide the information requested. Overall fasting plasma glucose levels, 2-hour postdextrose glucose concentrations, and glycosylated hemoglobin levels for 11,276 individuals were available. Only data for 8,984 patients undergoing hemoglobin A_{1c} (HbA_{1c}) measurement were analyzed, as the HbA_{1c} assay showed the least variance in glycosylated hemoglobin levels in healthy individuals.

Findings.—When the mean HbA_{1c} level plus 4 standard deviations was used as a cutoff point, this assay had a sensitivity and a specificity of 36% and 100%, respectively, compared with the OGTT. Because of the lack of agreement between OGTT findings and HbA_{1c} concentrations, models were developed for analyzing HbA_{1c} distribution in each study. Three subpopulations were identified, with the third likely to be patients with diabetes. When an HbA_{1c} level of 7% was used as a cutoff point, the assay had a sensitivity of 99.6% in this third subpopulation. When this cutoff point was reapplied to the OGTT findings, 89% of those with an HbA_{1c} level of at least 7% had diabetes, 7% had impaired glucose tolerance, and 4% were normal.

Conclusion.—The use of an HbA_{1c} concentration for diagnosing diabetes is more convenient than the OGTT. In addition, therapeutic decisions are based on this value, regardless of the OGTT results. Patients with a concentration of 7% or more—which is most often consistent with World Health Organization standards of a diagnosis of diabetes—frequently need pharmacologic intervention. Patients with an HbA_{1c} concentration of less than 7% are generally treated with diet and exercise, regardless of an OGTT diagnosis of impaired glucose tolerance or diabetes.

► I have heard repeatedly in continuing medical education talks by endocrinologists that we should not use glycated hemoglobin levels for the diagnosis of diabetes. I never got a satisfactory answer to my standard, "Why not?" (must have been written in stone somewhere). However, those of us who routinely used the glycated hemoglobin values are now vindicated; glycated hemoglobin is, indeed, a great test for diabetes, particularly when modestly or greatly elevated, and is more reproducible and convenient than the OGTT. Borderline results should encourage repeat and potentially more extensive testing.

M.A. Bowman, M.D., M.P.A.

Characteristics of Youth-onset Noninsulin-dependent Diabetes Mellitus and Insulin-dependent Diabetes Mellitus at Diagnosis

Scott CR, Smith JM, Cradock MM, et al (Univ of Arkansas, Little Rock; Arkansas Children's Hosp, Little Rock)
Pediatrics 100:84–91, 1997

3–4

Purpose.—Non–insulin-dependent diabetes mellitus (NIDDM) has traditionally been considered a disease of adults, in whom it has been extensively studied. There are few studies of NIDDM in young people, however. The term *youth-onset NIDDM* describes the occurrence of NIDDM in patients younger than 21. The characteristics of patients with youth-onset NIDDM at diagnosis were assessed and compared with those of young people with insulin-dependent diabetes mellitus (IDDM).

Methods.—Medical records of patients referred to a pediatric tertiary care center for evaluation of diabetes were reviewed. This review found 50 patients with youth-onset NIDDM, and a comparison group of patients with IDDM. The patients met National Diabetes Data Group criteria for type of diabetes, and the 2 groups were matched for age, sex, and area of residence. Their characteristics at diagnosis of diabetes were compared.

Results.—The number of cases of new-onset diabetes diagnosed at the children's hospital increased steadily during the 1990s. The patients with youth-onset NIDDM were 31 girls and 19 boys, mean age 14 years. Seventy-four percent of the patients with NIDDM were black, compared with just 18% of the IDDM comparison group. Mental retardation was found in the histories of 12% of patients with NIDDM and none of those with IDDM. The most frequent presenting symptoms were comparable in the 2 groups, though weight loss was more common in the IDDM group (Table 1). Almost all of the patients with NIDDM were obese; their mean body mass index was 35 kg/m^2, compared with 20 kg/m^2 in the IDDM group (Fig 3). Hypertension was present at diagnosis in nearly one third of the youths with NIDDM, and more than one fourth had diabetic ketoacidosis. Eighty-six percent of the patients with NIDDM had acanthosis

TABLE 1.—Presenting Symptoms for Patients With Youth-Onset Diabetes

Symptoms	% IDDM (n = 48)	% NIDDM (n = 40)	*P* Value
Abdominal pain	46	33	>.10
Dizziness	15	33	>.10
Headache	33	43	>.10
Nocturia	71	65	>.10
Polydypsia	96	85	>.10
Polyphagia	69	60	>.10
Polyuria	94	88	>.10
Visual disturbance	17	20	>.10
Weight loss	71	40	.005

(Courtesy of Scott CR, Smith JM, Cradock MM, et al: Characteristics of youth-onset noninsulin-dependent diabetes mellitus and insulin-dependent diabetes mellitus at diagnosis. *Pediatrics* 100:84–91, 1997. Reproduced by permission of *Pediatrics*, Vol 100, page 87. Copyright 1997.)

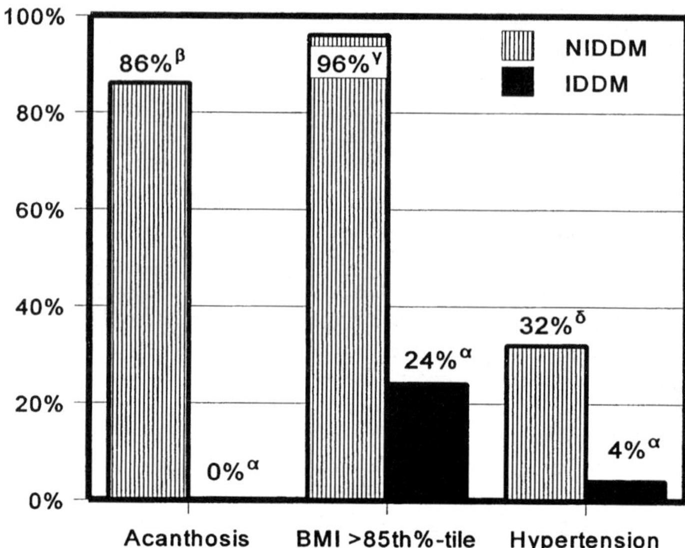

FIGURE 3.—Physical characteristics at diagnosis in youth-onset diabetes. Patients with IDDM α, N = 48 for all three characteristics; patients with NIDDM β, N = 35; γ, N = 49; δ, N = 44. (Courtesy of Scott CR, Smith JM, Cradock MM, et al: Characteristics of youth-onset noninsulin-dependent diabetes mellitus and insulin-dependent diabetes mellitus at diagnosis. *Pediatrics* 100:84–91, 1997. Reprinted by permission of *Pediatrics*, Vol 100, page 87. Copyright 1997.)

nigricans, compared with none of the IDDM group. The 2 groups were similar in their hemoglobin A_{1C} levels.

Conclusions.—This study compared the characteristics at diagnosis of pediatric patients with NIDDM versus those with IDDM. The major distinguishing factors of youth-onset NIDDM are lack of history of weight loss, obesity, acanthosis nigricans, and hypertension. Young people with new-onset diabetes who have these characteristics should be evaluated for NIDDM.

▶ Youth-onset NIDDM is increasingly recognized; in the past, we thought that all youth-onset diabetes was IDDM. Furthermore, it is sometimes difficult to figure out whether an individual patient has NIDDM or IDDM, particularly early after presentation. Diabetic ketoacidosis is a frequent presenting condition for NIDDM as well as IDDM, perhaps because we do not screen for NIDDM in adolescents. I suspect that many adolescents, particularly those who are obese, are black, and have a family history of diabetes, have mild, undetected diabetes. This report suggests that acanthosis nigricans and hypertension are two additional cues to screening for diabetes. The increased rate of NIDDM among patients with mental retardation was unexpected to me.

M.A. Bowman, M.D., M.P.A.

Insulin-dependent Diabetes Mellitus

Self-monitoring of Blood Glucose in Type I Diabetic Patients: Comparison With Continuous Microdialysis Measurements of Glucose in Subcutaneous Adipose Tissue During Ordinary Life Conditions

Bolinder J, Ungerstedt U, Hagström-Toft E, et al (Huddinge Hosp, Sweden; Karolinska Inst, Stockholm)
Diabetes Care 20:64–70, 1997   3–5

Background.—Preliminary findings have shown that true glycemic variations in some patients with type I diabetes may be too great to be detected by conventional self-monitoring of blood glucose (SMBG). A novel microdialysis glucose-monitoring technique was used to determine whether frequent self-recording of capillary blood glucose provides enough information about the diurnal changes in glucose control under the ordinary conditions of daily life.

Methods.—Twenty-four type I diabetic patients underwent continuous monitoring of adipose tissue glucose under ambulatory conditions. Each patient had a microdialysis probe implanted subcutaneously and perfused by a portable microinfusion pump. One-hour to 2-hour dialysate fraction samples were obtained on 3 consecutive days. Diurnal microdialysis glucose profiles were compared with SMBG recordings performed 7 times daily.

Findings.—Compared with the continuous microdialysis glucose recordings, the SMBG profiles revealed marked aberrations in 7 patients.

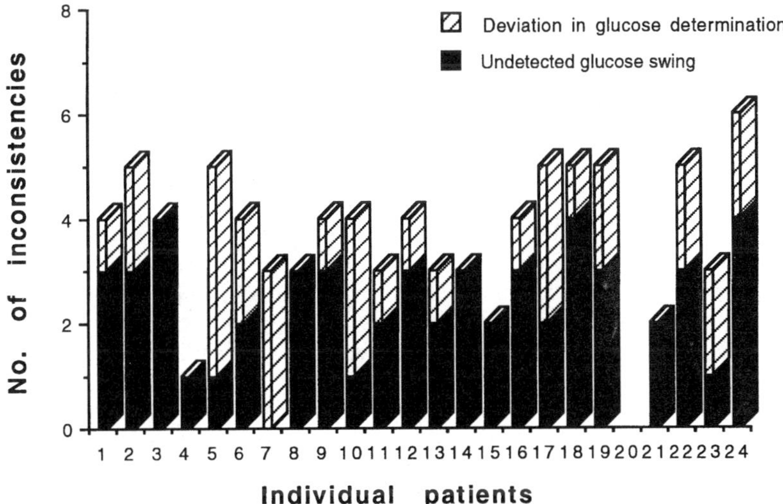

FIGURE 4.—Causes of significant discrepancies between self-monitoring of blood glucose and continuous microdialysis measurements of glucose in subcutaneous adipose tissue for more than 3 days in 24 type I diabetic patients. (Courtesy of Bolinder J, Ungerstedt U, Hagström-Toft E, et al: Self-monitoring of blood glucose in type I diabetic patients: Comparison with continuous microdialysis measurements of glucose in subcutaneous adipose tissue during ordinary life conditions. *Diabetes Care* 20:64–70, 1997.)

For these patients, five to 6 inconsistencies were registered during the 3-day study. A valid reflection of the diurnal glucose profile by SMBG was provided in only 4 patients. In 13 patients, the SMBG recordings paralleled the diurnal adipose tissue glucose profiles in an intermediate way. The inaccuracy of SMBG data was more often a result of unrecognized wide glucose swings than erroneous testing methods. This was more evident at night (Fig 4).

Conclusion.—Conventional SMBG recordings, even when done often, may not sufficiently reflect the characteristics of an individual's true diurnal blood glucose profile. Microdialysis of subcutaneous adipose tissue has great potential for the continuous recording of glucose levels, although the manual sampling method used in this study cannot be used in routine care.

▶ This is sad but may explain some of the difficulties we have in controlling type I diabetics. Essentially, even frequent home monitoring of blood glucose levels misses many of the high and low points in the blood sugar levels of diabetics, particularly at night. These misses are caused by a mixture of mistiming of the sampling and incorrect readings. In practice, high glycated hemoglobin levels, in spite of relatively normal home readings, should suggest the need for checking technique and trying sampling at different times.

M.A. Bowman, M.D., M.P.A.

The Safety of Injecting Insulin Through Clothing

Fleming DR, Jacober SJ, Vandenberg MA, et al (Wayne State Univ, Detroit; Univ of Michigan, Ann Arbor)
Diabetes Care 20:244–247, 1997

3–6

Objective.—Typical antiseptic practices for injecting insulin are time-consuming and complicated. Although many insulin users inject the drug through their clothing, there have been no studies on the safety of this practice. A 20-week single-blinded prospective crossover trial compared the safety and perceived benefits of injecting insulin through clothing vs. conventional subcutaneous injection practice.

Methods.—At enrollment and at 10 weeks and 20 weeks of the study, blood work was done for 50 patients randomly allocated to the conventional thigh injection technique or the through-clothing thigh injection technique and crossed over at 10 weeks. White blood cell counts, differential counts, and glycated Hb counts were statistically compared for the 2 groups. Patients were to record problems, perceived benefits, and other comments in log books.

Results.—Forty-two patients (21 women), aged 23 to 63 years, completed the study. The average duration of diabetes was 14 years. There were 7,275 injections through clothing made. No significant differences were found in white blood cell or neutrophil counts or percent glycated Hb between groups at any time point. Perceived benefits according to log entries were convenience of injecting through clothing, particularly when away from home, and less constraint in rotating injection sites. Difficulty in injecting through thick clothing and small bloodstains on clothing were listed as disadvantages.

Conclusion.—Injecting insulin through clothing does not appear to pose a safety risk.

▶ Anything to make compliance easier. I suspect this is a case of researchers following patients rather than researchers leading. Many patients have injected through their clothes, whether or not we knew it. In fact, the authors found a patient who reported having used the injection-through-clothing technique for 59 years!

Although the study included a reasonable number of individuals and lots of injections (13,720), I suspect there might be a rare complication. Thus, I would like to see a prospective, longer trial that continued to monitor for complications. In the meantime, I think we should offer this option to our patients.

M.A. Bowman, M.D., M.P.A.

Hypoglycemia in the Diabetes Control and Complications Trial
The Diabetes Control and Complications Trial Research Group (Bethesda, Md)
Diabetes 46:271–286, 1997   3–7

Introduction.—Hypoglycemia is the most frequently occurring adverse effect of intensive diabetes management in patients with insulin-dependent diabetes mellitus (IDDM). The Diabetes Control and Complications Trial (DCCT) was a multicenter, randomized clinical trial conducted to determine the effects of intensive therapy on the risk of hypoglycemia, but not the physiologic mechanisms by which hypoglycemia occurs. The risk factors for severe hypoglycemia based on the entire cohort of 1,441 DCCT patients over the full duration of follow-up in the trial (range, 3.5 to 9 years) were reported.

Methods.—All 1,441 patients with IDDM were randomly assigned to receive either intensive or conventional diabetes therapy (711 and 730 patients, respectively). During an average follow-up period of 6.5 years, participants were asked to report all episodes of suspected severe hypoglycemia. They also were questioned about severe episodes of hypoglycemia at quarterly follow-up visits.

Results.—Of 3,788 reported episodes of severe hypoglycemia, 1,027 were associated with coma or seizure. A total of 65% and 35% of patients in the intensive and conventional groups, respectively, had at least 1 episode of severe hypoglycemia. At trial end, the rates of severe hypoglycemia per 100 patient-years were 61.2 and 18.7, respectively, for patients in the intensive and conventional groups (Table 2). A high risk for severe hypoglycemia was observed in both groups for patients who were male, adolescent, had a prior history of hypoglycemia, and had no residual

TABLE 2.—Hypoglycemic Events in the Diabetes Control and Complications Trial by Treatment Group*

| | Conventional ($n = 730$) | | | | Intensive ($n = 711$) | | | | | |
| | Percentage of patients with an event | | | | Percentage of patients with an event | | | | | |
	At study end	Cumulative at 9 years	Number of events	Rate	At study end	Cumulative at 9 years	Number of events	Rate	Relative risk	95% CI
Hypoglycemic events										
Requiring assistance	34.9	41.3	892	18.7	64.6	72.8	2,896	61.2	3.28‡	(2.65, 4.05)
Coma and/or seizure	18.8	25.5	257	5.4	38.1	47.4	770	16.3	3.02‡	(2.36, 3.86)

*Rates were defined as episodes per 100 years of follow-up. Nine-year cumulative data were estimated by life-table methods. Relative risk (intensive/conventional) computed as ratio of event rates, was significant at $P < 0.001$.

(Courtesy of The Diabetes Control and Complications Trial Research Group: Hypoglycemia in the Diabetes Control and Complications Trial. *Diabetes* 46:271–286, 1997.)

C-peptide. Intensive treatment was associated with an increased risk of multiple episodes; 22% and 5% of patients in the intensive and conventional groups, respectively, experienced 5 or more episodes of severe hypoglycemia within the first 5 years of follow-up. Nearly 30% of patients experienced a second episode of severe hypoglycemia within 4 months of an initial episode. The strongest predictors of severe hypoglycemia in both groups were a previous episode, followed closely by a change in current HbA_{1c} value.

Conclusion.—Intensive treatment of IDDM is associated with a significantly increased risk of hypoglycemia, even after adjustment for HbA_{1c} levels.

▶ This is a statistically ponderous article. Because serious hypoglycemia was so much more frequent with intensive treatment, the authors tried to learn as much as possible about the causes. Serious hypoglycemia was more common with higher doses of insulin and with lower HbA_{1c} levels. Males, adolescents, and those with previous hypoglycemia were more likely to have hypoglycemia requiring assistance. Patients with some residual insulin secretion had less hypoglycemia. The authors estimated the risk of increased hypoglycemia for each 1% decline in HbA_{1c} level. The authors estimated that about 60% of the increased risk of hypoglycemia with intensive treatment is accounted for by the lowered HbA_{1c} level. Overall, the rate of hypoglycemia requiring assistance, such as coma and seizures, is significant and must be considered by each physician and patient.

M.A. Bowman, M.D., M.P.A.

Chronic Administration of Levosulpiride and Glycemic Control in IDDM Patients With Gastroparesis

Melga P, Giusti R, Mansi C, et al (Univ of Genoa, Italy)
Diabetes Care 20:55–58, 1997
3–8

Background.—Diabetic gastroparesis occurs in about 25% of patients with long-standing diabetes mellitus and in up to 50% of those who do not have dyspeptic symptoms. Autonomic neuropathy or blood glucose concentration may be involved in gastroparesis. Hyperglycemia impairs gastric emptying in healthy individuals and those with diabetes, but in healthy individuals, the rate of gastric emptying strongly affects carbohydrate absorption and blood glucose homeostasis. In individuals with diabetes, delayed gastric emptying may impair glycemic control. It is unclear whether gastrokinetic drugs may be useful in these individuals.

Methods.—Forty patients had insulin-dependent diabetes mellitus with signs of autonomic neuropathy and delayed gastric emptying. Gastric emptying time and glycemic parameters were examined before and after administration of placebo or levosulpiride 25 mg 3 times daily for 6 months.

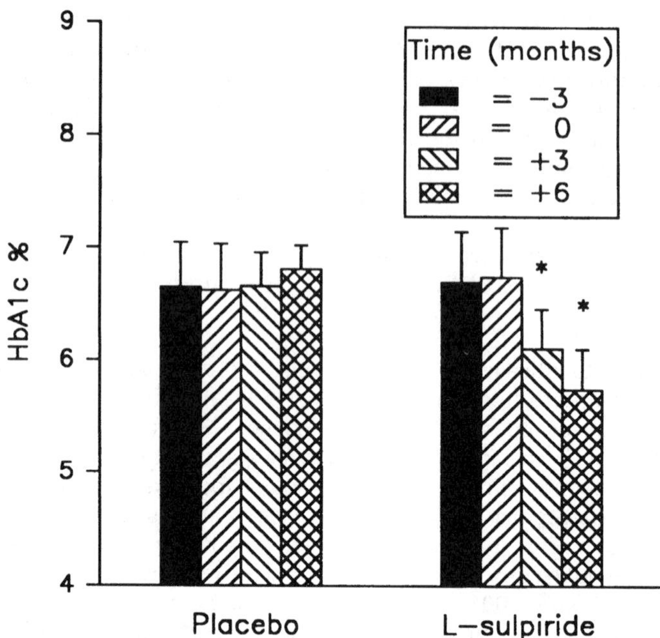

FIGURE 1.—Hemoglobin A_{1c} values (%) in the 2 groups of patients with diabetes before and after placebo (group 1) or levosulpiride (group 2) administration. * $P < 0.01$ vs. 0 and vs. placebo. (Courtesy of Melga P, Giusti R, Mansi C, et al: Chronic administration of levosulpiride and glycemic control in IDDM patients with gastroparesis. *Diabetes Care* 20:55–58, 1997.)

Results.—After 6 months, there were no significant differences in glycemic and HbA_{1c} values in patients who were given placebo. In patients given levosulpiride, glycemic control improved after 6 months (Fig 1). The dosage of insulin and the number of severe hypoglycemic episodes did not change. Also, gastric emptying time significantly decreased and dyspeptic symptoms improved.

Discussion.—In these patients with insulin-dependent diabetes mellitus and gastroparesis, treatment with levosulpiride for 6 months decreased gastric emptying time and significantly improved glycemic control. Insulin dosages did not change and the number of hypoglycemic episodes did not increase. Individuals with insulin-dependent diabetes mellitus who have unexplained poor glycemic control should be examined for gastric emptying abnormalities.

▶ This is 1 of a series of recent articles indicating that delayed emptying of the stomach in patients with diabetes inhibits our ability to control their blood sugar levels. (For example, see Lyrenas et al.[1] This article notes the peak blood sugar is delayed about 30 minutes in patients with diabetes who have delayed gastric emptying.) Although levosulpiride is not available in the United States, it is an established gastric kinetic agent in Europe.

The results of giving levosulpiride on improving the HbA$_{1c}$ in this study were impressive. However, of note, all patients were using regular insulin—perhaps regular insulin given 30 minutes before meals is okay until gastric emptying delay develops, then its onset of action is too fast. I wonder whether it makes sense to give a second agent (such as the levosulpiride or erythromycin), or to try giving the regular insulin concurrent with the meal? Of note, all of these patients had type I diabetes, but delayed gastric emptying also is known to occur in type II diabetes. In any case, in these patients with unexplained glucose variations, consider delayed gastric emptying as a possible cause.

M.A. Bowman, M.D., M.P.A.

Reference

1. Lyrenas EB, Olsson EHK, Arvidsson VC, et al: Prevalence and determinants of solid and liquid gastric emptying in unstable type I diabetes. *Diabetes Care* 20:413–418, 1997.

Self-reported Changes in Capillary Glucose and Insulin Requirements During the Menstrual Cycle
Lunt H, Brown LJ (Christchurch Hosp, New Zealand; Univ of Wollongong, Australia)
Diabetic Med 13:525–530, 1996

3–9

Introduction.—Women with insulin-dependent (type 1) diabetes mellitus have alterations of glycemic control associated with the menstrual cycle, which may require changes in insulin dose. The prevalence and pattern of self-reported perimenstrual changes in capillary glucose level and insulin dose were evaluated in a population-based study of women with type 1 diabetes.

Methods.—The population-based sample included 124 women, aged 18 to 40, with type 1 diabetes. They were asked about any changes in self-monitored capillary blood glucose levels and insulin requirements around the time of their menstrual periods. In addition, glycated hemoglobin levels were compared for women who did and did not adjust their insulin dose in the perimenstrual period.

Results.—Sixty-one percent of women reported perimenstrual changes in their capillary blood glucose level, most commonly an increase. Thirty-six percent adjusted their insulin dose in response to these changes. The mean glycated hemoglobin level was similar for women who did and did not adjust their insulin dose, 79 and 73 mmol mol^{-1} haem, respectively. Perimenstrual blood glucose changes were observed in 67% of women taking fixed-dose estrogen/progesterone oral contraceptives.

Conclusions.—Most women with type 1 diabetes report some perimenstrual alteration in their capillary blood glucose level. About half this group make changes in their insulin dose around this time, although the adjustments do not seem to make a significant difference in glycemic control. Prospective studies with objective measurements of glycemic control should be performed before women with diabetes are advised to make routine perimenstrual adjustments in their insulin dose.

▶ It is common for my insulin-dependent patients and I to struggle to determine what causes their many variations in blood sugar. Thus, this article is useful in showing that about half of all type I diabetic women observed increased blood sugar levels before the menses, and decreased levels during and after the menses. There was no difference in glycated hemoglobin measures between women who did or did not make perimenstrual changes in insulin, but this may suggest that the women who made the changes needed to do so to stay as controlled as the others.

M.A. Bowman, M.D., M.P.A.

Non–insulin-dependent Diabetes Mellitus

The Occurrence of Diabetic Ketoacidosis in Non–insulin-dependent Diabetes and Newly Diagnosed Diabetic Adults
Westphal SA (Maricopa Med Ctr, Phoenix, Ariz)
Am J Med 101:19–24, 1996

3–10

Introduction.—The occurrence of diabetic ketoacidosis (DKA) had been thought to indicate the underlying significant, irreversible β-cell damage that is a characteristic of type I, or insulin-dependent, diabetes. Yet certain adult patients without a history of type I diabetes also have exhibited DKA, and some are able to be treated without insulin after recovering sufficient β-cell function. The clinical characteristics of such patients were examined.

Methods.—Medical records were examined for all adult patients admitted to a medical ICU from January 1987 to January 1993 with a diagnosis of DKA. Patients with continuous insulin treatment and a history of DKA were classified as having type I diabetes. Those with no previous history of DKA and who had been treated with diet or an oral agent were classified as having type II, or non–insulin-dependent diabetes (NIDDM). A third group of patients was newly diagnosed with diabetes. An attempt was made to determine the status of diabetic treatment after the episode of DKA in patients with no history of type I diabetes.

Results.—Of the 226 patients included in the study, 106 were classified as having type I diabetes and 58 as having type II diabetes. Sixty-two patients had DKA as the initial manifestation of diabetes. The mean ages at the time of the episode of DKA were 30.3 for patients with type I diabetes, 41.2 for those with type II diabetes, and 32.2 for those with newly diagnosed diabetes. As a group, patients with type I diabetes had the lowest body mass index. Non-Hispanic whites accounted for 78.3% of patients with type I diabetes, 50% of those with type II diabetes, and 30.6% of those with newly diagnosed diabetes. Hispanics had a greater representation in the type II (29.3%) and newly diagnosed (33.9%) groups than in the type I group (11.3%). Whereas omission of insulin treatment was the most common cause of DKA in type I diabetes, infection was the most common cause identified in type II; no cause of DKA was identified in 43% of new-onset cases. Of those patients who were followed up for at least 12 months, about 24% of the newly diagnosed and 8% of those with a history of NIDDM were not taking insulin.

Discussion.—The categorizing of patients with diabetes as type I or II may not be precise, because DKA can occur in NIDDM. Adults with no previous history of diabetes or with a history of type II diabetes may have an episode of DKA and later require treatment with diet only or oral hypoglycemic agents. In the cases of newly diagnosed diabetes reviewed, immunologic characteristics typical of type I usually were absent. Thus, adult-onset diabetes must be viewed as a heterogeneous disorder.

▶ I have long thought that the characterization of many diabetics as type I or type II was unclear and imprecise. Some are obviously type I, some are obviously type II, and some have features of both. Further, the distinction is not very useful in practice; we use whatever we need to obtain control based on the individual patient's course of disease. Sure, type I patients may benefit from insulin pumps, but that is based on their glucose control needs, not on the title of their diabetes. However, another memory note is that insulin once does not mean insulin always; many can revert, at least temporarily, to other means of control.

M.A. Bowman, M.D., M.P.A.

Effects of Breakfast Cereals Containing Various Amounts of β-Glucan Fibers on Plasma Glucose and Insulin Responses in NIDDM Subjects

Tappy L, Gügolz E, Würsch P (Polyclinique Médicale Universitaire, Lausanne, Switzerland; Nestlé Research Centre, Lausanne, Switzerland)
Diabetes Care 19:831–834, 1996   3–11

Objective.—The glycemic and insulinemic response to a carbohydrate load depends greatly on the type of food consumed. The addition of viscous fibers can reduce the glycemic response to a meal, and this has been shown to be beneficial in diets supplemented with various polysaccharide gums. Oat contains a viscous fiber that is a linear polysaccharide, β-glucan. The association between the amount of β-glucan present in breakfast cereal on the glycemic and insulinemic response was studied in patients with non–insulin-dependent diabetes mellitus (NIDDM).

Methods.—The study included 8 patients with NIDDM, most of whom were receiving oral hypoglycemic agents. Their responses to 4 different meals were studied. On 3 occasions, they received a breakfast prepared with cooked extruded oat bran concentrate. Each of these breakfasts provided a 35-g carbohydrate load, but with a β-glucan content increasing from 4 to 8.4 g. They also were studied after eating a continental breakfast, consisting of bread, milk, cheese, and ham. The plasma glycemic and insulinemic responses to these meals were compared.

TABLE 3.—Metabolic Effects*

	Continental	4.0 g β-glucan	6.0 g β-glucan	8.4 g β-glucan
Plasma glucose (mmol/l)				
Basal	9.4 ± 1.0	9.5 ± 1.3	9.5 ± 1.1	9.5 ± 1.1
Delta max	3.8[a] ± 0.4	2.6[b] ± 0.5	1.6[c] ± 0.2	1.5[c] ± 0.3
	(100[a])	(67[b] ± 10)	(42[c] ± 4)	(38[c] ± 7)
Area under curve (4 h)	6.8[a] ± 1.2	4.7[a] ± 1.1	2.8[b] ± 0.6	2.5[b] ± 0.6
(above basal value)	(100)	(71 ± 15)	(41 ± 6)	(35 ± 7)
Plasma insulin (mU/l)				
Basal	22 ± 5	24 ± 6	20 ± 6	22 ± 6
Max	69[b] ± 14	46[c] ± 10	43[c] ± 10	41[c] ± 10
	(100)	(67 ± 14)	(62 ± 14)	(59 ± 14)

*Data are means ± standard error. Numbers in parentheses indicate the relative values compared with the continental breakfast. Values with different superscripts are significantly different: [a,b]$P < 0.05$; [b,c]$P < 0.01$; [a,c]$P < 0.001$.

(Courtesy of Tappy L, Gügolz E, Würsch P: Effects of breakfast cereals containing various amounts of β-glucan fibers on plasma glucose and insulin responses in NIDDM subjects. *Diabetes Care* 19:831–834, 1996.)

Results.—The oat cereal breakfasts were associated with a lower peak increase in plasma glucose than the continental breakfast: 67% of the control value at the 4-g dose of β-glucan, 42% at the 6-g dose, and 38% at the 8.4-g dose (Table 3). The β-glucan dose showed a linear inverse relation with the plasma glucose peak or the area under the glucose curve. The increase in plasma insulin after the β-glucan meals was only 59% to 67% of the values observed after the continental breakfast.

Conclusions.—At a carbohydrate load of 35 g, the addition of 5 g of β-glucan will produce a 50% reduction in the plasma glycemic response. Adding oat bran concentrate to food products can achieve this dose of β-glucan without affecting the taste of the food. Eating β-glucan–enriched foods, particularly at breakfast, could help to reduce hyperglycemia and insulin requirements in patients with diabetes, and postprandial insulin in patients with obesity and dyslipidemia.

▶ Decreasing the glycemic response to a meal can improve overall control for diabetics, as is true with the relatively new drug acarbose. A decreased glycemic response also lowers the peak insulin, which may be important because of theories that insulin may worsen atherosclerosis. Decreases in glycemic response also can be obtained by dietary measures. Psyllium and oat bran, both soluble fibers, reduce the glycemic response. This article used 50 to 67 g of cereal with mixed amounts of β-glucan (found in oat bran). Rolled oats have β-glucan, but only about 2 to 3 g in the serving size used in this report, compared to the better effects the authors observed with 4 to 8 g of β-glucan. Thus, although eating rolled oats would help, more effect could be achieved by supplementing the cereal with more fiber or eating a larger portion.

M.A. Bowman, M.D., M.P.A.

Motivational Interviewing to Improve Adherence to a Behavioral Weight-control Program for Older Obese Women With NIDDM: A Pilot Study

Smith DE, Kratt PP, Heckemeyer CM, et al (Univ of Alabama, Birmingham)
Diabetes Care 20:52–54, 1997   3–12

Objective.—Weight control among obese patients with non–insulin-dependent diabetes mellitus (NIDDM) is important. Motivational interviewing is designed to enhance adherence to weight-control programs. Motivational interviewing was added to a behavioral weight-control program for obese women with NIDDM to determine whether it enhances adherence to the program and improves posttreatment glycemic treatment.

Methods.—Either a 16-session group behavioral weight-control program or no intervention was conducted with 22 women with NIDDM (41% black), aged 50 years and older, whose weight was 120% to 200% of ideal. In the sessions, ambivalence about behavior change, personal goals, and problems to solve were examined. The difference between stated goals and exhibited behavior was evaluated in a way that increased the patient's motivation. Treatment outcome and treatment adherence were analyzed statistically.

Results.—The average duration of diabetes was 6.7 years. The mean baseline BMI was 34.7, and the mean baseline GHb was 10.25%. Sixteen women completed the study. There was no difference between groups with respect to dropouts. The intervention group had better adherence and glycemic control although weight loss did not differ significantly (Table 1).

Conclusions.—Whereas motivational intervention enhanced adherence to weight-reduction programs for a small sample of obese women with NIDDM, it did not significantly alter weight loss.

▶ What these authors call motivational interviewing is what many of us call routine investigation and counseling for noncompliance, albeit the authors spent more time with the patients than is available to many of us. However,

TABLE 1.—Mean Posttreatment Characteristics of Weight-Reduction Groups

	Standard	Motivational	*P* value
n	10	6	
Treatment sessions attended	8.9 ± 2.9	13.3 ± 2.0	0.01*
Food diaries submitted	10.1 ± 2.6	15.2 ± 1.8	0.01*
Self-monitored blood glucose (days)	32.2 ± 10.2	46.0 ± 16.1	0.05*
Reported exercise (days)	23.7 ± 11.6	35.2 ± 13.2	0.07*
Recorded calories (days)	55.7 ± 24.7	76.8 ± 15.2	0.07*
Glycemic control (% GHb)	10.8 ± 3.1	9.8 ± 1.3	0.05†
Weight loss (kg)	4.5 ± 2.2	5.5 ± 3.9	—†

Note: Data are means ± standard deviation.
*Kruskal-Wallis test.
†Analysis of covariance adjusted for baseline.
(Courtesy of Smith DE, Kratt PP, Heckemeyer CM, et al: Motivational interviewing to improve adherence to a behavioral weight-control program for older obese women with NIDDM: A pilot study. *Diabetes Care* 20:52–54, 1997.)

this is one of the few studies that has shown that this style of individualized behavioral change counseling is better than group education classes alone.

The results were more impressive in lowering of glycated Hb than is found with most drugs. Admittedly, 1 weakness is the study length of only 4 months (instead of the many years that patients with diabetes have their disease); will the results last? Despite this drawback, I believe we need to continue to investigate an individual's willingness to change, their barriers to change, and the perceived costs and benefits to them, and have the patient problem-solve alternatives, and consider the family, because I believe that is the only hope for long-term change.

M.A. Bowman, M.D., M.P.A.

Cardiac and Glycemic Benefits of Troglitazone Treatment in NIDDM

Ghazzi MN, Perez JE, Antonucci TK, et al (Parke-Davis Pharmaceutical Research, Ann Arbor, Mich; Washington Univ, St Louis)
Diabetes 46:433–439, 1997

3–13

Objective.—Although troglitazone, a thiazolidinedione for treatment of non–insulin-dependent diabetes mellitus (NIDDM) and other insulin-resistant diseases, improves the glycemic profiles of patients in human clinical trials, its cardiac safety in humans has not been determined. Left ventricular mass and function and the potential benefits of troglitazone on hyperglycemia, hyperinsulinemia, dyslipidemia, and hypertension in NIDDM were studied.

Methods.—In a multicenter parallel study, after a 3-week screening period including a 2-week washout period, 154 patients with NIDDM, mostly white males of average age 54 years, were randomly allocated to receive 800 mg troglitazone (n = 77) or as much as 20 mg daily or twice daily glyburide (n = 77) for 48 weeks. Primary cardiac parameters, left ventricular mass index, cardiac index, and stroke volume index were measured at baseline and 12, 24, 36, and 48 weeks by 2-dimensional echocardiography and pulsed Doppler. Glycemic, lipid, chemistry, and cardiovascular parameters were assessed. Parameters for the 2 groups were compared statistically.

Results.—The duration of diabetes ranged from 0 to 24 years. There were 114 patients who completed the study. There were 18 patients receiving troglitazone and 3 receiving glyburide who withdrew for lack of efficacy. Because of inaccurate echocardiographic analyses, 15 patients receiving troglitazone and 16 receiving glyburide were excluded from the left ventricular mass index analysis. Left ventricular mass index results were similar between groups and no patients had abnormal values. Confidence intervals increased significantly in patients receiving troglitazone but not in those receiving glyburide. Stroke volume index increased significantly in patients receiving troglitazone at all time points but in patients receiving glyburide only at weeks 36 and 48. Peripheral resistance and blood pressure decreased significantly for patients receiving troglitazone

TABLE 3.—Glycemic and Lipid Parameters

Parameter	Baseline	Week 12	Week 24	Week 36	Week 48
FSG (mmol/l)					
Troglitazone	12.7 ± 4.04	10.3 ± 3.42*	10.2 ± 3.46*	9.8 ± 3.20*	10.5 ± 3.28*
Glyburide	13.9 ± 3.85	10.4 ± 3.37*	10.4 ± 3.15*	11.0 ± 2.99*	11.2 ± 3.36*
HbA$_{1c}$ (%)					
Troglitazone	8.8 ± 1.60	8.9 ± 1.90	8.5 ± 1.80	8.3 ± 1.90‡	8.3 ± 1.80
Glyburide	9.0 ± 1.40	8.3 ± 1.60*	8.5 ± 1.50†	8.7 ± 1.60	8.8 ± 1.60
Insulin (pmol/l)					
Troglitazone	112.32 ± 98.76	64.44 ± 35.76*	71.46 ± 47.88*	67.74 ± 37.32*	82.68 ± 65.64‡
Glyburide	92.88 ± 60.90	127.44 ± 83.88†	114.36 ± 77.28‡	114.9 ± 69.54	113.22 ± 76.92
C-peptide (nmol/l)					
Troglitazone	0.91 ± 0.43	0.74 ± 0.24†	0.75 ± 0.26†	0.70 ± 0.26*	0.71 ± 0.24*
Glyburide	0.93 ± 0.40	1.00 ± 0.41	1.04 ± 0.48†	0.96 ± 0.38	0.91 ± 0.40
Total cholesterol (mmol/l)					
Troglitazone	5.64 ± 1.25	5.82 ± 1.15	5.87 ± 1.26	6.04 ± 1.21†	5.93 ± 1.13‡
Glyburide	5.76 ± 1.50	5.58 ± 1.11	5.62 ± 1.15	5.86 ± 1.43	5.80 ± 1.36
Triglycerides (mmol/l)					
Troglitazone	3.15 ± 3.91	2.06 ± 1.20*	2.29 ± 1.40†	2.16 ± 1.24*	2.14 ± 1.38‡
Glyburide	3.40 ± 4.80	2.79 ± 2.33‡	2.98 ± 2.87	3.28 ± 4.68	3.01 ± 2.97
HDL (mol/l)					
Troglitazone	1.02 ± 0.32	1.08 ± 0.29	1.08 ± 0.32	1.16 ± 0.36†	1.18 ± 0.33*
Glyburide	0.93 ± 0.25	0.96 ± 0.25	0.98 ± 0.26	1.00 ± 0.26	0.98 ± 0.27
LDL (mmol/l)					
Troglitazone	3.48 ± 0.92	3.80 ± 1.04‡	3.81 ± 1.26‡	3.87 ± 1.10*	3.77 ± 0.98‡
Glyburide	3.56 ± 0.93	3.46 ± 0.90	3.49 ± 0.95	3.63 ± 0.92	3.58 ± 0.92

Note: Data are means ± standard deviation for patients who completed 48 weeks of treatment. All tests were done on adjusted means.
*Statistically significant change from baseline ($P < 0.001$).
†Statistically significant change from baseline ($P < 0.01$).
‡Statistically significant change from baseline ($P < 0.05$).
(Courtesy of Ghazzi MN, Perez JE, Antonucci TK, et al: Cardiac and glycemic benefits of troglitazone treatment in NIDDM. *Diabetes* 46:433–439, 1997.)

but not for those receiving glyburide. Troglitazone had a more beneficial effect on glycemic and lipid parameters than did glyburide (Table 3). The adverse event profile for the 2 drugs was similar except that infection was reported more frequently with glyburide than with troglitazone (40% vs. 19%).

Conclusion.—Troglitazone had a beneficial effect on blood pressure, cardiac index, and vascular resistance, as well as a positive effect on the glycemic profile of patients with NIDDM.

▶ I am always suspicious of the new wonder drugs, because so many of them have not panned out to be much more than slight variations of old drugs. Thus, I have been suspicious of the hype about troglitazone, a new drug for NIDDM. However, I must say the literature thus far looks quite promising. This is but 1 article of many showing glucose benefits and few side effects of the insulin sensitizer.

This particular study also suggests improvement in cardiac output, lower diastolic blood pressures, lower insulin levels, increased levels of high-density lipoprotein cholesterol, and lower levels of triglycerides, all of which suggest potential for improved cardiac outcomes. The 48-week trial period, longer than many, also adds credence to the drug's safety.

The apparent increases in low-density lipoprotein levels were complicated by the use of a calculated low-density lipoprotein, which is considered unreliable at high triglyceride levels. I was personally not impressed with the small drop in glycated Hb levels.

It will take a while to determine the specific role of troglitazone, but its strength would appear to be its ability to lower insulin levels or lower the need for insulin. It is not yet adequately tested for patients with diabetes who are not already receiving insulin.

M.A. Bowman, M.D., M.P.A.

Diabetes Follow-up and Complications

Retinal Examination Intervals in Diabetic Patients on Diet Treatment Only

Hansson-Lundblad C, Agardh E, Agardh C-D (Univ Hosp, Lund, Sweden)
Acta Ophthalmol Scand 75:244–248, 1997   3–14

Introduction.—Successful treatment of diabetic retinopathy relies on early recognition of sight-threatening changes. This is usually achieved through regular retinal examinations performed every year or 2. It may be possible to extend this interval for patients considered at low risk for sight-threatening retinopathy. This 4-year follow-up study assessed the development of sight-threatening retinopathy among patients with type II diabetes that was under good metabolic control with dietary therapy only.

Methods.—The retrospective study included 117 patients with type II diabetes managed by diet only. They were identified on referral to a department of ophthalmology for fundus photography. Fundus photographs were performed at baseline and repeated at 2 and 4 years. The patients underwent yearly recording of mean blood glucose and hemoglobin A_{1C} levels.

Findings.—The patients' mean age at baseline was 62, and they had had diabetes for a mean of 3 years. During the 4-year follow-up period, 41% of patients continued with dietary therapy only, 49% switched from dietary control to oral hypoglycemic agents only, and 8% switched from dietary control to insulin alone or in combination with oral agents. At baseline, 91% of the patients were free of retinopathy and 9% had only minimal background retinopathy.

After 4 years, 79% of patients still had no signs of retinopathy and 19% had minimal background retinopathy. Just 2 patients had moderate background retinopathy. Just 10% of patients who were still being treated by dietary control at follow-up had minimal background retinopathy. During the follow-up period, mean blood glucose and hemoglobin A_{1C} levels were usually higher in patients treated with oral agents or insulin than in patients treated with dietary control only. These measures were not different for patients who received oral agents and those who received insulin.

Conclusions.—Patients with type II diabetes managed by dietary therapy alone have a low rate of development of diabetic retinopathy during 4 years of follow-up. For patients who have no or minimal retinopathy at initial diagnosis of type II diabetes and remain under good control with dietary treatment only, ophthalmologic follow-up can be delayed at least 4 years, the findings suggest. If metabolic control deteriorates, the risk of diabetic retinopathy must not be ignored.

▶ A small but significant minority of patients with type II diabetes have retinopathy when the diagnosis is made, probably resulting from a delay in diagnosis. However, in this study with excellent follow-up rates, those whose condition was well controlled with dietary intervention alone infrequently acquired retinopathy within the next 4 years. Those whose conditions were not well controlled received additional treatment, such as oral medications or insulin, and had a rate of development of retinopathy of 35%. This is a reminder that good control is associated with lower rates of retinopathy. Perhaps, however, we do not need to send our patients with early, mild, well-controlled diabetes to the ophthalmologist every year.

M.A. Bowman, M.D., M.P.A.

Serum Total Renin Is Increased Before Microalbuminuria in Diabetes
Allen TJ, Cooper ME, Gilbert RE, et al (Univ of Melbourne, Parksville, Victoria, Australia)
Kidney Int 50:902–907, 1996   3–15

Background.—Patients with insulin-dependent diabetes mellitus (IDDM) and microvascular complications have elevated serum prorenin. The link between the increase in prorenin and renal, retinal, or microvascular complications is uncertain. This study sought to determine if an increase in serum total renin concentration (TRC) can predict subsequent microalbuminuria in patients with IDDM.

Methods.—The longitudinal study included 78 patients with IDDM. Serum TRC and albumin excretion rates (AER) were measured over a 10-year follow-up period. The findings were compared for 12 patients with progressively increasing albuminuria and 66 patients whose albuminuria did not change.

Results.—At baseline, the patients with and without progressive albuminuria were similar in terms of duration of diabetes, age, follow-up, glycemic control, and blood pressure. At a diabetes duration of 5–10 years, geometric serum TRC was 350 mIU/L in the patients with increasing albuminuria vs. 189 mIU/L in those without increasing albuminuria. By the time diabetes duration reached 20 years, mean serum TRC in the progressors was 923 mIU/L. Serial TRC and AER measurements in the progressors showed a significant rise in TRC as long as 5 years before the onset of microalbuminuria.

Conclusions.—An increase in serum TRC occurs before microalbuminuria in patients with IDDM, suggesting that TRC could be a useful marker of developing diabetic nephropathy. Patients identified in this way could be targeted for more aggressive treatments, such as strict glycemic control or renoprotective drug therapy. Larger studies with longer follow-up and a formal cost-benefit analysis will be needed before TRC can be recommended as a screening marker.

▶ This study epitomizes to me why it is so important to stay abreast of developments in our field—and the difficulty of doing so. While following up total renin concentrations in our diabetic patients may or may not become a standard of care (this article certainly provides evidence that it might), it is indicative of how rapidly our management strategies can evolve. It has only been a few years since Dr. Berg reviewed the effects of angiotensin-converting enzyme (ACE) inhibitors on diabetic nephropathy.[1] Since that time, it has become a standard of care to check our patients for microalbuminuria and to institute ACE-I therapy to prevent the progression of micro-angiopathic nephropathy. However, these practices have not been uniformly incorporated in diabetic management, particularly at the primary care level. Now, here is an even newer and potentially more powerful screening tool to monitor our patients with diabetic complications. We all need to stay tuned and, it seems, be permanently contemplating change in our clinical practices.

W.W. Dexter, M.D.

Reference

1. 1995 YEAR BOOK OF FAMILY PRACTICE, p 58.

Electrical Spinal-cord Stimulation for Painful Diabetic Peripheral Neuropathy
Tesfaye S, Watt J, Benbow SJ, et al (Walton Hosp, Liverpool, England; Pain Research Inst, Liverpool, England)
Lancet 348:1696–1701, 1996   3–16

Background.—Conventional treatment for painful peripheral diabetic neuropathy is often ineffective and has unacceptable adverse effects. Electrical spinal cord stimulation was investigated as a treatment for chronic neuropathic pain.

Methods.—Ten diabetic patients unresponsive to conventional treatment were included in the study. After implantation of electrodes in the thoracic/lumbar epidural space, immediate neuropathic pain relief was assessed by connection to a percutaneous electrical stimulator or a placebo stimulator. Exercise tolerance was evaluated by treadmill testing.

Findings.—Eight patients had significant pain relief with the electrical stimulator and were converted to a permanent system. Significant relief of background and peak neuropathic pain was observed at 3, 6, and 14 months. Another patient died of unrelated causes 2 months after the start of the study while still benefiting from treatment. The last patient did not benefit from treatment past 4 months. Exercise tolerance was significantly improved in 7 patients at 3 months and in 6 patients at 6 months.

Conclusion.—Electrical spinal cord stimulation provides a new, effective way to relieve chronic diabetic neuropathic pain and improve exercise tolerance. This treatment should be considered for patients unresponsive to conventional treatment of neuropathic pain.

▶ Whatever luck of the draw, I have not had a patient with severe diabetic peripheral neuropathy that could not be reasonably controlled with medication. This study shows that an electrical spinal cord stimulator can be used successfully for these patients, although it is not without risk and did not work for everyone. Because the pain was no longer an inhibitor, patients' ability to walk improved, which should, in turn, be good for their overall health.

M.A. Bowman, M.D., M.P.A.

Diabetic Muscle Infarction
Umpierrez GE, Stiles RG, Kleinbart J, et al (Emory Univ, Atlanta, Ga)
Am J Med 101:245–250, 1996   3–17

Objective.—Patients with diabetes mellitus may develop diabetic muscle infarction (DMI), a rare complication. Only 22 cases of DMI have been reported. These 22 cases are reviewed, along with 3 new cases, to describe the clinical, histologic, and radiologic findings in DMI.

Findings.—Two thirds of the patients were women, and the mean age was 39 years. The typical patient had a long history of insulin-dependent diabetes mellitus with multiple end-organ microvascular complications. An abrupt onset of thigh pain and tenderness, with a palpable, painful mass, was the usual presentation. The tissue around the mass was swollen and indurated, but no systemic signs were present. The lesion persisted for a period of weeks, sometimes with exacerbations of symptoms. The lesion then gradually resolved over a period of weeks to months. About half of the patients had recurrences. The vastus lateralis, thigh adductor muscles, and biceps femoris were commonly involved. The calf muscles were affected in 2 of the 3 new patients. T2–weighted MRI scans showed high intensity in the infarcted muscle. Histologic examination revealed large areas of muscle necrosis and edema, sometimes with regenerating muscle fibers and lymphocytic interstitial infiltration.

Conclusions.—The rare complication of DMI can usually be diagnosed on the basis of the characteristic clinical findings and MRI picture. The histologic findings are nonspecific; muscle biopsy is not always necessary but is indicated in atypical or progressive cases. Being aware of this syndrome and performing early MRI should permit correct diagnosis and shorter hospitalization in patients with DMI. Treatment is nonsurgical and includes pain and glucose management and rest.

▶ I do not believe I have ever seen this complication in practice, and, given that only 22 have ever been reported, it is likely to be rare. However, I would want to recognize it if I saw it. Three things surprised me when I thought about the diagnosis of diabetic muscle infarction—cases were often bilateral, cases were often recurrent, and the creatinine phosphokinase level was often not elevated. The authors' only explanation for the last finding is that the levels may be measured late in the course and may only be elevated soon after the infarction. An MRI scan can be strongly suggestive, but biopsy is sometimes needed.

M.A. Bowman, M.D., M.P.A.

Thyroid Disorders

Treatment of Hypothyroidism With Once Weekly Thyroxine
Grebe SKG, Cooke RR, Ford HC, et al (Mayo Found and Clinic, Rochester, Minn; Wellington Hosp, New Zealand)
J Clin Endocrinol Metab 82:870–875, 1997

3–18

Background.—Therapy with T_4 for hypothyroidism restores euthyroidism in most patients. Noncompliance can be a problem in individuals who require daily lifelong treatment. The elimination half-life of T_4 is about 7 days, but it may have a longer biological effect. Weekly doses may improve patient compliance and also may benefit caregivers who must administer T_4 to others. Studies have shown that single doses of T_4 up to 3 mg are well tolerated by many patients. The safety and efficacy of weekly doses of T_4 were studied.

Methods.—In 12 patients with hypothyroidism, daily and weekly treatment with T_4 were compared. The mean age of patients was 50.8 years; 10

patients were women. Patients continued their daily dose of T_4 or took 7 times the daily dose once per week. The mean daily dose was 1.6 µg of T_4 per kilogram of body weight. Serum free T_4, free T_3, rT_3, TSH, and other markers of thyroid hormone effects were measured.

Results.—At baseline, mean serum TSH was higher and mean free T_4 was lower in patients who were assigned to weekly administration of T_4. A slightly higher serum total cholesterol level in patients taking T_4 once per week was the only sign of hypothyroidism at the tissue level. Mean peak free T_4 and mean peak free T_3 were significantly higher in patients taking weekly doses of T_4. No change was seen in the tissue markers of thyroid hormone effect. There was no treatment toxicity, including cardiac toxicity.

Discussion.—Weekly administration of T_4 in these individuals with hypothyroidism was safe, effective, and well tolerated. A weekly dose slightly greater than 7 times the normal daily dose may be needed to maintain complete euthyroidism. This weekly regimen may be unsafe in some patients if several doses are missed.

▶ One study of 12 patients is not sufficient to switch all patients with hypothyroidism to once-weekly therapy. There is enough evidence to suggest using once-weekly therapy for patients with compliance difficulty. Although it might be tempting to use once-weekly therapy for convenience in business travelers or those who must have their medication administered (such as patients in nursing homes), caution should be taken. There was a higher T_4 concentration within hours after administration of the weekly dose, and the possibility of the development of cardiac dysrhythmia cannot be excluded.

M.A. Bowman, M.D., M.P.A.

Resting Energy Expenditure Is Sensitive to Small Dose Changes in Patients on Chronic Thyroid Hormone Replacement

Al-Adsani H, Hoffer LJ, Silva JE (McGill Univ, Montreal)
J Clin Endocrinol Metab 82:1118–1125, 1997   3–19

Background.—Controversy exists over whether to treat subclinical hypothyroidism and hyperthyroidism and, if so, when and how. There is no solid support for the decision to fine-tune thyroxine dose in patients receiving chronic treatment with this hormone. The effects of modifying thyroxine dose on resting energy expenditure (REE) and on the thermic effect of glucose (TEG) were investigated in 9 patients treated chronically.

Methods and Findings.—The initial dose was adjusted twice at 6- to 8-week intervals to achieve a normal, slightly reduced, or slightly increased serum thyrotropin (TSH) level. Serum free thyroxine (T_4) and TSH were associated with dose. Serum triiodothyronine (T_3) levels were affected minimally and not correlated with dose, free T_4, or TSH. Serum free T_4 and T_3 remained within the normal range on most occasions. In each patient,

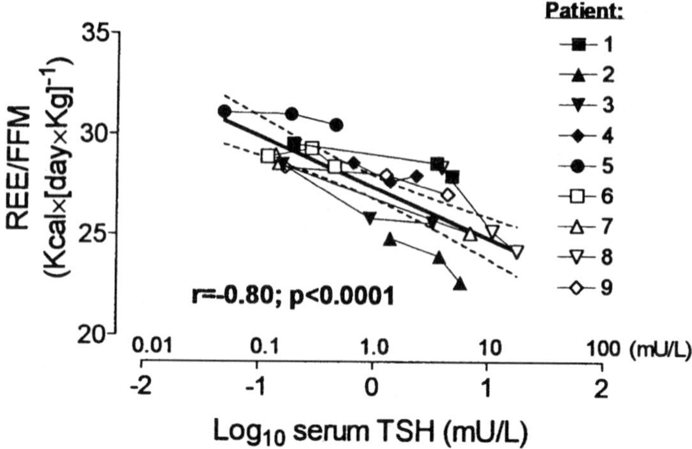

FIGURE 3A.—Effect of the induced changes in thyroid status, as reflected by thyrotropin (TSH), on resting energy expenditure (REE) and thermic effect of glucose normalized by fat-free mass (FFM). Each symbol connected by *lines* depicts 1 patient at the 3 thyroxine doses. A, the pooled, log-transformed TSH and REE/FFM data were submitted to linear regression analysis. The regression equation obtained was REE/FFM = 27.4 − 2.53 × logTSH and is plotted with its S_{yx}. The coefficient of correlation and the corresponding *P* value are shown. (Courtesy of Al-Adsani H, Hoffer LJ, Silva JE: Resting energy expenditure is sensitive to small dose changes in patients on chronic thyroid hormone replacement. *J Clin Endocrinol Metab* 82(4):1118–1125, copyright 1997, The Endocrine Society.)

REE was negatively correlated with TSH. Initial REE and its change between the highest and lowest dose were correlated with, respectively, initial serum TSH and the change in serum TSH between the highest and lowest T_4 dose. When TSH increased to 0.1 to 10 mU/L, REE declined by about 15%. In 6 patients, TEG rose as the dose was reduced, and higher values were associated with greater TSH levels, although nonsignificantly so (Fig 3A).

Conclusion.—In patients receiving chronic thyroxine therapy, REE is influenced significantly by the dose in a dose range encompassing serum TSH levels considered acceptable in the treatment of hypothyroidism. These REE changes may be clinically relevant in the absence of physiologic or behavioral compensations.

▶ Small changes in thyroid dosing within the normal range were associated with changes in TSH and resting metabolic rate. The authors estimate that this could make up to 150 kcal/day difference in energy needs (this could result in 15 pounds of weight gained a year). These results strongly suggest that we should not just aim for a normal TSH, but the normal TSH that seems best for the patient in terms of overall well being. If possible, it would make sense to try to avoid weight gain. The results also suggest that patients with slight elevations in TSH may benefit from thyroid replacement hormone.

M.A. Bowman, M.D., M.P.A.

Estimation of Tissue Hypothyroidism by a New Clinical Score: Evaluation of Patients With Various Grades of Hypothyroidism and Controls

Zulewski H, Müller B, Exer P, et al (Univ Hosp of Basel, Switzerland)
J Clin Endocrinol Metab 82:771–776, 1997   3–20

Background.—Sensitive and precise methods of measuring total and free thyroid hormones make it easy to diagnose thyroid dysfunction. Such methods also can detect subclinical forms of hypothyroidism and hyperthyroidism. Abnormal laboratory results can occur in patients taking drugs that interfere with hormone metabolism. In such cases, the decision to treat the patient frequently is determined by clinical assessment of the disease. It would be useful to have a symptom rating scale to evaluate the clinical status of such patients.

Methods.—Thyroid function tests were used to evaluate the signs and symptoms of hypothyroidism in 332 female patients; 50 had overt hypothyroidism, 93 had subclinical hypothyroidism, 67 had hypothyroidism and were treated with T_4, and 189 were euthyroid. The clinical score was the sum of the 2 best discriminating signs and symptoms. Serum thyrotropin and thyroid hormones were measured, as well as ankle reflex relaxation time, total cholesterol level, and other parameters that reflect tissue manifestations of hypothyroidism.

TABLE 2.—Scoring of Symptoms and Signs of Hypothyroidism

	On the basis of	New score Present	Absent
Symptoms			
Diminished sweating	Sweating in the warm room or a hot summer day	1	0
Hoarseness	Speaking voice, singing voice	1	0
Paraesthesia	Subjective sensation	1	0
Dry skin	Dryness of skin, noticed spontaneously, requiring treatment	1	0
Constipation	Bowel habit, use of laxative	1	0
Impairment of hearing	Progressive impairment of hearing	1	0
Wt increase	Recorded weight increase, tightness of clothes	1	0
Physical signs			
Slow movements	Observe patient removing his clothes	1	0
Delayed ankle reflex	Observe the relaxation of the reflex	1	0
Coarse skin	Examine hands, forearms, elbows for roughness and thickening of skin	1	0
Periorbital puffiness	This should obscure the curve of the malar bone	1	0
Cold skin	Compare temperature of hands with examiner's	1	0
Sum of all symptoms and signs present		12	0

Note: For clinical judgment, add 1 point to the sum of symptoms and signs in women younger than 55 years. Hypothyroid, more than 5 points; euthyroid, less than 3 points; intermediate, 3 to 5 points.
(Courtesy of Zulewski H, Müller B, Exer P, et al: Estimation of tissue hypothyroidism by a new clinical score: Evaluation of patients with various grades of hypothyroidism and controls. *J Clin Endocrin Metab* Vol 82, No. 3, pp. 771–776, 1997. Copyright The Endocrine Society.)

Results.—Only patients with severe overt hypothyroidism and low T_3 had classic signs of hypothyroidism (Table 2). These signs were rare or absent in patients with normal T_3, but low free T_4, and in patients with subclinical hypothyroidism. Results were similar in patients who were euthyroid and in those treated with T_4. In patients with overt hypothyroidism, the new clinical score had excellent correlation with ankle reflex relaxation time and total cholesterol level, but not with serum thyrotropin. In patients with subclinical hypothyroidism, the best correlation was seen between the new clinical score and free T_4 and serum thyrotropin.

Discussion.—This new clinical score combined with thyroid testing is useful for assessing signs and symptoms of hypothyroidism, thyroid failure, and treatment.

▶ Despite the title, this article is basically about the sensitivity and specificity of symptoms and signs of hypothyroidism. Slow ankle reflex time was clearly the best, with both high sensitivity (77%) and specificity (94%). Puffiness had a sensitivity of 60% and a specificity of 96%, much better than I would have expected. Slow movements (observed by the physician) and progressive impairment of hearing were the most specific but were not sensitive (36% and 22%, respectively). However, the scoring system the authors developed correctly classified only 62% of the hypothyroid patients. Because many of the symptoms and signs of hypothyroidism can be nonspecific, the authors' findings can be useful in deciding which patients should be tested for hypothyroidism.

M.A. Bowman, M.D., M.P.A.

4 Infectious Diseases

Introduction

Research on common upper respiratory infections is back in fashion, with interesting articles presented here on common cold risk and treatment, and practice-based research on sore throat. The articles in the following section on otitis mostly address antibiotic treatment, but there is also an especially interesting study on recurrent otitis and language skills at age 9.

The section on sinusitis opens with an important study of MRI findings in normal individuals, raising questions about the test in the diagnosis of sinus disease; and follows with an article showing unimpressive results of maxillary sinusitis treatment in a European general practice setting.

Sexually transmitted disease this year means chlamydia—3 articles on screening and diagnosis. The final miscellaneous section contains some very interesting studies on lowering fever in children, on *E. coli* infections, and on the emergence of drug-resistant *S. pneumoniae*. This year there is only a single article on HIV infection—on use of human growth hormone. I made the editorial decision that, quick as the Year Book process is, anti-retroviral treatment of HIV infection is changing so rapidly that even the Year Book couldn't keep up!

Randomized controlled trials: Abstracts 4–3, 4–5, 4–6, 4–8, 4–9, 4–10, 4–15, 4–19, 4–21, 4–22, and 4–24.

Alfred O. Berg, M.D., M.P.H.

Respiratory Infections

Social Ties and Susceptibility to the Common Cold
Cohen S, Doyle WJ, Skoner DP, et al (Carnegie Mellon Univ, Pittsburgh, Pa; Univ of Virginia, Charlottesville)
JAMA 277:1940–1944, 1997   4–1

Background.—Evidence suggests that susceptibility to common colds is increased among smokers and reduced among moderate drinkers. However, little is known about the role of other health practices, levels of catecholamines, cortisol, or normal variations in cellular immune function. The importance of network diversity for susceptibility, the importance of these behavioral and biological markers for susceptibility, and the

Open Randomised Trial of Prescribing Strategies in Managing Sore Throat

Little P, Williamson I, Warner G, et al (Southampton Univ, England)
BMJ 314:722–727, 1997

Background.—There is ongoing debate regarding the management of sore throat, which is a common problem in managed care. Double-blind trials effectively control for the placebo effect, but open trials provide a better reflection of everyday practice. An open, randomized, controlled trial of 3 different prescribing strategies for sore throat is reported.

Methods.—The study included 716 patients with sore throat from 11 English general practices. All patients were older than 4 years. All had an abnormal physical sign—usually tonsillitis or pharyngitis—in addition to sore throat. The patients were randomly assigned to 3 different prescribing strategies. Patients in group 1 received antibiotics for 10 days, those in group 2 received no prescription, and those in group 3 received antibiotics only if their symptoms had not started to resolve within 3 days. Outcomes—including duration of symptoms; satisfaction with, compliance with, and perceived efficacy of antibiotic treatment; and time off from school or work—were evaluable in 582 patients.

Results.—The median duration of antibiotic use was 10 days in group 1 versus 0 days in groups 2 and 3. Only about 30% of patients in group 3 took antibiotics. There were no differences in the proportion of patients who were better within 3 days: 37% in group 1, 35% in group 2, and 30% in group 3. Neither were there any differences in the duration of illness or

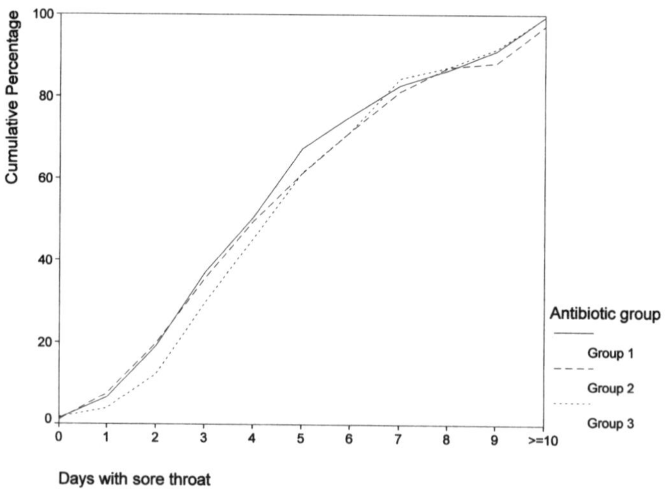

FIGURE 1.—Duration of sore throat after consultation in patients with sore throat randomly assigned to 1 of 3 treatment groups. (Courtesy of BMJ Publishing Group, from Little P, Williamson I, Warner G, et al: Open randomised trial of prescribing strategies in managing sore throat. *BMJ* 314:722–727, 1997.)

number of days off from work or school (Fig 1). Patients in group 1 had 1 less day of fever. At least 90% of patients in each group expressed satisfaction with their treatment.

Eighty-seven percent of patients in group 1 believed that the antibiotics were effective, compared with 55% in group 2 and 60% in group 3. Seventy-nine percent of patients in group 1 said that they would return to see the physician if they had a future attack, compared with 54% in group 2 and 57% in group 3. Patient reports suggested that the need to legitimize the illness to work, school, family, or friends was an important reason for seeing the physician. More-satisfied patients got better more quickly. Patient satisfaction was strongly affected by the way in which the physician dealt with the patient's concerns.

Conclusions.—For patients with sore throat seen in general practice, antibiotics have little impact on symptom resolution. However, antibiotic therapy tends to strengthen belief in the effectiveness of antibiotics, as well as the patients' intentions to see the physician again for future episodes. The decision to see the physician and the duration of illness are both affected by psychosocial factors. No prescription and delayed prescription are both acceptable strategies for dealing with sore throat in primary care.

▶ Add another log to the fire. I like the open randomized method and the use of a primary care office-based research network to get at outcomes for a commonly seen office problem. I also am attracted by the "real world" approach to the problem—take on all comers. One of the outcomes of this study was particularly interesting. Despite no difference in the duration of symptoms (see Fig 1), which is in contrast to other open studies that have demonstrated benefit for the antibiotic group, patients given antibiotics *believed* that they got better more quickly and were more likely to ask for antibiotics again. Thus, a vicious cycle is perpetuated: we (physicians) complain that patients expect antibiotics, but we (often) reinforce their expectations!

In this particular study, one area of potential bias was practitioner expectations and the possibility of selection bias. Though this was not well-addressed, patient response data seem solid. Perhaps in a future YEAR BOOK, I will be able to comment on the authors' contention that antibiotics are of only marginal benefit in preventing complications of group A streptococcus pharyngitis. Bearing in mind that this study did not consider etiology of the pharyngitis (group A streptococcus was only one etiology), with a bit of effort in educating our patients, this is one more upper respiratory tract infection in which antibiotic use can be reduced. For now, despite its limitations, I concur with the conclusions from this study.

W.W. Dexter, M.D.

Antibiotic Prescribing for Adults With Colds, Upper Respiratory Tract Infections, and Bronchitis by Ambulatory Care Physicians

Gonzales R, Steiner JF, Sande MA (Univ of Colorado, Denver; Univ of Utah, Salt Lake City)
JAMA 278:901–904, 1997

4–4

Introduction.—The emergence of antibiotic-resistant bacteria in our communities is due to the excessive use of antibiotics in ambulatory practice. Whereas before 1980, more than 99% of all *Streptococcus pneumoniae* were sensitive to penicillin, there has been an increasing percentage of *S. pneumoniae* isolates with high-level resistance to penicillin and cephalosporins in the last 10 years. Calls for health care providers to limit inappropriate and unnecessary antibiotic prescribing have been renewed in response to this growing community epidemic of drug-resistant *S. pneumoniae.* For seasonal respiratory illnesses, such as colds, upper respiratory infections, and bronchitis, antibiotics have no clinical benefit and are the most important targets for reducing unnecessary antibiotic use. The rates and predictors of antibiotic prescribing for colds, upper respiratory infections, and bronchitis were determined.

Methods.—In all, 1,529 physicians were surveyed to determine their rate of prescribing antibiotics for colds, upper respiratory tract infections, and bronchitis.

Results.—In 1992, about 21% of all antibiotic prescriptions to adults were the result of office visits for colds, upper respiratory tract infections, and bronchitis. Antibiotics were prescribed to 51% of patients diagnosed with colds, 52% diagnosed with upper respiratory tract infections, and 66% of those diagnosed with bronchitis, which accounted for 43% of antibiotic prescriptions in this group. Greater antibiotic prescription rates were associated with female sex and rural practice location. Lower antibiotic prescriptions rates were associated with black race.

Conclusion.—Colds, upper respiratory tract infections, and bronchitis account for a sizable proportion of total antibiotic prescriptions for adults by office–based physicians in the United States. However, research has shown that antibiotics have little or no benefit for these conditions. Across geographical areas, medical specialties, and payment sources, overuse of antibiotics is widespread. Broad-based strategies are needed to change prescribing behavior for these conditions.

▶ The emergence of antibiotic–resistant pathogens, particularly *Streptococcus pneumoniae*, was commented on last year[1] in relation to acute otitis media. This problem persists and is worsening, as evidenced by recent data from the CDC, which found a 60–fold increase in isolate resistance to penicillin from 1979 to 1992![2] One of the principal reasons for this frightening trend is the widespread use (abuse?) of antibiotics by ambulatory/primary care physicians. The authors present hard and overwhelming data illustrating the pervasive and profligate use of antibiotics by physicians and patients for conditions that are primarily viral (> 90% of the cases) and thus self-limited.

Why does this occur? An editorial accompanying this article points to such factors as patient expectations, insufficient time for educating patients, and inadequate knowledge.[3] Last year I looked at another potential source: drug company research supporting this practice.[4] A case I saw recently points to all of these. A youngster presented with a simple cold, and Dad demanded antibiotics because (a) they always work, and (b) that is what all the other doctors have done. A chart review confirmed my fears: 4 colds in the past 6 months (no evidence described in the chart supporting any bacterial infection), all treated with antibiotics, by 3 residents and 1 attending. One note even went so far as to document an assessment of viral upper respiratory infection, but the stated plan was to cover with antibiotics!

We must all work to change our practice behaviors in this respect. Yes, patients demand antibiotics. Yes, it is often the easy way out on a Friday afternoon in a busy clinic. We all can do better. I must admit to a wee bit of proselytization on the topic. In our residency, we are currently working with one of our community faculty (thank you, Burt) to develop guidelines and standards that we can use and maybe even fall back on when confronted by entrenched parental expectations. Together we can reverse these trends and improve the care we give our patients and our community.

W.W. Dexter, M.D.

References

1. 1997 YEAR BOOK OF FAMILY PRACTICE, pp 262–263.
2. Butler JC, Hofmann J, Cetrone MS, et al: The continued emergence of drug-resistant *Streptococcal pneumoniae* In the United States: An update from The Centers for Disease Control and Prevention's Pneumococcal Sentinel Surveillance System. *J Infect Dis*, 174:986–993, 1996.
3. Schwartz B, Bell DM, Hughes JM: Preventing the emergence of anti-microbial resistance: A call for action by clinicians, public health officials, and patients. *JAMA* 278:944–945, 1997.
4. 1997 YEAR BOOK OF FAMILY PRACTICE, p 117.

A Randomized Controlled Trial of Antibiotics on Symptom Resolution in Patients Presenting to Their General Practitioner With a Sore Throat
Howe RW, Millar MR, Coast J, et al (Univ of Bristol)
Br J Gen Pract 47:280–284, 1997   4–5

Background.—The appropriate use of antibiotics in the treatment of sore throat has not been established. The efficacy of penicillin, cefixime, and placebo on symptom resolution in patients seen with a sore throat in a general practice was tested in a randomized, controlled trial.

Methods.—Twenty-two general practitioners enrolled 154 patients in the study. The patients aged 16–60 years initially sought medical care for a sore throat and would have normally been given an antibiotic. The patients received 5 days of treatment with penicillin V, 250 mg 4 times a day; cefixime, 200 mg a day; or placebo. They were asked to keep a 7-day diary of symptom resolution. In addition, eradication of group A beta-hemolytic streptococcus (GABHS) was assessed.

Findings.—One hundred three patients (67%) completed the symptom diaries. Forty had been assigned to receive penicillin; 29, cefixime; and 34, placebo. Overall, symptom resolution by day 3 was greater in the patients taking cefixime than in those taking placebo. Penicillin was not significantly better than placebo, and cefixime did not differ significantly from penicillin. The proportion of patients using analgesia on day 3 differed significantly, the proportion being lowest in the cefixime group. Findings in the subgroup of patients without GABHS were comparable. Although the numbers were too small for statistical significance, the effects of penicillin and cefixime were similarly higher than placebo in patients with GABHS.

Conclusions.—Compared to placebo, cefixime appears to improve the rate of symptom resolution in patients with sore throat selected for antibiotic treatment by their general practitioner. The current findings also suggest that bacteria other than GABHS may be important in the pathogenesis of sore throat.

▶ "Well, doctor, we have two add-ons to your schedule this morning, both with sore throats. You'll have to hurry with them because we have a full schedule." How many times have we all heard that? We enter the examining room hoping that this is only a simple sore throat. The usual scenario is that over-the-counter medications have already been tried, the patient is very uncomfortable, not sleeping well, and states the need to get back to work as quickly as possible. Your examination confirms that this appears to be a pharyngitis and you now ponder what to do. An office beta-hemolytic streptococcus antigen test? A throat culture? Symptomatic treatment only? Symptomatic treatment plus antibiotics?

Experienced clinicians intuitively have learned that giving antibiotics in this situation does have certain risks, but the patients usually feel better faster. This was an interesting study of 22 general practitioners in Great Britain involved in a randomized prospective trial of typical patients with sore throat given penicillin, an oral cephalosporin, or placebo. Lo and behold, patients who received antibiotics had symptom resolution faster than the placebo group. This was unrelated to whether the patient had positive culture for GABHS. The broader spectrum cephalosporin antibiotic gave the greatest symptom relief, suggesting secondary bacterial infection other than streptococcus that was contributing to the symptoms.

This study does not take away the problem described earlier in this comment, but it does objectively document our collective experience that people get better faster when they receive antibiotics.

R.C. Davidson, M.D., M.P.H.

Six–Day Amoxicillin *vs.* Ten–Day Penicillin V Therapy for Group A Streptococcal Tonsillopharyngitis
Cohen R, Levy C, Doit C, et al (Robert Debré Hosp, Paris; CHI, Créteil, France)
Pediatr Infect Dis J 15:678–682, 1996   4–6

Introduction.—More than 42 years ago, treatment for group A streptococcal tonsillopharyngitis was established and consisted of administration of penicillin for 10 days. With the arrival of new cephalosporins, shorter treatments of 3 to 6 days showed comparable rates of eradication. A 6-day regimen of amoxicillin was compared with a 10-day regimen of penicillin for biologic efficacy in eradicated group A streptococcal tonsillopharyngitis.

Methods.—Three hundred eighteen children with group A streptococcal tonsillopharyngitis received either amoxicillin (160) or penicillin (158). Upon completion of treatment, the children returned after 4 days and after 1 month to be assessed clinically and bacteriologically. To compare pre- and post-treatment group A streptococcal isolates, total DNA restriction fragment length polymorphism was used.

Results.—In 118 of 141 children receiving amoxicillin (83.7%) and in 116 of 136 children receiving penicillin (85.3%), pretreatment group A streptococcus was eradicated at 4 days after the completion of treatment. In 9.9% of the children receiving amoxicillin and in 5.7% of the children receiving penicillin, bacteriologic relapses were observed 1 month after the outset of treatment. Four children in the amoxicillin group and 8 in the penicillin group had adverse events related to the study medications; 3 in the penicillin group had to discontinue treatment. In the amoxicillin group, compliance was significantly better based on diary cards and the weight of study drugs returned.

Conclusion.—In the treatment of group A streptococcal tonsillopharyngitis, the efficacy and safety of penicillin at 45 mg/kg/d 3 times a day for 10 days were not statistically different from those of amoxicillin at 50 mg/kg/d 2 times a day for 6 days.

▶ It makes sense to me. A shorter course of therapy equals less antibiotic use (in keeping with the theme of reducing antibiotic use), less cost, and better compliance, but without a drop in clinical efficacy. The length of antibiotic treatment for many infections has been based empirically. We are now finding that shorter courses are often effective, as for example, in the treatment of cystitis. The authors conclude that more efficacy data are needed. Probably so. Stay tuned and start to consider shortening the course of antibiotic therapy for group A streptococcal tonsillopharyngitis. [I certainly favor this approach over IM ceftriaxone—discussed in Abstract 4–9.] An even more heretical approach is alluded to in Abstract 4–3.

W.W. Dexter, M.D.

A Prediction Rule to Identify Low-risk Patients With Community-acquired Pneumonia

Fine MJ, Auble TE, Yealy DM, et al (Univ of Pittsburgh, Pa; Massachusetts Gen Hosp, Boston; Harvard Med School, Boston; et al)
N Engl J Med 336:243–250, 1997   4–7

Background.—About 4 million new cases of adult community-acquired pneumonia are seen in the United States each year. Hospital admission rates vary from region to region, which indicates that admission criteria may be inconsistent. Physicians tend to overestimate the risk of death, and patients at low risk are often hospitalized. Accurate, objective models for identifying low-risk patients with pneumonia may improve decisions about hospitalization.

Methods.—A prediction rule for patients with community-acquired pneumonia was derived from analyzing data from almost 14,200 adult inpatients. Patients were categorized into 5 classes by risk of 30-day hospital mortality. The prediction rule was validated with data from more than 38,000 inpatients and almost 2,300 additional inpatients and outpatients. In step 1 of the prediction rule, patients at low risk of death are identified from history and findings from physical examination (Fig 1). In step 2, the other patients are classified by findings from step 1 plus laboratory and radiographic data (Table 2).

Results.—Mortality rates were similar in the 5 risk classes in the 3 patient cohorts. Mortality was 0.1% to 0.4% in class I, 0.6% to 0.7% in class II, and 0.9% to 2.8% in class III. There were only 7 deaths among 1,575 patients in the 3 lowest risk classes from the group of almost 2,300 inpatients and outpatients; only 4 of these 7 deaths were pneumonia related. Risk class was significantly associated with risk of hospitalization among outpatients and with use of intensive care and number of days admitted among inpatients.

Discussion.—This prognostic model accurately identified patients with community-acquired pneumonia with a low risk of death. This rule may help physicians make better decisions about hospitalizing patients with pneumonia. The predictor variables are well defined and can be evaluated at the initial examination, and patients can be assigned to the lowest risk class by information from the history and initial examination.

▶ This is one of the most helpful articles I have reviewed this year. The authors used a retrospective review of 14,000 adult inpatients with community-acquired pneumonia. Using these data, they derived a prediction rule to be able to identify low-risk patients. They identified a number of variables (see Table 2), with severity points assigned to each positive finding.

The obvious implications of this study are that patients who are class I or class II by their scale and are therefore identified as low-risk patients could be treated as outpatients. However, as the authors point out, this study was

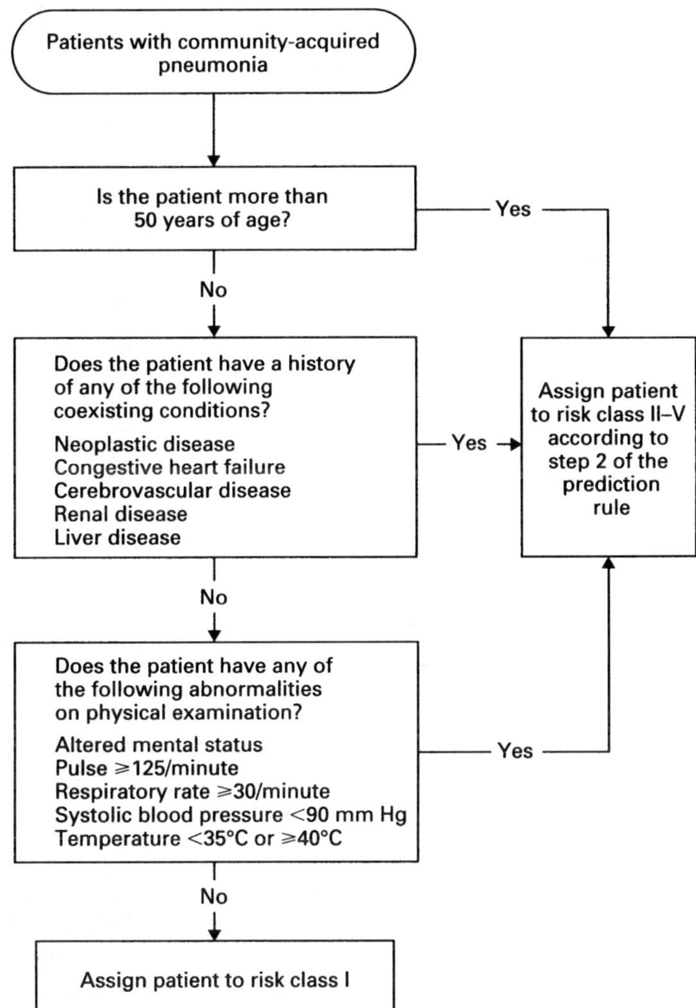

FIGURE 1.—Identifying patients in risk class I in the derivation of the prediction rule. In step 1, the following were independently associated with mortality: age older than 50 years, 5 co-existing illnesses (neoplastic disease, congestive heart failure, cerebrovascular disease, renal disease, and liver disease), and 5 findings from physical examination (altered mental status, pulse greater than or equal to 125 per minute, respiratory rate greater than or equal to 30 per minute, systolic blood pressure less than 90 mm Hg, and temperature less than 35°C or greater than or equal to 40°C). In the derivation cohort, 1,372 patients (9.7%) with none of these 11 risk factors were assigned to risk class I. All 12,827 of the other patients were assigned to risk class II, III, IV, or V according to the sum of the points assigned in step 2 of the prediction rule (see Table 2). (Reprinted by permission of *The New England Journal of Medicine*, from Fine MJ, Auble TE, Yealy DM, et al: A prediction rule to identify low-risk patients with community-acquired pneumonia. *N Engl J Med* 336:243–250, Copyright 1997, Massachusetts Medical Society. All rights reserved.)

not designed to study the efficacy of outpatient treatment in this low-risk population. In the Discussion section, they seem to hedge by describing a number of other variables not studied, which might limit their ability to use this scale to predict successful outpatient treatment.

However, this is based on a small number of studies (8) with an average number of subjects per study of 16. Not much to bank on here. The only conclusion I can draw is that I will be left struggling again this winter and waiting for more evidence.

W.W. Dexter, M.D.

Otitis

Comparison of Ceftriaxone and Trimethoprim-Sulfamethoxazole for Acute Otitis Media

Barnett ED, and the Greater Boston Otitis Media Study Group (Boston City Hosp)

Pediatrics 99:23–28, 1997

4–9

Background.—Almost two thirds of children will have 1 episode of acute otitis media by their first birthday. In the United States, standard treatment is 10 days of an oral antibacterial agent, although shorter and longer treatment courses have been studied. Ceftriaxone is a third-generation cephalosporin that has in vitro activity against *Streptococcus pneumoniae*, *Haemophilus influenzae*, and *Moraxella catarrhalis*. Previous studies have compared the effectiveness of a single dose of ceftriaxone and amoxicillin or cefaclor for acute otitis media, but those studies were limited by a small sample size. The efficacy of ceftriaxone and of trimethoprim-sulfamethoxazole for acute otitis media was examined in a prospective, randomized, single-blind trial.

Methods.—A single IM dose of ceftriaxone (maximum, 50 mg/kg) or trimethoprim-sulfamethoxazole (8 mg trimethoprim and 40 mg sulfamethoxazole/kg/day for 10 days) was administered to 484 children with

TABLE 2.—Clinical Outcome of Children Treated for Acute Otitis Media With Ceftriaxone vs. Trimethoprim-Sulfamethoxazole

| Day | No. | Ceftriaxone | | No. | TMP-SMZ | | P^* (95% CI)*† |
		Cured No. (%)	Failed No. (%)		Cured No. (%)	Failed No. (%)	
3	241	223 (92.5)	18 (7.5)	243	231 (95.1)	12 (4.9)	.42 (−1, .06)‡
14	197§	158 (80.2)	39 (19.8)	212	174 (82.1)	38 (17.9)	.02 (−1, .08)
28	136¶	108 (79.4)	28 (20.6)	155	124 (80.0)	31 (20.0)	.02 (−1, .08)

*Test of equivalence of successful treatment.

†One-sided confidence interval (*CI*) on difference in success rates, trimethoprim-sulfamethoxazole (*TMP-SMZ*) minus ceftriaxone.

‡Hypothesized δ = 0.03.

§Includes children followed from days 4 to 14 after elimination of children who failed on or before day 3 and those lost to follow-up or changed to a different antibacterial agent for a nonotitis condition during days 4 to 14; includes some children not seen at the day 14 visit but seen at the day 28 visit, reported having been well during the study period and classified as cured.

¶Includes children followed from days 15 to 28 after elimination of children who failed on or before day 14 and those lost to follow-up or who were changed to a different antibacterial agent for a nonotitis condition on days 15 to 28.

(Reproduced by permission of *Pediatrics* courtesy of Barnett ED, and the Greater Boston Otitis Media Study Group: Comparison of ceftriaxone and trimethoprim-sulfamethoxazole for acute otitis media. *Pediatrics* 99:23–28, copyright 1997.)

TABLE 5.—Adverse Events Reported at Day 3, by Drug

	Ceftriaxone No. (%)	TMP-SMZ No. (%)	P
Pain at injection site on day 3	19/225 (8.4)		
Diarrhea*	46/195 (23.6)	19/207 (9.2)	<.001
Rash*	21/206 (10.2)	14/201 (7.0)	.245

*Present at day 3 but not at day 0, as reported by caretaker.
Abbreviation: TMP-SMZ, trimethoprim-sulfamethoxazole.
(Reproduced by permission of *Pediatrics* courtesy of Barnett ED, and the Greater Boston Otitis Media Study Group: Comparison of ceftriaxone and trimethoprim-sulfamethoxazole for acute otitis media. *Pediatrics* 99:23–28, copyright 1997.)

acute otitis media. Children were between 3 months and 3 years of age. The children were evaluated periodically for 28 days.

Results.—On day 3, 92.5% of children given ceftriaxone and 95.1% of children given trimethoprim-sulfamethoxazole were improved or cured. On day 14, 80.2% of children given ceftriaxone and 82.1% of children given trimethoprim-sulfamethoxazole were cured. On day 28, 79.4% of children given ceftriaxone and 80.0% of children given trimethoprim-sulfamethoxazole were cured (Table 2). The peristence of middle ear fluid was similar for both groups at days 14 and 28. At day 3, 8.4% of children given the injection of ceftriaxone still had pain at the injection site. New diarrhea was more common in children given ceftriaxone (Table 5).

Discussion.—A single dose of ceftriaxone was as effective as 10 days of trimethoprim-sulfamethoxazole at days 14 and 28 for otitis media in these children. There were few adverse effects. Ceftriaxone was compared with trimethoprim-sulfamethoxazole rather than with amoxicillin because it appeared that the rate of β-lactamase–producing resistance of *H. influenzae* and *M. catarrhalis* might limit the usefulness of amoxicillin for acute otitis media. In another study of a single injection of ceftriaxone compared with 10 days of oral antibacterial therapy, parents were very satisfied with the assigned treatment when their child improved, but expressed a strong preference for the single-dose parenteral regimen both before and after treatment.

▶ I was struck by the use of ceftriaxone for acute otitis media. Not so long ago, in my training institution, this drug was reserved for serious bacterial infections and used only with permission. Has familiarity bred contempt or have resistant pathogens led us to more widespread use of this drug? There is certainly appeal in using a single IM dose of antibiotics instead of a 10-day course of oral treatment.

The authors and the study design addressed problems inherent in evaluating acute otitis media, such as factoring in spontaneous resolution of the illness and treatment protocols, and the results are quite solid. Note, however, that this treatment was comparably effective with, not better than, the alternative and was accompanied by an increase in side effects. Is this a viable alternative to traditional oral antibiotic therapy for acute otitis media?

It would appear so. Perhaps a more compelling question is, Do we need to be this aggressive in treating an illness that can resolve spontaneously?

W.W. Dexter, M.D.

Efficacy of Antimicrobial Prophylaxis for Recurrent Middle Ear Effusion
Mandel EM, Casselbrant ML, Rockette HE, et al (Children's Hosp of Pittsburgh, Pa; Univ of Pittsburgh, Pa)
Pediatr Infect Dis J 15:1074–1082, 1996   4–10

Objective.—Whereas antimicrobial prophylaxis for recurrent acute otitis media (AOM) has been shown to be effective, the role of prophylaxis for asymptomatic middle ear effusion (otitis media with effusion [OME] is equivocal. The efficacy of antimicrobial prophylaxis in preventing recurrent episodes of OME and AOM in at-risk children was examined.

Methods.—At Children's Hospital of Pittsburgh, 111 children aged 7 months to 12 years, who were effusion free but who had histories of chronic or recurrent middle ear effusions (MEE), received amoxicillin (20 mg/kg once daily) or placebo for 1 year. Patients were examined and had tympanometry monthly. Any ear, nose, or throat symptoms were recorded. Patients had a throat culture and audiometry performed at entry, 4, 8, and 12 months and after a new episode. Patients with new episodes of AOM received 40 mg/kg/d of amoxicillin clavulanate or erythromycin sulfisoxazole.

Results.—Compared with the placebo group, the amoxicillin group had significantly fewer episodes of MEE (3.18 vs. 1.81), AOM (1.04 vs. 0.28), and OME (2.15 vs. 1.53). The average length of time amoxicillin patients had MEE was 19.7% vs. 33.2% for placebo patients (P=0.002). The median time to the first episode of MEE was significantly longer in the amoxicillin group than in the placebo group (5.1 vs. 2.7 months). The percentage of cultures in the amoxicillin group with beta-lactamase-positive or *Streptococcus pneumoniae* organisms were similar throughout the study.

Conclusion.—Amoxicillin prophylaxis decreased recurrence of MEE, AOM, and OME in at-risk children.

▶ At first glance, the results from this study seemed to lend weight to prior data supporting the use of prophylactic antibiotics. On closer inspection, though, I am not as confident in the findings. The entry criteria were revised (loosened), the abstract reports N=111, but this includes the placebo group, and the stratification scheme resulted in 12 subgroups! The authors, to their credit, looked at some culture data to assess drug resistance. Overall, though, I do not believe the data support any definitive conclusion on the use of antibiotics for prophylaxis against middle ear effusions. Take-home message: you can't judge a study by its cover (abstract).

W.W. Dexter, M.D.

Safety of Topical Ear Drops Containing Ototoxic Antibiotics

Rakover Y, Keywan K, Rosen G (Central Emek Hosp, Afula, Israel)
J Otolaryngol 26:194–196, 1997   4–11

Introduction.—For the treatment of chronic suppurative otitis media with tympanic membrane perforation or as preventive treatment after tube insertion, topical application of ear drops is commonly used. The question of ototoxicity was raised after cochlear damage caused by polymyxin B and neomycin occurred after experimental topical use in a baboon. The safety of topical ear drops in clinical use was evaluated because of the common use of topical ear drops and their ototoxic potential.

Methods.—Myringotomy and the insertion of tympanostomy tubes were performed on 446 children, 3–8 years of age. After the operation, preventive treatment with polymyxin B (10,000 U/mL), B-neomycin (2.5 mg/mL), and dexamethasone (0.5 mg/mL) ear drops was administered for 2 weeks to 358 children. No ear drops were administered to 88 children. Before the operation and up to 3 months after the operation, audiometric tests were performed.

Results.—Before and after operation, all 446 children had a normal sensorineural hearing threshold. In the group that was treated with drops, there was no sensorineural hearing loss.

Conclusion.—For a short period of time (2 weeks), topical ear drops with ototoxic antibiotics are clinically safe. An explanation may be that serious otitis media thickens the middle ear mucosa, blood supply is increased, and ototoxic agents are removed relatively quickly, thereby protecting the cochlea.

▶ When faced with the all-too-common problem of a child with the signs and symptoms of otitis externa, the prevailing thought in this community is that otic drops containing an antibiotic and steroid combination should not be used if a tympanic membrane perforation is present or cannot be ruled out. This presents a major problem to the clinician. Because the child's ear is exquisitely tender from the infection and swelling in the ear canal, it is often impossible to achieve adequate visualization of the tympanic membrane. The antibiotic steroid drops are usually very effective in bringing about resolution of the problem, assuming the infection has not advanced to the stage that the drops cannot get into the canal secondary to swelling. The scenario is all too familiar. The child is crying, the mother is demanding something be done, you know you have an easily applied medication that will help, but you have this nagging reservation that there just might be a tympanic perforation and maybe the drops might cause some type of permanent damage to the otic bones of the middle ear.

This was an interesting study of 446 children who underwent myringotomy and insertion of tympanostomy tubes. Eighty percent received a postoperative course of the standard polymixin-B, neomycin, dexamethasone ear drops for 2 weeks whereas the other 88 did not receive any ear drops. Audiometric tests were performed before the operation and for up to 3 months afterward. The authors could find no evidence of ototoxicity in any of the children who had received drops. So at least in this study with a known man-made hole in the tympanic membrane, there was no adverse effect from treating with ear drops.

Because previous studies have raised the issue of ototoxicity, I still will not treat a child with otitis externa and a known tympanic membrane perforation with these drops. However, this article makes me feel a little more comfortable faced with the scenario I described above in prescribing these drops for acute otitis externa without visualization of the tympanic membrane.

R.C. Davidson, M.D., M.P.H.

Efficacy of Ototopical Ciprofloxacin in Pediatric Patients With Otorrhea
Wintermeyer SM, Hart MC, Nahata MC (Ohio State Univ, Columbus; Children's Hosp, Columbus, Ohio)
Otolaryngol Head Neck Surg 116:450–453, 1997   4–12

Introduction.—Otorrhea is a common occurrence among patients with tympanostomy tube placement. The bacteriology of ear fluid in such cases varies according to patient age, and opportunistic pathogens increase with the duration of the otorrhea. Ciprofloxacin, the only available oral antibiotic with antipseudomonal coverage, is not approved for pediatric use in its oral form. A study of 29 children with otorrhea and confirmed *Pseudomonas aeruginosa* in ear fluid evaluated the efficacy and safety of topical ciprofloxacin.

Methods.—The patient group ranged in age from 1 to 14 years (mean age, 4.8 years). All had a history of tympanostomy tube placement. The mean duration of a history of ear disease was 3.3 years, and the mean duration of ear drainage for the current ear infection was 5 months. Excluded were patients with a documented hypersensitivity to quinolone antibiotics. Treatment consisted of 3 ciprofloxacin drops 3 times daily for 14 days in the affected ear or ears. Aural irrigation was performed twice daily before drop administration. The effectiveness of the therapy was assessed on days 7 and 14. Patients with a complete cessation of drainage, a dry cavity, and no signs of infection were considered clinically cured.

Results.—After 14 days of treatment with ciprofloxacin drops, 18 of the 29 patients were cured, 8 had improvement (a 50% reduction in days with drainage and/or minimal moisture in the cavity), 2 were cured after change to an alternate therapy, and 1 had no improvement. Two additional children were cured after 3 weeks of treatment. Six of the cured patients had been only partially compliant with the treatment regimen. There were no adverse effects from ototopical ciprofloxacin, and the number of ear infections in these patients was significantly reduced in the year after the study.

Conclusion.—The use of topical ciprofloxacin in pediatric patients with otorrhea achieved a cure rate of nearly 70% and a cure improvement rate of 90%. The outcome was not significantly affected by age, gender, duration of acute drainage, use of aural irrigations, or the presence of multiple pathogens.

▶ Good things come in small packages! This appears to be an effective treatment for children and adults with unresponsive otorrhea. I was impressed that the authors thought to check for serum levels of the drug (it was unmeasurable), as well as looking carefully for ototoxicity (it did not occur). Topical ciprofloxacin seems to be a very safe treatment and appears to be quite effective. I will give this one a try in my patients, large and small, with otorrhea that has not responded to more standard therapy.

W.W. Dexter, M.D.

Recurrent Otitis Media During Infancy and Linguistic Skills at the Age of Nine Years

Luotonen M, Uhari M, Aitola L, et al (Univ of Oulu, Finland)
Pediatr Infect Dis J 15:854–858, 1996   4–13

Background.—Because otitis media in infancy is so common, its adverse effects may have important practical significance. The possible relationship between early recurrent acute otitis media and linguistic performance among second graders was investigated.

Methods.—Data were collected retrospectively from the parents of 394 children in 18 second grade classes selected at random in a medium-sized city in Finland. Auditory, picture vocabulary, morphologic competence, and reading comprehension were assessed.

Findings.—The reading comprehension scores of children who had had more than 4 otitis episodes before 3 years were significantly lower than those of children who had had fewer episodes of otitis media. Early otitis media was associated with impaired reading comprehension test scores after adjustment for confounding variables in a multiple-regression analysis. It was also significantly correlated with teacher assessment of the child's reading comprehension. Otitis episodes after 3 years were not associated with abnormal test findings.

Conclusions.—Middle-ear disease in infancy appears to have a significant adverse effect on reading comprehension among 9-year-olds, even when such episodes were treated effectively. The prevention of otitis media in the first 3 years is stressed.

▶ One of the rationales behind aggressive treatment of otitis media has been to prevent the possible speech and language difficulties. This retrospective correlation of current reading ability with past episodes of otitis media is not convincing. Although the authors demonstrate no demographic differences between the study groups, they do not account for other possible confounders. For instance, they found that recurrent otitis impairs girls more than boys and speculate that this is attributable to inherent gender differences. I don't buy it. There is something else at work here, not yet

treatment does not improve their clinical course, these patients do not require an initial radiographic examination. Whether antibiotics should be given when symptoms persist beyond 2 to 3 weeks remains to be determined.

▶ Add this article to the growing body of literature documenting the ineffectiveness and inappropriateness of using antibiotics for upper respiratory infections (see Abstract 4–4). The methodology used in this study was a bit quirky but, I think, reasonably sound. I would agree with the authors that, if anything, only the more severe cases were selected, and there might have been a bias to treat in follow-up. The conclusions are ones I can support: x-ray studies are not necessary and neither are antibiotics. However, I suspect that the latter might be a harder sell to our patients. Nevertheless, I recommended adding acute sinusitis to the list of upper respiratory infections that do not necessarily require or benefit from antibiotic treatment.

W.W. Dexter, M.D.

Sexually Transmitted Disease

Genital *Chlamydia* Infections in Sexually Active Female Adolescents: Do We Really Need to Screen Everyone?
Mosure DJ, Berman S, Fine D, et al (Ctrs for Disease Control and Prevention, Atlanta, Ga; James Bowman Associates, Seattle; Family Health Internatl, Research Triangle Park, NC; et al)
J Adolesc Health 20:6–13, 1997   4–16

Objective.—Screening for *Chlamydia* infections in women is important because the infection is usually asymptomatic and can result in the spread of infection and long-term complications. Sexually active female adolescents have demonstrated an infection rate of about 10%. Whereas guidelines recommend screening for all sexually active female adolescents, they do not address predictors of infection. Results of an assessment of trends in *Chlamydia* prevalence and prevalence by risk group, and of development and testing of a predictive model are presented.

Methods.—Data from the Region X Chlamydia Screening Project from 1988–92 collected in Alaska, Idaho, Oregon, and Washington included *Chlamydia* screening information for sexually active females aged 15 to 19 undergoing a pelvic examination. Trends in *Chlamydia* prevalence were stratified by demographic, clinical, and behavioral risk factors including multiple sexual partners in the last 30 days, new sexual partner in the last 60 days, a sexual partner with multiple sexual partners, or a symptomatic sexual partner. Logical regression analysis was used to identify predictive variables. Predictive models were developed for all years combined. Individual probabilities of infection were calculated.

Results.—Of 148,650 female adolescents screened, 46% were younger than 18, 90% were white, 8% were currently pregnant, 26% had been pregnant, and 31% reported no contraceptive use. The prevalence of *Chlamydia* was 10%, with 73% of these showing no signs of infection.

TABLE 4.—Predictor Models for Chlamydial Infection in Females, Ages 15–19 Years, Region X Chlamydia Project, 1989–92

Prevalence	1989 OR (95% CI)[a] 11%	1992 OR (95% CI)[a] 8%	Total OR (95% CI)[a] 10%
Race			
White	Referent	Referent	Referent
Black	2.1 (1.7–2.5)	2.1 (1.7–2.5)	2.1 (1.9–2.3)
Hispanic	1.3 (1.1–1.6)	1.4 (1.1–1.7)	1.2 (1.1–1.3)
Other	1.3 (1.1–1.6)	1.3 (1.1–1.6)	1.3 (1.2–1.4)
Currently pregnant	1.4 (1.3–1.6)	1.6 (1.4–1.9)	1.4 (1.3–1.5)
Contraceptive method			
None	*	*	Referent
Oral contraceptives	*	*	0.8 (0.8–0.9)
Barrier	*	*	0.7 (0.7–0.8)
Other	*	*	0.7 (0.6–0.9)
Clinical findings			
MPC	2.8 (2.5–3.2)	2.5 (2.1–3.1)	2.7 (2.5–2.9)
Friable cervix	2.4 (2.1–2.7)	2.4 (2.1–2.8)	2.5 (2.3–2.7)
Reported sexual behavior			
New sex partner	1.4 (1.2–1.5)	1.3 (1.2–1.5)	1.4 (1.3–1.5)
Symptomatic partner	1.9 (1.5–2.3)	2.3 (1.7–3.1)	2.1 (1.9–2.4)
Multiple sex partners	*	1.8 (1.4–2.2)	1.4 (1.3–1.6)
Partner with multiple sex partners	1.5 (1.3–1.7)	*	1.2 (1.1–1.3)

[a]Odds ratio (95% confidence intervals).
*Variables not significant, therefore not included in the model.
(Reprinted by permission of Elsevier Science Inc. from Mosure DJ, Berman S, Fine D, et al: Genital Chlamydia infections in sexually active female adolescents: Do we really need to screen everyone? *J Adolesc Health* 20:6–13, 1997. Copyright 1997 by the Society for Adolescent Medicine.)

Black patients were twice as likely to be infected as white patients. Teens previously or currently pregnant had an infection prevalence of 12% and 13%. Risk of infection increased for subjects reporting any of the 4 sexual risk behaviors or those who had clinical findings (Table 4). The prevalence of infection decreased by 42% of the study period. The 9 independent predictors of *Chlamydia* identified were race, currently pregnant, current contraceptive method, mucopurulent cervicitis, presence of cervical friability, and the 4 behavioral risk factors. Individual year predictor models were similar to the overall predictor model. A prevalence below 6% could not be identified by screening criteria. This type of screening program is cost effective for a population with a 2% or higher prevalence of *Chlamydia* infection. The youngest age group had an infection prevalence of 6% because youth is a predictor of infection.

Conclusion.—The need for reevaluation of screening guidelines is important as new tests for *Chlamydia* are developed. These results support the national recommendation for screening of sexually active female adolescents during pelvic examination.

▶ In our clinic, screening for *Chlamydia*, although almost routine, is still debated. This study should end the debate. Although there is potential bias in this study in that only Title X family planning clinics were used, the scope of the study (N=148,650) lends weight to the evidence. Of particular note are the authors' conclusions that no risk factors were reliable as screening indicators (see Table 4), and no population had less than a 6% prevalence—a number consistent with other studies. The good news? This study supports previous evidence indicating that the use of oral contraceptives does not increase the risk of *Chlamydia* infections, and there seems to be a trend toward declining prevalence. Screening is easy and relatively inexpensive (about $25 for a urine or urethral swab DNA probe) and should be a routine part of our care.

W.W. Dexter, M.D.

Diagnosis of *Chlamydia Trachomatis* Infections in Asymptomatic Men and Women by PCR Assay

Toye B, Peeling RW, Jessamine P, et al (Ottawa Gen Hosp, Ont, Canada; Univ of Ottawa, Ont, Canada; Regional Municipality of Ottawa-Carleton, Ottawa, Ont, Canada; et al)
J Clin Microbiol 34:1396–1400, 1996   4–17

Background.—*Chlamydia trachomatis* infections are the most prevalent sexually transmitted bacterial disease in North America. Screening for genital chlamydial infection is, therefore, a high priority in public health. The ability of a polymerase chain reaction (PCR) assay to detect this infection in asymptomatic men and women was investigated.

Methods.—Urethral swab specimens were collected from 472 men for culture and PCR assay. First-void urine (FVU) samples were collected from 379 of these men and assessed by enzyme immunoassay (EIA) and PCR assay. Cervical swab specimens were also obtained from 242 women for culture, EIA, and PCR assay. Infection was diagnosed when patients tested culture positive or positive by PCR with both plasmid-based and major outer membrane protein–based primers.

Findings.—The prevalence of infection was 7.6% among men and 7.9% among women. In men, the sensitivities of urethral swab specimen culture and PCR assay were 61% and 72%, respectively, and of FVU specimen EIA and PCR, they were 55% and 91%, respectively. The specificities of all the assays were 99.8% or better. The positive and negative predictive values for PCR testing of FVU specimens were 100% and 99.4%, respectively. For PCR of urethral swab specimens, the corresponding values were 96.3% and 97.8%. Cervical swab specimen culture and PCR testing had sensitivities of 42% and 90%, respectively, and specificities of 100% and 99.3%, respectively. The results of EIA were negative for all cervical swabs.

Conclusion.—A greater number of infected asymptomatic women will be identified with PCR testing of cervical swab specimens than with culture or EIA. In asymptomatic men, PCR testing of FVU specimens is noninvasive, sensitive and specific. If found to be cost-effective, PCR testing of FVU specimens may prove useful as a method of screening asymptomatic men to improve case finding and decrease the reservoir for infection transmission.

▶ Screening of women for *Chlamydia* is discussed in this YEAR BOOK in Abstract 4–18. Screening men is equally, perhaps more, important as a significant percentage of infected men are asymptomatic. Limitations of testing in asymptomatic men have included a lack of sensitivity of the test and reluctance of men to undergo testing as it is quite uncomfortable. Techniques for DNA amplification of FVU specimens seem to be the way to go, either by PCR or ligase chain reaction.

W.W. Dexter, M.D.

The Vaginal Introitus: A Novel Site for *Chlamydia Trachomatis* Testing in Women
Wiesenfeld HC, Heine RP, Rideout A, et al (Univ of Pittsburgh, Pa)
Am J Obstet Gynecol 174:1542–1546, 1996   4–18

Background.—The identification of *Chlamydia trachomatis* has been done by tissue culture or antigen detection methods. Recently, the polymerase chain reaction (PCR) has been reported in the diagnosis of *C. trachomatis*. Because of the limitations of urine testing by DNA amplification methods and the need for noninvasive sampling procedures, the vaginal introitus was evaluated as a sampling site for *C. trachomatis* testing.

Methods.—Three hundred women attending a sexually transmitted diseases clinic were studied. Swabs were obtained from the vaginal introitus and tested by PCR. Two hundred women also self-collected an additional introitus swab and provided a urine sample for PCR testing.

Findings.—Vaginal introitus swabs obtained by health care providers had a sensitivity of 92% in the detection of urogenital *C. trachomatis*, which is higher than PCR, culture, or enzyme immunoassay of the cervix or urethra. Polymerase chain reaction testing of swabs collected by the patients had an 81% sensitivity. The sensitivity of urine sample–testing by PCR was 73%.

Conclusion.—Obtaining samples from the vaginal introitus for *C. trachomatis* testing by PCR is highly effective. Sampling by patients and health care providers were both as effective as commonly used diagnostic tests requiring vaginal speculum examination.

▶ A good case has been made in Abstract 4–16 for screening for *Chlamydia trachomatis*. If you are still performing the "gold standard" test with a cervical swab for tissue culture or antigen detection, think again. Obtaining the sample by this method is invasive, inconvenient, and costly, although still the way to go if you are doing a thorough pelvic examination. In our institution, we are using a urine sample to screen for *Chlamydia* via DNA ligase chain reaction, and we have been quite pleased with our results. Here is another easy, noninvasive method of screening for *Chlamydia*.

W.W. Dexter, M.D.

Miscellaneous

The Efficacy of Tepid Sponge Bathing to Reduce Fever in Young Children
Sharber J (Univ of Arizona, Tucson)
Am J Emerg Med 15:188–192, 1997   4–19

Introduction.—Fever is one of the most common complaints in children presenting to the emergency department. For children with fever, antipyretic medications and tepid sponge baths are prescribed commonly in the urgent care and emergency department settings. While the efficacy of antipyretic medications to reduce fever has been well established, the efficacy of tepid sponge baths remains to be determined. Sponge baths are time-consuming for staff, and children complain of discomfort during the bath. The efficacy and amount of discomfort between febrile children receiving antipyretic medication alone and antipyretic medication with a tepid sponge bath were evaluated.

Methods.—Twenty children, ages 5 to 68 months, with a fever of $\geq$ 38.9°C received 15 mg/kg acetaminophen alone or acetaminophen and a 15-minute tepid sponge bath. Tympanic temperature was monitored every 30 minutes for 2 hours. The children were monitored for any signs of discomfort, such as goosebumps, shivering, and crying.

Results.—During the first hour, sponge-bathed children cooled faster, but after 2 hours, there were no temperature differences between the 2 groups. Significantly higher discomfort scores were found in the children who had the sponge baths.

Conclusion.—Parents anxiety about febrile children can be relieved with reassurance, accurate information about fever, and appropriate management.

▶ I can remember receiving sponge baths from my mom as a youngster and I carried that bit of medicine, as Mom taught me, forward into my practice and home. Fever is common, fever is natural, and, probably, fever is beneficial. We often feel, as parents and physicians, that we should be "doing something" for febrile patients. In my attempts to "treat" fevers, I have often recommended tepid baths despite my own (mostly unpleasant) personal experience as the bather and the bathee. There were certainly some holes in the methodology here: use of tympanic thermometer, single investigator, difficulty standardizing protocol, and the subjective nature of the monitoring. Nevertheless, after reading this study, I will have to caveat my recommendations to parents regarding tepid baths for fever reduction. Perhaps our drive to "do something" should be focused on active empathetic listening and simple reassurance.

W.W. Dexter, M.D.

***Escherichia coli* O157:H7 Diarrhea in the United States: Clinical and Epidemiologic Features**

Slutsker L, for the *Escherichia coli* O157:H7 Study Group (Natl Ctr for Infectious Diseases, Atlanta, Ga)

Ann Intern Med 126:505–513, 1997   4–20

Background.—*Escherichia coli* O157:H7 is increasingly recognized as an important cause of bloody diarrhea, and infection with the pathogen is a major cause of postdiarrheal hemolytic syndrome in children in the United States and Canada. A population prevalence study was conducted in 10 United States hospitals to determine the frequency of isolation of *E. coli* O157:H7 and to identify the clinical and epidemiologic features of infection.

Methods.—The 10 hospitals selected represented all 4 census divisions in the United States. Nine served general patient populations and 1 was a pediatric center. Each institution screened a median of 1,300 stool specimens annually. A clinical data form was completed for all patients from whom *Campylobacter, Salmonella* or *Shigella* species or *E. coli* O157:H7 were isolated and for every 25th patient from whom no pathogen was isolated.

Results.—Overall, 1,708 of the specimens (5.6%) examined during the study period (October 1990 to October 1992) yielded at least 1 of the 4 major bacterial enteric pathogens (Table 2). Dual infections were present in 11 patients. *Escherichia coli* O157:H7 was isolated from 0.39% of 30,463 tested fecal specimens; it was found most frequently during the summer months, and represented the highest isolation proportions in hospitals in Maine and Wisconsin. In addition, *E. coli* was more likely to be isolated from visibly bloody stool specimens than from specimens without visible blood; it was the pathogen most commonly isolated from visibly bloody stool specimens that yielded a bacterial enteric pathogen, accounting for 39%. The largest number of *E. coli* O157:H7 isolates was obtained from children aged 1 to 4 years (18 specimens) and adults aged 60 to 69 years (17 specimens).

All 118 *E. coli* O157:H7 isolates produced at least 1 Shiga toxin and 10 (8.5%) were resistant to at least 1 antimicrobial agent. Diarrhea was an almost universal finding with each pathogen, but bloody diarrhea was significantly more common among those with *E. coli* O157:H7 infection. Other clinical signs or symptoms independently associated with *E. coli* compared with the remaining 3 pathogens were visibly bloody stool specimens, no reported fever, a peripheral leukocyte count greater than 10×10^9/L, and abdominal tenderness.

Conclusion.—Isolation proportions from fecal specimens for *E. coli* O157:H7 surpassed those of other common enteric pathogens in certain geographic areas and age groups. Patients with a history of acute bloody

TABLE 2.—History, Physical, and Laboratory Findings in Patients From Whom *Escherichia coli* O157:H7, *Campylobacter* Species, *Salmonella* Species, or *Shigella* Species Were Isolated at 10 Hospitals in the United States, 1990 to 1992

Characteristic*	Patients with *Escherichia coli* O157:H7 (*n* = 104)	Patients with *Campylobacter* Species (*n* = 568)	Patients with *Salmonella* Species (*n* = 389)	Patients with *Shigella* Species (*n* = 232)	Patients with Any of the Four Pathogens
			%		
History					
Diarrhea	98.0	96.9	95.2	96.4	96.3
Bloody diarrhea	91.3	37.0	33.8	54.3	44.1
Abdominal cramps	90.5	79.5	69.7†	77.9	77.7
Reported fever	35.0	58.7	72.0	78.6	64.2
≥7 bowel movements per day†	65.5	61.1	54.8	53.6	58.3
Vomiting	35.6	34.4	41.0	49.0	39.0
Hospitalization	47.1	20.7	38.2	20.6	28.1
Physical and laboratory findings					
Objective fever	41.4	50.9	69.4	69.4	56.6
Abdominal tenderness	72.0	45.4	28.8	33.5	40.8
Visible blood in stool specimen	63.0	7.8	4.8	14.7†	11.8
Stool specimen positive for occult blood†	82.8	52.0	43.4	59.1	53.5
Any fecal leukocytes in stool specimens	70.5	42.9	29.4	37.8	39.5
≥10 fecal leukocytes per high-power field in stool specimen	23.9	16.0	10.2	11.1	13.9
Peripheral leukocyte count > 10×10^9/L	70.9	42.0	45.3†	58.0†	49.0

*Denominator for each characteristic includes only patients for whom information was available.
†This information was available for less than 65% of patients.
(Courtesy of Slutsker L, for the *Escherichia coli* O157:H7 Study Group: *Escherichia coli* O157:H7 diarrhea in the United States: Clinical and epidemiological features. *Ann Intern Med* 126:505–513, 1997.)

diarrhea should be cultured for *E. coli* O157:H7 because infection with this organism may result in serious disease.

▶ This particular bug has been getting a lot of press lately. This study caught my attention because of the locations evaluated. My home state (Maine) had the highest isolation proportion of this pathogen! The prevalence of *E. coli* O157:H7 is certainly on the rise. There are some limitations to this study, however. It is hospital based, not random, and patients already seeking care were selected by their physicians for inclusion in the study. Nevertheless, although these limitations exist (and there are also geographic differences), *E. coli* should figure prominently in your differential diagnosis in patients with crampy, bloody diarrhea, and the workup should reflect this. An excellent review of the epidemiology, clinical features, diagnosis, and treatment is provided in a recent article in the *American Family Physician.*[1]

W.W. Dexter, M.D.

Reference

1. Koutkia P, Mylonakis E, Flanigan T: Enterohemorrhagic *Escherichia coli* O157:H7: An emerging pathogen. *Am Fam Physician* 56:853–859, 1997.

Penciclovir Cream for the Treatment of Herpes Simplex Labialis: A Randomized, Multicenter, Double-blind, Placebo-controlled Trial
Spruance SL, for the Topical Penciclovir Collaborative Study Group (Univ of Utah, Salt Lake City; VIP Research Inc, Bryan, Tex; Westover Heights Clinic, Portland, Ore; et al)
JAMA 277:1374–1379, 1997   4–21

Background.—No antiviral drug has been found to be consistently effective in large, well-controlled clinical trials involving otherwise healthy patients with herpes labialis. Topical 1% penciclovir cream was compared with vehicle control cream in this randomized, double-blind patient-initiated, 2–arm parallel clinical study of immunocompetent patients with recurrent herpes simplex labialis.

Methods.—Thirty-one ambulatory U.S. clinics enrolled a total of 2,209 patients, 1,573 of whom initiated treatment for a recurrence. Treatment consisted of topical 1% penciclovir cream or placebo applied every 2 hours during waking hours for 4 consecutive days.

Findings.—In the patients receiving active treatment, classical lesions (such as vesicles, ulcers, and/or crusts) healed 0.7 day faster than those in the placebo recipients. In addition, pain and lesion virus shedding resolved more rapidly in the penciclovir recipients. Penciclovir cream was effective whether treatment was initiated early or late. The incidences of adverse events were comparable in the 2 groups.

Conclusions.—Penciclovir cream is the first treatment to have a clear impact on the course of recurrent herpes labialis in immunocompetent patients. All clinical and laboratory measures of the disease were improved with this treatment. Faster healing and pain resolution were evident in patients applying the cream in the prodrome and erythema stages, as well as in those starting treatment in the papule and vesicle lesion stages.

▶ "Just be patient, they will go away on their own." This is advice we often dispense, is not often welcome, and at least for cold sores, perhaps is no longer necessary. Oral medications such as acyclovir and famciclovir can often be used in treating herpes simplex (HSV) lesions to great effect but are expensive, inconvenient, and sometimes not well tolerated. In this large multicenter study, treatment was demonstrated to be effective, safe, well-tolerated, and seemed to help even if treatment was begun late in the outbreak. The drawbacks—it is inconvenient (the cream is applied every 2 hours) and the benefit (only marginally faster healing), may not warrant its use. I should note that the study population was quite skewed, nearly all subjects were white women. However, it is relatively inexpensive ($20 to $25 for 2 g in pharmacies in our area), and these may be minor issues for those with recurrent HSV. I will offer this treatment with these caveats.

W.W. Dexter, M.D.

Post-intercourse Versus Daily Ciprofloxacin Prophylaxis for Recurrent Urinary Tract Infections in Premenopausal Women

Melekos MD, Asbach HW, Gerharz E, et al (Univ of Patras, Greece; Phillips Univ, Marburg, Germany; Elisabeth Hosp, Straubing, Germany)
J Urol 157:935–939, 1997   4–22

Introduction.—Recurrent, uncomplicated lower urinary tract infections (UTIs) occur in up to 10% of women of all ages. An enhanced adherence of gram-negative Enterobacteriaceae to the vaginal and urethral mucosa is one of the factors that may promote infection. The management of recurrences is a major problem in women prone to UTIs. A substantial decrease in recurrence has occurred with daily prophylactic administration of co-trimoxazole, nitrofurantoin, cinoxacin, and cephalosporins. The effectiveness of newer 4–fluoroquinolones, such as ciprofloxacin, has not been tested for its long-term results in guarding against recurrences, nor has there been a comparison of daily application with postcoital application.

Methods.—Following a curative, conventional treatment of the initial acute UTI, 70 women began a prophylactic regimen of 125 mg ciprofloxacin after intercourse and 65 women took ciprofloxacin on a daily basis. Urine and introital samples were taken during the 12–month follow-up period, when the patients were followed bacteriologically and clinically. After the end of preventive treatment, the women were followed for an additional year.

Results.—During prophylaxis there was 0.043 infection per patient in the post-intercourse group compared with 0.031 in the daily group. Before the start of the corresponding prophylactic regimen, there were 3.67 UTIs per patient in the post-intercourse group and 3.74 UTIs per patient in the daily group. Gram-negative Enterobacteriaceae were equally distributed in both groups and were found in 86% of the vaginal vestibule cultures before prophylaxis. During prophylaxis, there was 5.6% gram-negative Enterobacteriaceae in the postcoital group and 2.5% in the daily group. After the end of prophylaxis, the overall improvement of the incidence of UTIs per patient and the rate of introital colonization with enteric gram-negative bacteria were maintained. Abnormal introital colonization was found in 36% of all women, and infection occurred in 34%.

Conclusion.—Long-term post-intercourse prophylaxis with ciprofloxacin was as effective as daily prophylaxis and had the advantage of requiring only one third the amount of the drug used in daily prophylaxis.

▶ Urinary tract infections (UTIs) are exceedingly common; the symptoms are often painful and aggravating; and, particularly with recurrent infections, there is a risk of significant sequelae. If you have been using daily antibiotic prophylaxis, read this study and think about using postcoital prophylaxis instead. The authors' conclusions, equal effectiveness, better compliance, and significant decrease in amount of antibiotic usage compared with daily prophylaxis, are very well supported. However, given rising concerns about excessive use of antibiotics and emerging resistant organisms, even less use might be a laudable goal. Let me do some math: daily prophylaxis = 365 doses of antibiotic per year; postcoital prophylaxis (based on this study) = 130; 3 doses per day twice-daily dosing; for recurrent UTI (4 per year per patient) = 24. I tend to favor the latter approach (though perhaps a slightly riskier gambit). Empiric treatment of dysuria, particularly in our patients with history of recurrent UTIs might be a way to go. It has certainly been shown to be a cost-effective strategy.[1] However, I am convinced by this study and will include this strategy in my recommendations to patients.

W.W. Dexter, M.D.

Reference

1. Barry HC, Ebell MH, Hinchner J, et al: Evaluation of suspected urinary tract infection in ambulatory women: A cost utility analysis of office based strategies. *J Fam Pract* 44:49–60, 1997.

The Continued Emergence of Drug-resistant *Streptococcus pneumoniae* in the United States: An Update From the Centers for Disease Control and Prevention's Pneumococcal Sentinel Surveillance System
Butler JC, Hofmann J, Cetron MS, et al (Ctrs for Disease Control and Prevention, Atlanta, Ga)
J Infect Dis 174:986–993, 1996   4–23

Introduction.—The most common cause of purulent meningitis, community-acquired pneumonia, bacteremia, and acute otitis media is *Streptococcus pneumoniae*. Although penicillin had been prescribed for treat-

nonsusceptible or resistant to penicillin, erythromycin, and trimethoprim-sulfamethoxazole, whereas those nonsusceptible or resistant to tetracycline have remained constant (Fig 2).

Conclusion.—In the United States, the proportion of isolates with reduced susceptibility and the number of serotypes of nonsusceptible strains are increasing. To treat and prevent disease caused by these strains, improved local surveillance for penicillin-resistant *S. pneumoniae* infections, judicious use of antibiotics, and development and use of effective pneumococcal vaccines will be required.

▶ As I reviewed this interesting study, I recalled a recent patient we admitted to the University hospital with community-acquired pneumonia. The initial gram stain of sputum was highly suggestive of *Streptococcus pneumoniae.* As the family practice resident and I discussed the antibiotic options for this patient, we quickly decided on a relatively expensive third-generation cephalosporin. We both were concerned with potential drug resistance to the more standard drugs such as penicillin or trimethoprim-sulfamethoxazole. This study gives strong evidence that we were right to not rely on first-line antibiotics. The U.S. Centers for Disease Control and Prevention monitors the drug resistance of pneumococcal strains in the United States. They have monitored these figures for a number of years with an unfortunate lapse between 1988 and 1991. When surveillance was reestablished in 1992, a surprising and frightening jump in resistance and nonsusceptibility was found in the pneumococcal isolates. This pneumococcal microbe is a formidable enemy and seems quite capable of adapting to build resistance against our antibiotics. One wonders how long it will take before we will see similar resistance figures for our current new and more powerful antibiotics.

R.C. Davidson, M.D., M.P.H.

Recombinant Human Growth Hormone in Patients With HIV-associated Wasting

Schambelan M, and the Serostim Study Group (San Francisco Gen Hosp)
Ann Intern Med 125:873–882, 1996   4–24

Introduction.—Body wasting is a frequent AIDS-defining condition. It is linked to impaired function and decreased quality of life and is an independent predictor of death. A previous study found that 1 week of treatment with growth hormone leads to weight gain and nitrogen retention in patients with HIV-associated body wasting. However, the long-term effects of treatment are unknown. The long-term effects of growth hormone treatment on body weight, body composition, functional performance, and quality of life were assessed.

Methods.—The randomized, double-blind, placebo controlled trial included 178 patients with HIV-associated body wasting. All had unintentional weight loss of 10% or more of body weight or weight less than 90% of the lower limit of ideal. The patients were randomized to receive 12 weeks of treatment with recombinant human growth hormone, 0.1 mg/kg/day, or placebo. The average dosage in the growth hormone group was 6 mg/day. Clinical and laboratory outcome measures included weight, body fat, lean body mass, bone mineral content, total body water, extracellular water, work output, and quality of life.

Results.—Weight increased significantly in the growth hormone group, by a mean of 1.6 kg. Lean body mass increased by 3.0 kg whereas body fat decreased by 1.7 kg. None of these measures was significantly changed in the placebo group. The differences between groups were significant at 12 weeks. Treadmill work output increased by a greater amount in the growth hormone group. There were no apparent differences in quality of life, days of disability, or use of medical resources. Growth hormone treatment was well tolerated, with no increase in clinical events, AIDS progression, CD4+ or CD8+ cell count, or viral burden.

Conclusion.—Treatment with recombinant human growth hormone appears to be beneficial for patients with HIV-associated body wasting. It increases body mass, lean body mass, and work output while reducing fat body mass. The treatment is well tolerated; the cost remains to be determined.

▶ This is 1 of 2 excellent randomized, controlled trials on growth hormone treatment in patients with AIDS published in the same issue of the *Annals of Internal Medicine*. The study abstracted here had the better design for studying the effect of growth hormone by itself. The second article reported a more complex study that also tested insulin-like growth factor–1 singly and in combination with growth hormone.[1] The message from both is clear: growth hormone provides net benefit, but the length of follow-up—12 weeks—is, unfortunately, too short to tell whether the treatment's benefits are long lasting. The treatment is well tolerated. The costs (which are substantial) are not addressed in either study.

A.O. Berg, M.D., M.P.H.

Reference

1. Waters D, Danska J, Hardy K, et al: Recombinant human growth hormone, insulin-like growth factor 1, and combination therapy in AIDS-associated wasting. *Ann Int Med* 125:865–872, 1996.

5 Asthma and Allergic Rhinitis

Introduction

Five articles in this chapter on asthma focus on children, with a useful study on the relationship of URI symptoms and later asthma, and a very important controlled trial of immunotherapy (showing no benefit). The single article on allergic rhinitis provides evidence that an inexpensive over-the-counter drug works just fine.

Randomized controlled trials: Abstracts 5–3, 5–4, and 5–6.

Alfred O. Berg, M.D., M.P.H.

Early Childhood Respiratory Symptoms and the Subsequent Diagnosis of Asthma
Dodge R, Martinez FD, Cline MG, et al (Univ of Arizona, Tucson)
J Allergy Clin Immunol 98:48–54, 1996   5–1

Introduction.—Physicians often are reluctant to make a diagnosis of asthma in infants and very young children who are coughing or wheezing because these symptoms usually resolve. However, some believe that early childhood respiratory symptoms are a risk factor for asthma because older children and adults with asthma have reported a higher than expected frequency of coughing and wheezing when they were very young. The natural history of respiratory symptoms in a community-based sample of young children who were observed prospectively for up to 11 years was described.

Methods.—There were 786 children younger than 5 years who were studied with a parent-administered mail survey every 1 to 2 years for 3 to 11 years. About three fourths of the children enrolled were younger than 2 years. Questions on the survey asked whether the child usually coughs first thing in the morning in bad weather, whether the child coughs on most days for as much as 3 months of the year, whether the child has a cough when there is not a cold, and whether the child has seen a doctor for asthma. Calculations were made of odds ratios and confidence intervals.

Results.—The risk of a subsequent diagnosis of asthma showed no significant increase with any single respiratory symptom, such as coughing or wheezing only with a cold, among children younger than 1 year. Asthma was more likely to be diagnosed later, however, among 1- and 2-year-olds who had wheezing only with a cold and those who had attacks of shortness of breath with wheezing than among children without these symptoms. The odds ratio was 23.1 for the children who had wheezing only with a cold. Symptoms were even more strongly associated with subsequent asthma at the age of 3 to 4 years, with an odds ratio of 7.2 for attacks of shortness of breath with wheezing.

Conclusions.—Symptoms that begin at or persist through the age of 3 to 4 years are significantly associated with future asthma; however, respiratory symptoms reported by parents in the first year of life of their children are not significantly associated with future asthma. Children in whom asthma developed later were likely to have mothers with a history of asthma and to have elevated serum IgE levels. The risk of diagnosis of asthma is increased with persistent symptoms after the age of 3 years.

▶ When a child shows the first episode of respiratory symptoms suggestive of asthma, the parents obviously are concerned about the implications for long-term asthma. This interesting study followed up a group of children longitudinally to determine the predictive value of respiratory symptoms. They found that very young children, less than 1 year of age, showed a very poor correlation between symptoms and the subsequent diagnosis of asthma. However, as the children got older, certain symptoms became more predictive of a diagnosis of asthma. By the time the children were at least 3 years old, the relative risk began to mount significantly for an ultimate diagnosis of asthma in those with common respiratory symptoms related to asthma.

I think, from the findings of this study, that we are safe in telling the parents of our very young patients that we simply do not know whether their symptoms are a harbinger of later asthma. As the children get older, however, it is more likely that certain symptoms, such as wheezing, will be predictive of an ultimate diagnosis of asthma.

Regardless of the age of the child, the new onset of symptoms related to asthma in a young child should trigger vigorous reduction of risk factors in the environment. The most important of these is parental smoking.

R.C. Davidson, M.D., M.P.H.

Prevalence of Possible Undiagnosed Asthma and Associated Morbidity Among Urban Schoolchildren
Joseph CLM, Foxman B, Leickly FE, et al (Henry Ford Health System, Detroit; Univ of Michigan, Ann Arbor; James Whitecomb Riley Hosp for Children, Indianapolis, Ind)
J Pediatr 129:735–742, 1996   5–2

Purpose.—Asthma is the most common chronic disease of children and is more common in minority children than in white children. There is little information on the prevalence of undiagnosed asthma among minority children or on the consequences of failure to recognize these cases. The prevalence of undiagnosed asthma among urban schoolchildren was assessed.

Methods.—The population-based, cross-sectional study included 230 urban schoolchildren in grades 3, 4, and 5. They represented 61% of eligible children at 2 Detroit public elementary schools. Ninety-eight percent were African-American. The children were assessed by a caretaker survey and by in-school pulmonary function testing. Children with reported symptoms and/or bronchial hyperresponsiveness (BHR) were considered to have undiagnosed asthma. The definition of BHR was a decline of at least 15% in baseline forced expiratory volume in 1 second after an exercise challenge.

Results.—Seventeen percent of the children had a reported physician diagnosis of asthma. Eighty-three percent had reported wheezing in the previous year. Of the remaining 189 children, 6% had undiagnosed asthma on the basis of BHR. Another 8.5% met modified American Thoracic Society symptom criteria for asthma. In total, 14% of children met 1 or the other criterion.

Allergies and eczema were more likely to be reported for children with BHR than for children without asthma (no BHR, no symptoms, and no physician diagnosis of asthma); the odds ratio (OR) was 8.5 for allergies and 6.4 for eczema. Children meeting the symptom criteria for asthma were significantly more likely to have reported allergies (OR, 6.2), reported bronchitis (OR, 6.7), sleep disruption (OR, 7.1), and missed physical education classes (OR, 15.0).

Conclusion.—As many as 14% of urban school-aged children may have undiagnosed asthma, depending on the diagnostic criteria used. Compared with children without asthma, these children may be more likely to have allergies, bronchitis, sleep disruption, and missed physical education classes. It may be beneficial to target urban, predominantly African-American school-aged populations for asthma screening.

▶ This interesting study concerns schoolchildren between grades 3 and 5 in 2 elementary schools in the urban Detroit area who were screened for possible asthma. The authors found a surprisingly high incidence (14%) of children with a high probability of having previously undiagnosed asthma.

I am convinced that this study significantly overestimates the population of children with asthma. I was particularly concerned with the symptom score produced by a questionnaire to the childrens' caregivers. The pulmonary function tests performed in the schools are more objective measures than the symptom score. In spite of this concern, I do think the study sends a strong message that we need to maintain a high level of suspicion for young children in urban areas with symptoms of wheezing or cough.

R.C. Davidson, M.D., M.P.H.

A Controlled Trial of Immunotherapy for Asthma in Allergic Children

Adkinson NF Jr, Eggleston PA, Eney D, et al (Johns Hopkins Univ, Baltimore, Md)

N Engl J Med 336:324–331, 1997   5–3

Background.—Few clinical trials of multiple-allergen treatment for perennial allergic asthma have been performed. The additive benefit of broad-spectrum immunotherapy was investigated in the current randomized, placebo-controlled study.

Methods.—One hundred twenty-one allergic children with moderate-to-severe, perennial asthma were included. All were receiving daily medication for asthma. Subcutaneous injections of a mix of up to 7 aeroallergen extracts or placebo were given, with maintenance injections for 18 months or more. Medications were adjusted every 2 to 3 weeks based on peak flow rates and symptoms.

Findings.—Median medication scores decreased from 5.4 to 4.9 in the immunotherapy group and from 5.2 to 5 in the placebo group (a nonsignificant between-group difference). The number of days of oral corticosteroid use was comparable in the 2 groups. Thirty-one percent of the immunotherapy group and 28% of the placebo group had partial or complete remission of asthma. The groups did not differ in their use of medical care, symptoms, or peak flow rates.

Conclusions.—In these allergic children with perennial asthma receiving appropriate medical treatment, immunotherapy with injections of allergens for more than 2 years was not beneficial. These findings are not consistent with common clinical opinion and previous research.

▶ Asthma in allergic children is always seen as a perplexing problem. In addition to maximizing inhaled medications and reducing exposure to allergens, there is always the question of the efficacy of immunotherapy. This well-controlled study of 121 allergic children showed no evidence of benefit from immunotherapy for these children.

In addition to the contribution of the excellent study design, the credibility of this finding is increased, to my mind, by the identity of the researchers. This study came from the asthma and allergy center at a major university medical center. If there was any study bias, it would be toward the use of immunotherapy in children. I think this important study lends credence to inhalations. The authors therefore recommend that inhaled albuterol should be prescribed for patients with mild asthma on an as-needed basis.

I suspect that our patients already intuitively know this. Even if we set up a strict regular use schedule, my guess is they use it when needed more often than on a regular schedule. It is comforting to know that there is no major difference in efficacy between the 2 schedules. For mild asthma, I concur with these authors that an on-demand scheduling regimen is appropriate.

R.C. Davidson, M.D., M.P.H.

Chest Radiography in the Initial Episode of Bronchospasm in Children: Can Clinical Variables Predict Pathologic Findings?
Walsh-Kelly CM, Kim MK, Hennes HM (Med College of Wisconsin, Milwaukee)
Ann Emerg Med 28:391–395, 1996   5–5

Background.—Routine chest radiography in every child with an initial episode of wheezing may be too expensive. It was determined whether historical or clinical variables could accurately identify nonbronchospastic causes and complications of bronchospastic illness on chest radiography in children with an initial episode of wheezing.

Methods and Findings.—Six hundred thirty-three children seen in 1 emergency department with an initial episode of wheezing during a 16-month period were included in a prospective case series. The median age was 8 months. Thirty-nine children (6.2%) had abnormalities on radiography. Sixty-eight percent of the children had evidence of reactive airway disease on radiographs, and 25.4% had normal findings. No 1 variable could accurately predict all abnormal radiographic results. A model was constructed of 9 variables identified in a discriminant function analysis, but it did not accurately discriminate among patients with normal radiographic findings, abnormal radiographic findings, and evidence of reactive airway disease.

Conclusion.—No clinical variables, alone or in combination, could accurately identify patients with abnormal radiographic findings. Chest radiography should be included in the diagnosis of children with an initial episode of bronchospasm.

▶ Chest radiography has been under attack as an unnecessary test in primary care and emergency situations such as bronchitis and pneumonia. This study provides convincing evidence that in the pediatric emergency situation, chest radiography is important in properly diagnosing an initial episode of bronchospasm. Foreign bodies and vocal chord problems are just 2 of the conditions that mimic acute asthma, and chest radiography may be the only way to differentiate among these conditions. Children with an established diagnosis of asthma would not likely need chest radiography in

6 Gastroenterology

Introduction

This section opens with a state-of-the-art review on reflux disease and an interesting long-term follow up study of the same condition. The section on gallbladder disease includes a meta-analysis of complications based on studies totaling 90,000 patients. A decision analysis on testing for *H. pylori* follows, paired with a study of the economic and clinical consequences of various management strategies. Articles on risk and treatment make up a short section on inflammatory bowel disease. The final miscellaneous section includes a randomized trial on treatments for pancreatitis, a meta-analysis of treatments for hemorrhoids, and a caution regarding liver biopsy.

Randomized controlled trial: Abstract 6–11.

Alfred O. Berg, M.D., M.P.H.

Reflux

Gastroesophageal Reflux Disease
Kahrilas PJ (Northwestern Univ, Chicago)
JAMA 276:983–988, 1996   6–1

Introduction.—To describe any symptomatic condition or histopathologic alteration resulting from episodes of gastroesophageal reflux, the term gastroesophageal reflux disease was coined. About 7% of adults have daily heartburn, 14% have weekly heartburn, and 40% have monthly heartburn. Strategies for identifying and managing the complications of gastroesophageal reflux disease are reviewed.

Methods.—Controlled therapeutic trials on the management of gastroesophageal reflux disease in adults with esophageal complications were conducted to determine new developments in diagnosis and therapeutics. The review included esophagitis, acid-suppressive medications, prokinetic drugs, maintenance therapy, antireflux surgery, esophageal stricture, Barrett's metaplasia, and extraesophageal manifestations, such as reflux-induced asthma and otolaryngological manifestations.

Results.—Long-term antisecretory therapy usually is used to treat esophagitis, typically a chronic, recurring disorder. An alternative strategy is laparoscopic antireflux surgery, but there are no controlled trials com-

143

TABLE 4.—Diagnostic Validity of the I-GERQ Score

Cut-off value	Sensitivity	Specificity	Positive predictive value†	Negative predictive value†
>3	.94	.72	.20	.99
>5	.86	.85	.30	.99
>7	.74	.94	.48	.98
>13	.37	.99	.74	.95
>15	.14	1.00	1.00	.94

Score 1 point for each item marked with an *asterisk* in tables. Maximum possible score is 25.
†Assuming a GERD prevalence among infants of ~7%.
Aronow and Silverberg. *Pediatric Gastroenterology* 1983:214.
(Courtesy of Orenstein SR, Shalaby TM, Cohn JF: Reflux symptoms in 100 normal infants: Diagnostic validity of the infant gastroesophageal reflux questionnaire. *Clin Pediatr* (Phila) 35:607–614, 1996.)

Methods and Findings.—The 138–item I-GERQ was administered to the parents of 100 infants attending a well-baby clinic (comprising the control group) and to the parents of 35 infants referred to a gastroenterology division for GERD assessment and positive results on esophageal pH probe or biopsy. The healthy group was found to have a high prevalence of reflux symptoms. Daily regurgitation was documented in 40%, respiratory symptoms in 34%, daily hiccups in 36%, crying for more than 1 hour a day in 17%, and arching in 10%. Many symptoms were significantly more prevalent in the GERD group than in the control group, however, with odds ratios exceeding 3 for nearly 20 items (Table 4). The 25–point I-GERQ score had positive and negative predictive values of 1.00 and 0.94 to 0.098, respectively. Infant exposure to environmental smoke was not a statistically significant provocative factor for GERD.

Conclusions.—The prevalence of GERD symptoms among healthy infants is high. However, the I-GERQ is a valid diagnostic tool, with the potential to considerably reduce the costs of accurate diagnosis of infantile GERD.

▶ Administering questionnaires in the office can be somewhat cumbersome. This is one instance, though, where it could prove quite useful. All babies burp, hiccup, spit up, and cry. These are frequent complaints in the office, and our task is to sort out the few who may actually have GERD. The I-GERQ proved to be fairly quick and easy (15 to 20 minutes of parent time in the office) and was also reliable. Despite some limitations of the study, which the authors discuss, the I-GERQ, particularly in its shortened form, seems effective and efficient in the identification of infants who warrant further evaluation and perhaps therapy.

W.W. Dexter, M.D.

Gallbladder Disease

Presence of Fever and Leukocytosis in Acute Cholecystitis
Gruber PJ, Silverman RA, Gottesfeld S, et al (Albert Einstein College of Medicine, New Hyde Park, NY; Winthrop Univ, Mineola, New York)
Ann Emerg Med 28:273–277, 1996   6–4

Objective.—Despite textbook characterizations, many patients who come to the emergency department (ED) for acute cholecystitis (AC) do not have fever or an elevated white blood cell (WBC) count. The frequency of fever and leukocytosis in patients admitted with a diagnosis of AC who underwent cholecystectomy during the same hospitalization was retrospectively determined.

Methods.—Charts of 198 patients, aged 18–92 years, given a diagnosis of AC in the ED and operated on during the same hospitalization were reviewed for data regarding fever (oral temperature, 100°F or higher or rectal temperature, 100.4°F or higher) and elevated WBC count (11,000/mm^3 or greater).

Results.—Nongangrenous AC was diagnosed in 103 patients, chronic cholecystitis in 44, and gangrenous AC in 51. Approximately one third of patients had a fever, 61% had elevated WBC counts, 24% had both, and 31% had neither. Within 8 hours of arrival at the ED, 29% of patients with nongangrenous AC had fever, 68% had leukocytosis, 25% had both, and 28% had neither. Of patients with gangrenous AC, 41% had fever, 73% had leukocytosis, 29% had both, and 16% had neither. In patients with chronic AC, 27% had fever, 32% had leukocytosis, 14% had both, and 55% had neither. Time to surgery was significantly longer for patients with chronic cystitis than for those with nongangrenous AC (101 vs. 68 hours).

Conclusion.—Patients who arrive at the ED with AC, including gangrenous cystitis, frequently do not have fever or leukocytosis.

▶ The diagnosis of acute abdominal pain is always a challenge, and AC is a common part of the differential that is especially subtle. The patient history is the most important part of the diagnosis, and gallbladder symptoms often resemble gastric problems. The presence of fever and elevated WBC count are often used to differentiate the inflammation of the gall bladder from the acid conditions of the stomach. This study confirms what we have often experienced. We have many patients with AC who do not have fever or an elevated WBC count. The laboratory fails us again and reinforces the importance of a careful history and physical examination in patients with an acute abdomen.

J.E. Scherger, M.D., M.P.H.

more specific diagnosis is provided when endoscopy is used first; this strategy also rules out malignancy and reassures patients.

▶ I was surprised at the findings of this study. On balance, I am skeptical of conclusions based on theoretic models, not patient studies. It is difficult to broadly apply a purely mathematical finding to individuals with symptoms in the office. I do not believe I am alone in often opting for empiric treatment of dyspepsia and gastroesophageal reflux disease, recommending endoscopy only if compelled to do so by recurrent or other symptoms. At present, the clinical literature does not strongly support one management approach over another (see Abstract 6–1). This decision analysis study reinforces this from a cost-based approach. While I may not change my overall approach to this entity, this certainly removes one barrier to recommending initial endoscopy for my patients.

W.W. Dexter, M.D.

Management Strategies for *Helicobacter pylori*-seropositive Patients With Dyspepsia: Clinical and Economic Consequences
Ofman JJ, Etchason J, Fullerton S, et al (Univ of California, Los Angeles; Emory Univ, Atlanta, Ga; RAND, Santa Monica, Calif)
Ann Intern Med 126:280–291, 1997   6–7

Introduction.—Up to 40% of the adult population in the United States is affected by dyspepsia, or epigastric pain or discomfort that is represented by a gnawing or burning sensation. This condition results in indigestion with belching, bloating, and fullness, and is relieved by food, antacids, or antisecretory drugs. Ulcer therapy has been revolutionized with recognition of the role of *Helicobacter pylori* in the pathogenesis of peptic ulcer disease. The role of anti-*H. pylori* therapy in the management of non-ulcer dyspepsia is being debated because the association between *H. pylori* gastritis and non–ulcer dyspepsia is equivocal and dyspeptic symptoms have not been alleviated consistently by antibiotic treatment. Initial anti-*H. pylori* therapy is the alternative to initial endoscopy in *H.-pylori*-seropositive patients; however, the costs and benefits of these alternative strategies are still unknown.

Methods.—In *H. pylori*-seropositive patients with dyspepsia, the costs and outcomes of initial anti-*H. pylori* therapy and initial endoscopy were compared with decision analysis. The initial endoscopy strategy entailed biopsy and a rapid urease test of all ulcers. Patients with non-ulcer dyspepsia received a trial of ranitidine, 150 mg twice daily, for 8 weeks. Patients with esophagitis received omeprazole, 20 mg twice daily for 12 weeks. Surgery was performed on patients with gastric cancer.

Results.—Initial anti-*H. pylori* therapy averages $820 per patient compared with $1,276 per patient for initial endoscopy, representing an average savings of $456 per patient. The financial effect of a 252% increase in the use of antibiotics for initial *H. pylori* therapy is offset by reduction of the endoscopy workload by 53%. Before the 2 strategies become equally cost effective, endoscopy-related costs must be reduced by 96%. Varying the rates of *H. pylori* eradication, the complications of antibiotics, or the response of symptoms to cure *H. pylori* did not substantially affect the financial benefits of initial anti-*H. pylori* therapy in patients with nonulcer dyspepsia.

Conclusion.—The most cost-effective management strategy is initial anti-*H. pylori* therapy in *H. pylori*-seropositive patients with dyspepsia. This strategy can be used as a basis for management and policy decisions about *H. pylori*-seropositive patients with dyspepsia, unless physicians are concerned about resistance to antimicrobial agents or the lack of proven benefit of anti-*H. pylori* therapy in nonulcer dyspepsia. Randomized studies of the strategies that evaluate outcomes and patient preferences are needed to optimize management decisions.

▶ And now for the opposing view. In this decision analysis, the authors demonstrate a significant cost savings for medical treatment vs. initial endoscopy for this subset of dyspeptic patients. Certainly, if we begin recommending endoscopy to all our patients with dyspepsia, the overall cost of managing these patients might not increase by much (according to Silverstein et al.), but the workload would increase astronomically. Even if more family doctors and internists become proficient at and perform endoscopy, we could not get to everyone with dyspepsia. Thus, while I disagree with the conclusion that this model should dictate management and policy decisions, this certainly seems a reasonable middle ground. And, depending on whose numbers you believe, it might provide some cost savings along with expeditious and appropriate care. Ultimately, I think that well-designed clinical trials, not computer mathematical models, should shape our management recommendations in the office.

W.W. Dexter, M.D.

Prospective Study of Diet and the Risk of Duodenal Ulcer in Men
Aldoori WH, Giovannucci EL, Stampfer MJ, et al (Harvard School of Public Health, Boston; Harvard Med School, Boston)
Am J Epidemiol 145:42–50, 1997   6–8

Background.—Diet has long been suspected of being associated with duodenal ulceration. Geographic variations in this disease may be explained by dietary differences. Associations between dietary factors and risk of duodenal ulcer were assessed.

Methods and Findings.—A cohort of 47,806 men, 40 to 76, without diagnoses of gastric or duodenal ulcer or cancer, was studied prospectively. One hundred thirty-eight cases of duodenal ulcer were diagnosed during the 6-year follow-up. There was little evidence of an important effect of fat, type of fat, or protein consumption. A greater consumption of fruits and vegetables was correlated with a lower risk of duodenal ulcer after

7 Skin Conditions

Introduction

This short chapter opens with 2 articles on treatment and follow-up of patients with acne. It also includes a nice review of tinea versicolor, a new observation on irritant contact dermatitis, the linkage between stress and alopecia areata, and a wonderful historical perspective on suntanning.
Randomzed controlled trial: Abstract 7–2.

Alfred O. Berg, M.D., M.P.H.

Acne Vulgaris

Predictors of Severity of Acne Vulgaris in Young Adolescent Girls: Results of a Five-Year Longitudinal Study

Lucky AW, Biro FM, Simbartl LA, et al (Univ of Cincinnati, Ohio; Children's Hosp Med Ctr, Cincinnati, Ohio; Dermatology Research Associates, Cincinnati, Ohio)
J Pediatr 130:30–39, 1997   7–1

Background.—Despite the prevalence and physical and psychological effects of acne vulgaris, little is known about the natural history of this disease. Factors that may be useful in predicting the severity of facial acne in girls were investigated.

Methods.—Four hundred thirty nine black and 432 white fourth- and fifth-grade girls volunteered for the study with their legal guardians' permission. At annual examinations during a 5-year period, the degree of facial acne was classified as mild, moderate, or severe. In addition, blood samples were obtained at 1, 3, and 5 years.

Findings.—There were no racial differences in acne or hormone levels. The number of acne lesions increased progressively with age and maturation. Regardless of age, there were many more comedonal than inflammatory acne lesions. The girls with severe acne by year 5 had had significantly more comedones and inflammatory lesions than girls with mild or moderate acne, as early as 10 years of age, about 2.5 years before menarche, when their degree of acne was mild. Menarche onset occurred significantly later in girls with mild comedonal acne than in those with severe comedonal acne. Compared with girls with mild or moderate comedonal acne, girls in whom severe comedonal acne developed had significantly

---

TABLE.—Treatment Approaches for Tinea Versicolor

Agent	Suggested Dosing
Topical	
Ciclopirox olamine 1% cream*	Twice daily for 2 weeks
Ketoconazole 2% cream*	Twice daily until clinical improvement
Miconazole 2% cream*	Once daily for 2 weeks
Oxiconazole nitrate 1% cream	Once to twice daily until clinical improvement
Selenium sulfide 2.5% shampoo*	Once daily for 7 days
Terbinafine 1% cream	Twice daily for 2 weeks
Systemic	
Ketoconazole	200 mg/d for 10 days
Fluconazole	400 mg/d for 3 days
Itrraconazole	200 mg/d for 7 days

*Currently approved by the Food and Drug Administration for the treatment of tinea versicolor.
(Courtesy of Savin R: Diagnosis and treatment of tinea versicolor. *J Fam Pract* 43:127–132, 1996. Reprinted by permission of Appleton & Lange, Inc.)

---

similarly raised. The organism can be easily removed from the stratum corneum by lightly scraping the skin or stripping it with cellophane tape. A simple, inexpensive test—the potassium hydroxide preparation—can then be performed to confirm the presence of the organism.

Treatment.—Traditional topical agents, such as selenium sulfide, have been found to be effective, but recurrence is likely and often rapid. Therapeutic interest is currently focused on synthetic "-azole" antifungal drugs, which interfere with the sterol metabolism of the infectious agent. Ketoconazole is an imidazole that has been used successfully for years, both orally and topically, although it does not have Food and Drug Administration approval for this indication. Fluconazole and itraconazole are newer derivatives that appear to have minor and infrequent adverse effects. Oral antifungal agents (except for ketoconazole) carry a low risk of hepatotoxicity (Table).

Conclusion.—There are several good treatment options for patients with tinea versicolor. Patients may be given the option of topical or systemic therapy, although oral itraconazole and oral fluconazole have many advantages over topical agents.

▶ I still find this very common condition not diagnosed and improperly treated. Paradoxically, the more widespread the condition is, especially on the chest and back, the less often it seems to be correctly diagnosed and treated. Many clinicians believe that fungal infections are very localized. When the condition is diagnosed, the old-fashioned treatments such as selenium sulfide are still used. They are odorless and may stain clothing. Modern treatment of tinea versicolor involves oral treatment for widespread conditions and potent topical therapy for smaller, localized areas.

J.E. Scherger, M.D., M.P.H.

The Influence of Hard Water (Calcium) and Surfactants on Irritant Contact Dermatitis

Warren R, Ertel KD, Bartolo RG, et al (Procter and Gamble Co, Cincinnati, Ohio)
Contact Dermatitis 35:337–343, 1996　　　　　　　　　　　　　　　　　7–4

Background.—Irritant contact dermatitis is the most common occupation-associated disease. The most common cause is exposure to solvents and oils, and the second most common cause is exposure to soap and detergents. Studies have sought to identify the mechanisms of irritation of surfactants. Environmental factors, such as humidity, are also involved in irritant contact dermatitis. It was recently shown that the calcium content of water increases the adsorption of the major soap component, laurate, to skin. The calcium content of water can vary from place to place and may affect the development of irritant contact dermatitis.

Methods.—The effect of the calcium content of water (water hardness) on irritant contact dermatitis was studied by examining differences in skin reactions from exposure to 3 cleansing agents. Two washing methods were tested with sodium soap, triethanolamine soap, and synthetic detergent cleansers. Water hardness ranged from 0 grain to 11 grain. Skin dryness and redness were evaluated clinically, and hydration was measured with an instrument. Soap binding to the skin was measured using Fourier transform infrared reflectance spectroscopy.

Results.—After the more mild washing procedure, skin treated with hard, 11-grain water was significantly drier, had more erythema, and was less hydrated than skin treated with deionized 0-grain water. Results of the 3 cleansing agents were similar. The hardness of the rinse water had a greater effect on skin than the hardness of the wash water. The effect of water hardness on soap binding to skin showed a similar pattern. The relationship between water hardness and irritation did not hold true under more exaggerated washing procedures.

Discussion.—The calcium content of water affects erythema and dryness of skin caused by common skin cleansing agents. The hardness of the rinse water has the most profound effect. These effects were determined only after a mildly exaggerated washing procedure. All 3 cleansing agents were clinically mild when 0-grain water was used, but the effects were significantly different with hard water. The calcium content of water has a direct effect on the skin barrier and an indirect effect through its interaction with surfactants.

▶ I included this somewhat obscure study as a reminder of the importance of soap products in causing contact dermatitis. I often say that using soap brings more patients to the doctor for skin rashes than the absence of its use. The hardness of water may interact with soap products as a factor in contact dermatitis. The practical applicability of this study is questionable; however, it is informative to note that the hardness of water directly correlates with the propensity of soap to generate contact dermatitis. Further research must be done before an evidence-based recommendaton can be made to patients.

J.E. Scherger, M.D., M.P.H.

Microbiology of Infected Atopic Dermatitis

Brook I, Frazier EH, Yeager JK (Naval Hosp, Bethesda, Md)
Int J Dermatol 35:791–793, 1996   7–5

Purpose.—The skin lesions of patients with atopic dermatitis (AD) frequently become infected. Studies of the microbiology of secondary bacterial infection of AD lesions have been incomplete. The aerobic and anaerobic microbiology of these infections is studied.

Methods.—The retrospective study included 41 specimens of secondarily infected AD lesions from 41 patients. Each specimen was analyzed for the presence of aerobic and anaerobic bacteria.

Findings.—Thirty-six percent of patients had aerobic or facultative anaerobic bacteria only, 20% had anaerobic bacteria only, and 44% had mixed anaerobic–aerobic flora. A total of 72 isolates were recovered, including 34 aerobic or facultative species, 35 strictly anaerobic isolates, and 3 candidal species (Table 1). *Staphylococcus aureus* was the most frequent aerobic and facultative isolate, followed by group A β-hemolytic streptococci and *Escherichia coli*. *Peptostreptococcus* was the most frequent anaerobic genus, followed by pigmented *Prevotella, Porphyromonas,* and *Fusobacterium*. About one third of patients had single bacterial isolates, most commonly *S. aureus*. Sixteen patients harbored organisms that produced the enzyme β-lactamase, and they were mainly organisms residing in the mucous membranes close to the AD lesions. Lesions on the legs and buttocks tended to be infected with enteric gram-negative rods and *Bacteroides fragilis* organisms. Lesions of the fingers, scalp, face, and neck were more likely to have group A β-hemolytic streptococci, pigmented *Prevotella, Porphyromonas,* and *Fusobacterium*.

Conclusions.—The findings help to clarify which specific organisms are responsible for secondary infection of AD lesions. The causative bacteria vary by the anatomical site of the lesions. Cultures of secondarily infected AD lesions should be processed to recover aerobic as well as anaerobic bacteria.

▶ Be aware that allergic skin lesions frequently become infected. Unless appropriate antibiotic treatment is started, these lesions are resistant to the usual treatment for allergies. This study and the corresponding table indicate how multiple organisms from the skin are usually involved in the infection. A broad-spectrum antibiotic with sensitivity against β–lactamase-producing organisms is necessary, such as a first-generation cephalosporin. Such an antibiotic is also effective for lesions on the buttocks and legs, which are more often a result of gram-negative organisms.

J.E. Scherger, M.D., M.P.H.

TABLE 1.—Isolation of Organisms From 41 Secondarily Infected Eczema Lesions at Different Anatomical Locations

	Fingers	Hand	Leg	Trunk	Anatomic Location Scalp	Face and Neck	Buttocks	Total No. of Isolates
Total number of specimens	6	6	6	5	6	7	5	
Aerobic bacteria								
S. aureus	3	3	2	3	1			12
S. epidermidis	1					1		2
α Streptococcus	2							2
Group A Streptococcus	2	1	1			1		5
Group D Streptococcus			1					1
Escherichia coli			2				2	4
Enterobacter sp.				1			1	2
Proteus sp.			1	1			1	3
P. aeruginosa			1	1				2
K. pneumoniae						1		1
Total no. of aerobes	8	4	8	6	1	3	4	34
Anaerobic bacteria								
Peptostreptococcus spp.	3	2	1	3	1	2	1	13
P. acnes	1		1	1				3
Clostridium sp.			2				1	3
Eubacterium sp.						1		1
B. fragilis group			1				2	3
Pigmented Prevotella and Porphyromonas sp.	3				3	2		8
Fusobacterium sp.	1				1	2		4
Total no. of anaerobes	8	2	5	4	5	7	4	35
Fungi								
Candida sp.	1						1	
Candida albicans							1	
Total no. of isolates	17	6	13	10	6	10	10	72

(Courtesy of Brook I, Frazier EH, Yeager JK: Microbiology of infected atopic dermatitis. *Int J Dermatol* 35:791–793, 1996.)

Stress and Alopecia Areata: A Psychodermatologic Study

Gupta MA, Gupta AK, Watteel GN (Univ of Western Ontario, London; Univ of Toronto)
Acta Derm Venereol 77:296–298, 1997

7–6

Background.—Reports have linked psychosocial stress to the onset and exacerbation of alopecia areata (AA), with linkage rates ranging from 6.7% to 96%. Little is known clinically about stress-reactive AA, and the severity of the emotional stressor and that of the AA do not correlate directly.

Methods.—Stress reactivity of AA and psychosocial measures were studied among 16 patients with AA (or alopecia totalis) and 28 patients with alopecia universalis. Patients used a 10-point scale to rate alopecia exacerbation by stress. Relationships between psychosocial stress measures and AA severity were determined, and dermatologic and psychological characteristics of patients reporting an association between stress and AA were compared with those who did not.

Results.—Stress reactivity score was correlated with psychological measures ($P < 0.05$). Patients with higher depression scores were more likely to be high stress reactors. Stress reactivity correlated significantly ($P < 0.05$) with 9 of 17 psychosocial measures. A prevalence of high stress reactivity in AA of 15.9% was found.

Conclusions.—In patients with AA, high stress reactivity was significantly associated with depression scores in the range of major depressive disorders, which may affect immune status. Patients with stress-reactive alopecia may have depressive illness, an important management consideration.

▶ This small study done at the University of Michigan serves as a reminder that stress plays an important role in alopecia areata. Patients with this condition, and other skin conditions such a psoriasis and chronic eczema, should be screened for mental health problems, especially chronic stress and depression.

J.E. Scherger, M.D., M.P.H.

Treatment of Chronic Urticaria With Ketotifen

Egan CA, Rallis TM (Univ of Utah, Salt Lake City)
Arch Dermatol 133:147–149, 1997

7–7

Background.—Chronic urticaria is a difficult problem to treat. The lesions are caused by a local increase in capillary permeability, induced by histamine and other local mediators released from mast cells or basophils. Most patients have no specific allergic trigger for chronic urticaria. Most of the available treatments target the symptoms and block the end-point receptors. The potent antiasthma and antiallergic drug ketotifen was used to treat a highly resistant case of chronic, severe urticaria.

Case Report.—Woman, 43, had a 5-month history of urticaria and pruritus after influenza vaccination and a case of pneumonia. She had seen many dermatologists and received many drug treatments. She had episodes of breathing difficulty that led to several emergency department visits and had become depressed and suicidal. An extensive workup identified no underlying source of her urticaria. Her condition improved after receiving IV ranitidine hydrochloride and hydroxyzine hydrochloride in the hospital, along with an elemental diet. However, the urticaria recurred after discharge. After another severe exacerbation, the patient experienced moderate improvement in response to a course of high-dose pulse methylprednisolone acetate, but there was no response to a second course. She also had moderate improvement with plasmapheresis and supplemental oral cyclophosphamide, but she was unable to tolerate the cyclophosphamide.

The patient was then treated with ketotifen fumarate, which she had bought in Mexico. The dosage was 2 mg orally twice daily. All other drug treatments were withdrawn, except for fluoxetine and levothyroxine. This treatment rendered the patient free of urticaria for the first time in 9 months. Her pruritus resolved with time, and she was able to return to a normal diet. She has required no further hospitalizations since starting ketotifen. The authors have had similarly good results with ketotifen treatment in 3 other patients with chronic urticaria.

Discussion.—Ketotifen appears to be a safe and effective treatment for chronic urticaria that does not respond to other treatments. Unlike other drugs, which merely treat the symptoms, ketotifen acts to stabilize the mast cells and prevent the release of mediators. Although widely used elsewhere, ketotifen is currently unavailable in the United States. Double-blind trials of ketotifen treatment for chronic idiopathic urticaria are warranted.

▶ Anti-inflammatory therapy may be entering a new era. Leukotriene inhibitors are being released for the treatment of asthma and may reduce the use of corticosteroids. The drug reported here has a similar effect on the inflammatory process and may provide a practical alternative to steroids for chronic urticaria. As the biochemistry of the inflammatory process is better understood, more-specific medications will be available, and we may look back on steroids as a crude, sledge hammer approach to treating inflammation.

J.E. Scherger, M.D., M.P.H.

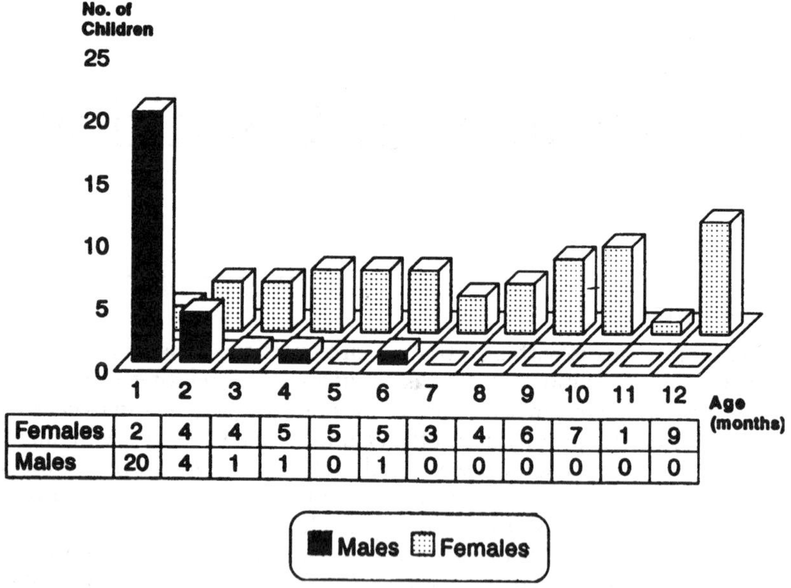

	1	2	3	4	5	6	7	8	9	10	11	12
Females	2	4	4	5	5	5	3	4	6	7	1	9
Males	20	4	1	1	0	1	0	0	0	0	0	0

FIGURE 1.—Age distribution of children younger than 1 year with urinary tract infection. (Courtesy of Goldman M, Barr J, Bistritzer T, et al: Urinary tract infection following ritual Jewish circumcision. *Isr J Med Sci* 32:1098–1102, 1996.)

Results.—By 2 weeks after the circumcision, 52% of urinary tract infection episodes were diagnosed. The incidence of urinary tract infection induced by *Escherichia coli* was significantly lower in boys than in girls. The incidence of urinary tract infection induced by *E. coli* was significantly lower in boys treated within 2 weeks after circumcision compared with infants treated before the procedure or more than 2 weeks after the procedure. In 6 of 27 boys and 2 of 55 girls, positive blood cultures of an identical microorganism were noted. The occurrence and severity of urinary tract malformations were similar in boys and girls.

Conclusions.—There may be an association between the high rate of urinary tract infection and ritual Jewish circumcision. A more sterile technique by the circumciser may lower the risk of urinary tract infection in male newborns.

▶ Circumcision appears to be here to stay, based on culture, religion, personal preference, and some medical benefits. Many techniques are widely available, and there has been interest in ritual Jewish circumcision methods. This report from Israel suggests that the ritual Jewish technique may be associated with a higher incidence of urinary tract infection. Other studies should be done comparing various circumcision techniques and the incidence of urinary tract infection.

J.E. Scherger, M.D., M.P.H.

Local Anesthesia for Circumcision: Which Technique Is Most Effective?

Lenhart JG, Lenhart NM, Reid A, et al (Univ of Nevada, Reno; Univ of North Carolina, Chapel Hill)
J Am Board Fam Pract 10:13–19, 1997   8–2

Background.—Several researchers have demonstrated the reliability and safety of local anesthetic in eliminating the pain associated with circumcision. However, there have been no studies determining which technique is most effective for decreasing the pain of the procedure.

Methods.—Fifty-six infants undergoing circumcision were assigned randomly to 1 of 3 groups: distal branch block, root block, and subpubic block. Cry responses and changes in heart rate and oxygen saturation were analyzed.

Findings.—The distal branch block technique was discontinued during the study because of concern about possible untoward outcomes. Thus only data from the circumcisions of 42 infants assigned to the other 2 groups were analyzed. The pain of circumcision was more reliably decreased by the dorsal penile nerve root block than by the subpubic technique. No serious complications occurred with any of the techniques studied (Fig 3).

Conclusions.—During circumcision, greater comfort can be provided by administering local anesthetic with blockade at the penile root; performing the procedure in a quiet, warm environment; leaving the upper extremities unrestrained; and allowing enough time for the anesthetic agent to take effect (at least 5 minutes, timed). Modifications in the design of restraining

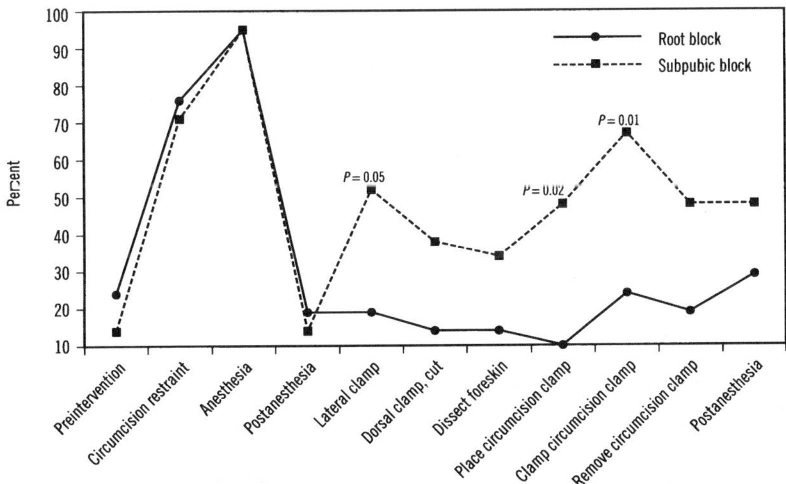

FIGURE 3.—Comparison of percentage of infants crying at specific points in the procedure by method of anesthesia (n = 21 for each group). (Courtesy of Lenhart JG, Lenhart NM, Reid A, et al: Local anesthesia for circumcision: Which technique is most effective? *J Am Board Fam Pract* 10:13–19, 1997.)

boards should be investigated, because hyperextension of the lower extremities during preparation caused a great deal of distress.

▶ I hope that very few physicians are doing circumcision without anesthesia. Two methods of subcutaneous injection, dorsal penile nerve block and local infiltration, are easily learned. Topical anesthetic creams also are becoming popular but are less effective. This article is an outstanding randomized controlled trial of the 2 local injection methods, and it shows that the dorsal penile nerve block is most effective. This technique can be taught right in the nursery, and I have even encouraged nursery nurses to motivate and sometimes instruct physicians in using the technique at the time they do circumcisions. Infants cannot speak, but their cries let us know that circumcision is painful without anesthesia.

J.E. Scherger, M.D., M.P.H.

Effect of Neonatal Circumcision on Pain Response During Subsequent Routine Vaccination

Taddio A, Katz J, Ilersich AL, et al (Hosp for Sick Children, Toronto; Toronto Hosp; Univ of Toronto)
Lancet 349:599–603, 1997

8–3

Background.—Preliminary research suggests that pain in the neonatal period may have long-lasting effects on future infant behavior. Whether neonatal circumcision affects pain responses at 4- or 6-month vaccinations compared with uncircumcised babies was investigated, and the effects of circumcision pretreatment with lidocaine–prilocaine cream (Emla) were determined.

Methods and Findings.—Eighty-seven infants were studied prospectively. One group was uncircumcised, 1 had been randomly assigned to Emla pretreatment for pain in circumcision, and 1 group had been assigned to placebo before circumcision. The 3 groups were comparable in birth and infant characteristics at the time of vaccination, including age and temperament scores. Multivariate analysis demonstrated significant differences in percentage facial action, percentage cry time, and visual analogue scale pain scores at vaccination. Univariate analyses were significant for all outcome measures. Babies receiving placebo before circumcision had higher difference scores than uncircumcised babies for percentage facial action, percentage cry duration, and visual analogue scale pain scores. All outcome measures showed a significant linear trend, that is, pain scores increased from uncircumcised infants to those pretreated with Emla to those given placebo before circumcision.

Conclusions.—Pain responses to routine vaccination are stronger in circumcised babies than in uncircumcised ones. Preoperative Emla treatment can attenuate this pain response. Such treatment is recommended to alleviate neonatal pain during circumcision.

▶ This interesting article suggests that the pain of circumcision, without anesthesia, is remembered by the infant as a conditioned response to pain. This is 1 more piece of evidence to support the use of local anesthesia for circumcision. Doing circumcision without anesthesia is barbaric and needs to be stopped. The methods of anesthesia are very simple to learn and are very safe.

J.E. Scherger, M.D., M.P.H.

Circumcision in the United States: Prevalence, Prophylactic Effects, and Sexual Practice
Laumann EO, Masi CM, Zuckerman EW (Univ of Chicago)
JAMA 277:1052–1057, 1997   8–4

Introduction.—There is little consensus regarding the significance of the foreskin in male sexual performance and satisfaction. Health and sexual outcomes of circumcision were evaluated to determine whether there are differences in contraction of sexually transmitted diseases (STDs) and differences in sexual function between circumcised and uncircumcised men.

Methods.—Data were collected from the National Health and Social Life Survey regarding sexual, attitudinal, and health-related experiences of circumcised and uncircumcised men. This probability sample included 1,410 American men aged 18–59 years. There was an oversample of black and Hispanic groups for comparative analysis.

Results.—There were no significant differences in circumcised and un-circumcised men regarding the likelihood of contracting STDs. There was a slight tendency for uncircumcised men to experience sexual dysfunction, particularly later in life. Circumcised men were more likely to participate in a more elaborated set of sexual practices. This pattern differed across ethnic groups, indicating the influence of social factors.

Conclusion.—Circumcision offers no discernable prophylactic benefit and may increase the likelihood of contracting STDs. Men, especially older men, who are circumcised may have a decreased chance of experiencing sexual dysfunction. Physicians and parents should understand the potential benefits and risks of circumcision before newborns are circumcised.

▶ The circumcision question is likely to rage on indefinitely. Steeped in religion, culture, advocacy for infants, cosmetics, and patient preference, the decision regarding circumcision is much more complex than simply weighing the medical risks and benefits. This review of a large population confirms other reports concluding that the medical evidence does not come down on either side of the question. Family physicians and other primary care physicians should be flexible and supportive in counseling regarding circumcision.

J.E. Scherger, M.D., M.P.H.

Prostate Cancer

Trends in Prostate Cancer Survival in Sweden, 1960 Through 1988: Evidence of Increasing Diagnosis of Nonlethal Tumors

Helgesen F, Holmberg L, Johansson J-E, et al (Örebro Med Ctr, Sweden; Univ Hosp, Uppsala, Sweden; Harvard School of Public Health, Boston)
J Natl Cancer Inst 88:1216–1221, 1996   8–5

Introduction.—Although the incidence of prostate cancer has increased over the past few decades, survival from prostate cancer also has increased. This is despite the lack of any major treatment advance. The observed trends could be related to increased detection of less aggressive prostate tumors. Trends in prostate cancer in Sweden were analyzed to see whether this is the case.

Methods.—The population-based cohort study included all 80,901 cases of prostate cancer detected in Sweden from 1960 through 1988. Follow-up information was available on 80,383 of these patients. Observed and relative survival rates were calculated for this cohort per 5-year age group in 5-year diagnostic periods and according to the diagnostic method used. The results were compared for geographic areas with differing incidence rates of prostate cancer.

Results.—The survival rates were 17.5% at 10 years and 3.5% at 20 years. The relative survival rates were 41% and 29%, respectively. The 10-year relative survival rates improved from 29% for patients whose prostate cancer was diagnosed from 1960 to 1964 to 45% for those whose cancer was diagnosed from 1975 to 1979. The relative survival rates plateaued after about 18 years, at 18% for patients whose cancer was diagnosed from 1960 to 1964 to 31% for those whose cancer was diagnosed from 1970 to 1974. Outcomes were better still for patients whose cancer was diagnosed later on.

The 10-year survival rates were 45% in areas with a high incidence of prostate cancer and 36% in areas with a low incidence. Men with cancer diagnosed from 1960 to 1964 lost an estimated 48% to 68% of life expectancy after diagnosis, depending on age. For men with cancer diagnosed from 1985 to 1988, loss of life expectancy decreased by more than 50% in all age groups.

Conclusions.—Most of the recent improvement in survival from prostate cancer probably results from improved detection of nonlethal tumors and from lead-time bias. Because of the increase in relative survival rates, time trends potentially could confound nonrandomized comparisons of prostate cancer treatments. Although increased diagnosis could lead to curative therapy for some patients with aggressive prostate cancer if diagnosed early, the detection of nonlethal tumors is potentially harmful to individual patients.

▶ This paper simply provides European data for an observation already firmly established in the United States: that with the enormous increase in screening activities (chiefly with prostate-specific antigen), survival from prostate cancer has increased. Of course, what is not clear with these new data or with the U.S. experience is whether the improvement is "real" (i.e., due to better diagnosis and treatment) or whether it is an artifact because the number of cancer deaths is diluted by the huge number of early cancers diagnosed through screening that might have been better left alone. This debate will extend long into the next century, and most of the relevant data are likely to be generated in Europe rather than the United States. The reason for this is that screening has become much more widespread in the United States than in Europe, so that clean epidemiologic data (such as those reported in this article) will be harder to obtain in this country. In the United States, the 2 major randomized trials testing the efficacy of screening are having trouble recruiting patients, because so many of them already have been screened. The main point I would emphasize is that practitioners should retain a modicum of skepticism about screening while the data are collected from whatever source.

A.O. Berg, M.D., M.P.H.

Fifteen-year Survival in Prostate Cancer: A Prospective, Population-based Study in Sweden
Johansson J-E, Holmberg L, Johansson S, et al (Örebro Med Centre, Sweden; Uppsala Univ, Sweden; Harvard Univ, Boston)
JAMA 277:467–471, 1997   8–6

Objective.—The course of prostate cancer is highly variable, and the prognosis of an individual patient is impossible to predict. With the rise of screening and aggressive treatment of early disease, the risk of overdiagnosis and overtreatment is expected to increase. The natural history of initially untreated early stage prostate cancer was studied, including an analysis of long-term survival by stage, grade, and patient age.

Methods.—The prospective cohort study included 642 consecutive patients in whom prostate cancer was diagnosed between 1977 and 1984. All cases were diagnosed at 1 Swedish hospital with a strictly defined catchment area. The patients' mean age was 72 years, and all were followed up until 1994. Three hundred patients had localized disease, T0 to T2. One hundred eighty-three had locally advanced prostate cancer, T3 to T4, and 159 had distant metastases at diagnosis. The proportion of patients who died of prostate cancer was calculated, with the 15-year survival rate corrected for other causes of death.

Results.—Of 541 deaths, 201 were of prostate cancer. Eleven percent of patients with localized disease died of prostate cancer. The corrected 15-year survival rate in this group was 81%, whether or not treatment was deferred (deferred in 223 of 300 patients). The corrected 15-year survival rate was 57% for patients with locally advanced disease and 6% for those with distant metastases.

Conclusions.—"Watchful waiting" is associated with good long-term survival for patients with localized prostate cancer. In this group, initial radical treatment appears to prevent few deaths. Taking such an aggressive approach to all patients would lead to considerable overtreatment of early stage prostate cancer. The situation is different for patients with locally advanced or metastatic disease, who need aggressive therapy in an attempt to improve their prognosis.

▶ This article certainly does not settle the debate about what to do with small, localized prostate cancers, but it provides more data for those who do not favor screening and advocate a "watchful waiting" attitude toward the small cancers that are often detected at screening or incidentally. The figure (in the original article) contains the clinical take-home message, showing that the survival curves for treated and untreated are virtually identical. Although this was not a randomized, controlled trial (and many despair of ever seeing one because of technical difficulties in the research), I find the results compelling. Certainly for a man older than 70, these findings show that watchful waiting is a perfectly acceptable alternative to treatment of whatever kind.

A.O. Berg, M.D., M.P.H.

Recent Developments in the Epidemiology of Prostate Cancer
Mettlin C (Roswell Park Cancer Inst, Buffalo, NY)
Eur J Cancer 33:340–347, 1997   8–7

Introduction.—Epidemiologic research in prostate cancer has shown that few of the many possible risk factors have a strong association with the disease. There are now greater opportunities to study the etiology of prostate cancer because the incidence of and mortality from the disease have increased. Much of the increased incidence reflects changes in detection technology, but increased mortality reflects other factors. Recent trends in patterns of occurrence, research of risk factors, public health implications for prevention, and early detection are discussed.

Incidence and Mortality.—There have been dramatic changes in the incidence of prostate cancer. In 1985, the age-adjusted incidence in North America was more than 50% higher than it was in Western Europe, 8 times higher than it was in Japan, and 50 times higher than it was in China. Recently, the incidence in Western countries has risen sharply. The rate of prostate cancer is significantly higher in African-American men than it is in white men, but rates have risen dramatically in both groups (Fig 3). Mortality from prostate cancer varies significantly from region to region. The highest mortality rates are in Switzerland, Sweden, and Norway. The lowest mortality rates are in Japan, Hong Kong, Singapore, and other Asian countries. In the United States, age-adjusted mortality from prostate cancers has increased by 28% in the last 35 years.

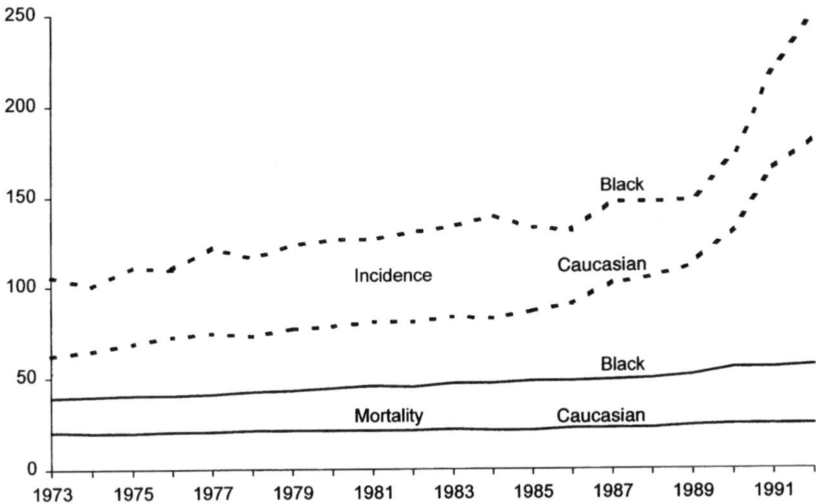

FIGURE 3.—Trends in age-adjusted prostate cancer incidence and mortality rates per 100,000 in black and white men in the United States, 1973 to 1992. (Modified from Kosary CL, Ries LAG, Miller BA, et al (eds): *SEER Cancer Statistics Review 1973–1992.* Bethseda, Md, National Cancer Institute, NIH Publication No 96–2789, 1996. (Courtesy of Mettlin C: Recent developments in the epidemiology of prostate cancer. *Eur J Cancer* 33:340–347, 1997. Reprinted with kind permission from Elsevier Science Ltd, The Boulevard, Langford Lane, Kidlington 0X5 1GB, UK.)

Race and Ethnicity.—The rate of prostate cancer varies greatly among different race and ethnic groups. The highest rates are among African-Americans, and the lowest rates are among native Japanese. The reasons for this are unclear. It has recently been shown that biomarkers of 5α-reductase activity are higher in black and white men than they are in Japanese men. These race-related differences may explain geographic differences in risk that are not explained by environmental or cultural factors.

Discussion.—Recent research of prostate cancer has focused on risk factors such as race, diet, lifestyle, vasectomy, and family history. As prostate cancer becomes a greater public health concern, monitoring incidence and mortality will be important. Identifying risk factors may help prevent the disease and may be useful for early detection interventions.

▶ This is one of those fascinating but profoundly puzzling articles which shows that prostate cancer incidence and mortality vary enormously worldwide and that we have few clues as to why. It is written by one of the world's best-respected epidemiologists. The incidence of prostate cancer is increasing dramatically in North America, almost certainly as a result of screening, whereas the slight updrift of the mortality trend line has not changed, implying that improved detection is not improving clinical outcome (see Fig 3). The cumulative effect of known risk factors does not come close to explaining the variations. At this point, the epidemiologic evidence does not provide physicians with much to use in primary prevention (e.g., race, ethnicity, family history, diet), and secondary prevention (screening) still has not been shown to work.

A.O. Berg, M.D., M.P.H.

Erectile Dysfunction

A Double-blind, Placebo-controlled Evaluation of the Erectile Response to Transurethral Alprostadil

Hellstrom WJG, Bennett AH, Gesundheit N, et al (Tulane Univ, New Orleans, La; Albany Med College, NY; VIVUS, Menlo Park, Calif)
Urology 48:851–856, 1996

8–8

Purpose.—The need for intracorporeal injection may limit the use of effective forms of drug therapy for erectile dysfunction. Recent studies have shown that vasoactive drugs may be effectively given topically to the urethral mucosa. At-home intraurethral treatment with alprostadil was evaluated for safety and efficacy in the treatment of erectile dysfunction.

Methods.—The multicenter, prospective, randomized controlled trial included 68 men with erectile dysfunction. The erectile dysfunction was primarily organic and had been present for a mean of 41 months. Patients completing the study self-administered alprostadil in 4 doses (125, 250, 500, and 1,000 μg) and placebo in random order over 2 to 4 weeks. Outcome measures, evaluated in double-blind fashion, included ability to have intercourse, patient ratings of erectile response, penile volume measurements, and patient reports of comfort and ease of use.

Results.—Full penile enlargement was obtained by 75% of patients. Erection sufficient for intercourse, as reported by the patient, was achieved by 49%. Penile pain was the main side effect, occurring in 9% to 18% of alprostadil treatments, and was more frequent at higher doses. The treatment was rated acceptably comfortable and easy to administer. None of the patients experienced priapism.

Conclusions.—For most patients with long-standing erectile dysfunction, at-home treatment with transurethral alprostadil can restore erections and enable sexual intercourse. The alprostadil dose required appears to be higher than used in direct injection therapy. The authors call for longer-term studies of the efficacy, safety, and patient acceptance of transurethral alprostadil.

Treatment of Men With Erectile Dysfunction With Transurethral Alprostadil

Padma-Nathan H, for the Medicated Urethral System for Erection (MUSE) Study Group (Univ of Southern Calif, Los Angeles; Tulane Univ, New Orleans, La; St Louis Univ; et al)
N Engl J Med 336:1–7, 1997

8–9

Introduction.—Erectile dysfunction in men compromises sexual performance, diminishes self-esteem, and disrupts personal relationships. The effectiveness of alprostadil (prostaglandin E_1) administered to the urethral mucosa was evaluated in this randomized, prospective, double-blind, placebo-controlled trial.

Methods.—All men had an erectile dysfunction with a primary organic cause. A total of 1,511 men from investigational sites in the United States were tested in the clinic for response to 125, 250, 500, and 1,000 µg of alprostadil. Men with sufficient responses were randomly assigned to receive either alprostadil or placebo self-administered to the distal urethra by means of a proprietary drug-delivery system. The penile response was evaluated by patient use of an Erection Assessment Scale. Duration of penile response and level of comfort were also recorded. Treatment time was 3 months.

Results.—During clinic testing, 996 of the 1,511 men evaluated had maximal responses on the Erection Assessment Scale without significant adverse effects with at least 1 of the 4 doses of alprostadil. The men were allowed to select their home dose of alprostadil. Doses selected were: 125 µg by 116 men, 250 µg by 171 men, 500 µg by 302 men, and 1000 µg by 407 men (Table 2). Maximal responses and duration of response were positively correlated with the dose. Of 996 men who underwent home treatment, 961 reported results of at least 1 administration. The completion rate after the 3-month treatment period was 87.7%. In the alprostadil and placebo groups, respectively, 64.9% and 18.6% of men reported having sexual intercourse at least once in the 3-month period. The re-

TABLE 2.—Responses to Alprostadil During In-Clinic Testing

Variable	Dose of Alprostadil			
	125 µg	250 µg	500 µg	1000 µg
No. of men*	1490	1492	1117	1140
Percentage with a maximal response of 4 or 5†	12.3	16.6	39.6	48.8
Mean time to onset of response (min)	7	7	7	7
Mean time to maximal response (min)	21	22	23	24
Mean time to return to nonerect state (min)	67	70	74	79
Rating of comfort level (% of men)‡				
Very comfortable	15.7	13.0	14.2	12.5
Comfortable	48.5	48.6	51.8	50.1
Neutral	26.8	26.8	24.5	26.1
Uncomfortable	8.7	10.7	8.9	9.0
Very uncomfortable	0.4	0.9	0.7	2.4

*Numbers shown are the total numbers of men in whom the indicated doses of alprostadil were tested; for each variable studied, data were collected on at least 95 percent of doses administered. None of the men received a given dose more than once during the resting period.

†Maximal penile responses were scored on the Erection Assessment Scale as described in the Methods section. Men who had maximal responses scored as 4 or 5 with more than one of the doses of alprostadil may be counted in more than one column.

‡Because of rounding, percentages do not all total 100 percent.

(Reprinted by permission of *The New England Journal of Medicine.* Padma-Nathan H, for the Medicated Urethral System for Erection (MUSE) Study Group: Treatment of men with erectile dysfunction with transurethral alprostadil. *N Engl J Med* 336:1–7, 1997. Copyright 1997, Massachusetts Medical Society. All rights reserved.)

ported orgasm rates were 63.6% and 23.5% for the alprostadil and placebo groups, respectively. Seven of 10 administrations of alprostadil were followed by intercourse in men in the alprostadil group who reported having sexual intercourse at least once. The response to alprostadil was similar regardless of age or organic cause of erectile dysfunction. Each dose of alprostadil was more effective than placebo. During clinic testing, 35.7% of men reported penile pain. Most men reported mild pain. Only 36 men quit the trial because of penile discomfort. During clinic testing, 3.3% and 0.4% of men experienced hypotension and syncope, respectively. The frequency of hypotension increased with dose. During home treatment, 10.8% of alprostadil administrations caused penile pain in 32.7% of men. There was no incidence of urethral stricture, penile fibrosis, or priapism during clinic testing or home treatment.

Conclusion.—Treatment with transurethral alprostadil resulted in erections and ability to perform sexual intercourse in a substantial number of men. The main side effect was penile pain, which was mild in most men.

▶ Erectile dysfunction is a common and vexing problem. As the population ages, it most likely will become even more common, though no less vexing. How vexing? In the study population described in Abstract 8–8, most men had tried one or more therapies, including cognitive therapy, without success. During the past several years, the YEAR BOOK OF FAMILY PRACTICE has reviewed a variety of approaches to the treatment of impotence. These treatment methods range from dealing with the psychologic causes with psychotherapy and medication, to the physical with injection, vacuum pumps, and implants. These treatment methods are all somewhat invasive and of modest benefit. In addition, studies supporting these techniques all seem to be small, and the initial study by Hellstrom et. al. (Abstract 8–8) is no exception. The study by Padma-Nathan, et al. (Abstract 8–9) however, was orders of magnitude more sizable with the same robust results—a very convincing follow-up. This technique appears to be fairly effective and reasonably well tolerated (see Table 2). Although those treated in these studies had primarily organic erectile dysfunction, this remains a problem that is multifactorial and this treatment should probably be used in that context. It does, though, seem to offer a safe and beneficial approach for the growing number of men in our practices who have erectile dysfunction.

W.W. Dexter, M.D.

Stress Incontinence

Morbidity and Mortality of Incontinence Surgery in Elderly Women: An Analysis of Medicare Data
Sultana CJ, Campbell JW, Pisanelli WS, et al (Case Western Reserve Univ, Cleveland, Ohio)
Am J Obstet Gynecol 176:344–348, 1997   8–10

Purpose.—An increasing proportion of operative procedures are performed in elderly persons. There are few data on gynecologic operations

TABLE 7.—Number of Deaths Within 30, 60, and 90 Days of Surgery

Age group (yr)	30 days		60 days		90 days	
	No.	% *	No.	% *	No.	% *
65–74	106	0.2	148	0.3	177	0.4
75–84	91	0.5	126	0.7	160	0.9
≥85	28	1.6	34	2.0	40	2.3
TOTAL	225	0.3	298	0.5	377	0.6

*Percentage of total in age group.

(Courtesy of Sultana CJ, Campbell JW, Pisanelli WS, et al: Morbidity and mortality of incontinence surgery in elderly women: An analysis of Medicare data. *Am J Obstet Gynecol* 176:344–348, 1997.)

and surgery to treat urinary incontinence in elderly women. For counseling purposes, it would be useful to have information on the mortality and risks of these procedures. Medicare data were used to assess the morbidity and mortality of surgical procedures to treat incontinence in elderly women.

Methods.—The study used Medicare data on surgical procedures performed for incontinence from 1984 to 1991. Secondary diagnosis codes were used to gather information on comorbid conditions and reasons for readmission. The analysis included the surgical mortality rate and causes of mortality in women 65 years or older undergoing retropubic suspension, needle urethropexy, and anterior vaginal repair (Table 7). Specific complications and causes of postoperative morbidity were assessed, as were the effects of comorbidity on duration of hospital stay, postoperative readmission, and mortality.

Results.—The analysis included 66,478 women, with a median age of 71 years. Incontinence surgery was associated with 30-day mortality of 0.33%. Mortality and duration of stay both increased linearly with age. Myocardial infarction was associated with 14% of deaths, stroke with 14%, thromboembolic events in 9%, and pneumonia in 3%. Diabetes and heart failure were more frequent among patients who died, but hypertension was not. Patients older than 80 years had a 30-day readmission rate of 5%. The most frequent reasons for readmission were urinary tract infection, 12%; hypertension, 16%; and other unspecified complications, 9%. Complications occurring in 1% of patients each were myocardial infarction, pulmonary embolism, stroke, deep vein thrombosis, and pneumonia.

Conclusions.—Experience demonstrates the safety of surgery for urinary incontinence in elderly women, particularly those younger than 80 years. Mortality and duration of stay both increased with older age. This, along with the effect of chronic disorders, should be taken into account in patient counseling.

▶ I have always looked at the conclusions drawn from this type of study with some skepticism. While certainly providing a broad overview of the issue, I am not sure I agree with the conclusions of the authors. First, it assumes that the procedures are all warranted in the first place. Perhaps more striking is that an acceptable death rate to the authors (or surgeons) (see Table 7), may not be acceptable to our patients, particularly our younger patients, contemplating an elective procedure. Certainly one's quality of life can suffer dramatically from incontinence, and the various surgical options may provide relief (Abstract 8–11). I do not hesitate to include surgery as an alternative in my recommendations to my patients when we discuss management options. However, the mortality and morbidity statistics are important factors to consider in helping our patients make an informed choice.

W.W. Dexter, M.D.

The Effectiveness of Surgery for Stress Incontinence in Women: A Systematic Review

Black NA, Downs SH (London School of Hygiene & Tropical Medicine)
Br J Urol 78:497–510, 1996

8–11

Introduction.—Various surgical procedures are performed to treat stress incontinence, but there is no consensus as to which is most effective. There have been no systematic reviews of the literature on this topic. Such a review was performed, with the goals of assessing the methodologic quality of studies of surgery performed to treat stress incontinence, the effectiveness of the procedures, and associated complications.

Methods.—A comprehensive search of the literature identified 11 randomized controlled trials, 20 nonrandomized trials or prospective cohort studies, and 45 retrospective cohort studies. The studies were systematically reviewed, with special attention to methodologic quality of the prospective studies. Additional information was provided by the retrospective studies in some cases.

Results.—The prospective trials were of generally low methodologic quality, with variable inclusion criteria, surgical management, and outcome assessments. These problems made meta-analysis of the data impossible. The weakness of the evidence for the effectiveness of surgery made it difficult to draw firm conclusions. Colposuspension appeared to provide a better and longer lasting effect than did anterior colporrhaphy and needle suspension. There were few data on the effectiveness of sling procedures. Outcomes were no different in comparisons of different techniques of performing each procedure, likely because of the methodologic weakness of the studies. There were few valid and reliable data on the frequency of postoperative complications, making it difficult to establish the safety of the procedures. There was some evidence that repeat operations may be less successful than the initial procedures.

Conclusions.—The current trial evidence does not provide a sound scientific basis for the surgical treatment of stress incontinence. Large, high-quality prospective studies are needed, with cases defined according to accepted criteria. The studies should use standard measures of the severity of stress incontinence, standardized surgical terminology, and valid and reliable outcomes. The outcomes should not be confined to the short term, and should include the patient's as well as the surgeon's assessments.

▶ In our residency program, we are making an effort to emphasize evidence-based medicine. This article illustrates one of the pitfalls: Often the evidence available is quite thin, even for treatments we might consider well-supported. It is sometimes startling, and often humbling, to have this fact pointed out. While the authors' literature search was quite thorough, the method by which they included or excluded studies is not well explained. Nevertheless, their findings certainly give one pause. Incontinence in women, stress incontinence in particular, is ubiquitous in our practices, and surgery to address this problem is frequently performed. To recommend a surgical treatment, particularly an elective one, it should have some reasonable chance for success with acceptably low risk. The authors correctly conclude that, based on the evidence they feel is acceptable, these two criteria are not well-demonstrated for surgical procedures to correct stress incontinence. Are better studies needed? Certainly. Should we stop recommending this procedure to our patients based on this study? No. Should we discuss with them the (often scanty) evidence regarding various recommendations we make? Absolutely.

W.W. Dexter, M.D.

Miscellaneous

Vasectomy Is Associated With an Increased Risk for Urolithiasis
Kronmal RA, Krieger JN, Coxon V, et al (Univ of Washington, Seattle)
Am J Kidney Dis 29:207–213, 1997   8–12

Background.—In a recent multicenter study of vasectomy as a potential risk factor of coronary artery disease, an unexpected finding was an increased risk of urolithiasis. This association was further investigated in a case-control study.

Methods and Findings.—The case patients were 244 men experiencing initial episodes of urolithiasis. The age-matched control subjects were 423 men with no history of urolithiasis. Logistic regression analysis showed that, among men younger than 46 years, men with vasectomies had a relative risk for urolithiasis of 1.9 compared with those without urolithiasis. Among men 46 years or older, the relative risk was 0.9 for men with vasectomies. Men with vasectomies had a 2.0 relative risk of urinary calculi up to 4 years before evaluation compared with men without vasectomies. This excess risk persisted for up to 14 years after vasectomy.

Conclusions.—In men younger than 46 years, vasectomy is associated with a 2-fold increased risk for urolithiasis, which may persist for up to 14 years after vasectomy. Given the widespread use of vasectomy for contraception, this increased risk for urolithiasis may result in substantial excess morbidity.

▶ In an interesting spin-off from the Coronary Artery Surgery Study (CASS), the authors report "discovering" a positive relationship between vasectomy and the risk of forming kidney stones. At first blush, these numbers seem compelling; CASS, after all, provides data on more than 11,000 men. On closer inspection, the actual population studied, men with vasectomies, was relatively small (N=667). The study was retrospective, based on recall, and the vasectomy "rate" of 33% is quite high, so I am at odds with the authors' conclusion that selection bias was not a factor. Causality was not shown, and no convincing physiologic or metabolic explanations were given. Vasectomy has been under fire lately with various studies reporting associations with disease entities including kidney stones and prostate and testicular cancer. The latter two were recently reviewed by Dr. Berg[1, 2], and the evidence does not seem to support an association between vasectomy and these disease entities. Likewise, with urolithiasis, I am not convinced. Vasectomy, in my mind, remains a cost-effective, safe, and simple approach to birth control.

W.W. Dexter, M.D.

References

1. 1996 Year Book of Family Practice, p 125.
2. 1996 Year Book of Family Practice, p 137.

Comparison of Dietary Calcium With Supplemental Calcium and Other Nutrients as Factors Affecting the Risk for Kidney Stones in Women
Curhan GC, Willett WC, Speizer FE, et al (Brigham and Women's Hosp, Boston; Harvard Med School, Boston; Harvard School of Public Health, Boston; et al)
Ann Intern Med 126:497–504, 1997   8–13

Background.—Calcium intake is thought to play an important role in kidney stone formation. However, little is known about the risk factors for stone formation in women. The association of dietary and supplemental calcium intake and the risk for kidney stones in women was examined.

Methods.—A prospective cohort study included 91,731 female participants in the Nurses' Health Study I, with a 12-year follow-up. The women were 34 to 59 years of age at study enrollment in 1980, with no history of kidney stones. Self-administered food-frequency questionnaires were completed in 1980, 1984, 1986, and 1990.

Findings.—Eight hundred sixty-four cases of kidney stones occurred during 903,849 person-years of follow-up. After potential risk factors were controlled, dietary calcium intake was found to be inversely associated with the risk for kidney stones, and supplemental calcium intake was positively associated with risk. Women in the highest quintile of dietary calcium intake had a 0.65 relative risk for stone formation, compared with women in the lowest quintile. Women taking supplemental calcium had a relative risk of 1.2, compared with women who did not. Sixty-seven percent of the women taking supplemental calcium either did not take it with a meal or took it with meals with an oxalate content that was probably low. In addition, compared with women in the lowest quintile,

TABLE 4.—Age-Adjusted and Multivariate Relative Risks for Symptomatic Kidney Stones According to Intake of Dietary Calcium

Variable	Intake of Dietary Calcium					Chi-Square Value (*P* Value for Trend)†
	Quintile 1	Quintile 2	Quintile 3	Quintile 4	Quintile 5	
Intake of dietary calcium, *mg/d*	<488	488–642	643–801	802–1098	>1098	
Quintile median, *mg/d*	391	567	716	912	1303	
Cases of stone formation, *n*	241	188	155	162	118	
Person-years, *n*	178 362	180 874	181 718	181 591	181 303	
Age-adjusted relative risk (95% CI)	1.0	0.78 (0.65–0.94)	0.66 (0.54–0.81)	0.70 (0.58–0.86)	0.49 (0.39–0.60)	−6.29 (<0.001)
Multivariate relative risk (95% CI)†	1.0	0.83 (0.68–1.01)	0.72 (0.58–0.89)	0.79 (0.64–0.99)	0.65 (0.50–0.83)	−2.80 (0.005)

Note: For illustrative purposes, quintile cutpoints and median for intake of dietary calcium were derived from responses to the 1986 dietary questionnaire. However, the period-specific quintile values were used for the 1980–1992 analyses. Relative risks are for the risk for stone formation compared with the group that had the lowest intake of dietary calcium.

*A chi-square value greater than 1.96 denotes a *P* value less than 0.05. The sign of the chi-square value indicates the direction of the trend.

†The multivariate model included age (in 5-year categories); alcohol (8 categories); body mass index (5 categories); and intake of supplemental calcium (4 categories), dietary calcium, animal protein, potassium, sodium, sucrose, and fluid (quintile groups for the last 5 variables).

(Courtesy of Curhan GC, Willett WC, Speizer FE, et al: Comparison of dietary calcium with supplemental calcium and other nutrients as factors affecting the risk for kidney stones in women. *Ann Intern Med* 126:497–504, 1997.)

women in the highest quintile of sucrose intake had a relative risk of 1.52; of fluid intake, 0.61; and of potassium intake, 0.65 (Table 4).

Conclusion.—High dietary calcium intake apparently reduces the risk for symptomatic kidney stones in women. Taking supplemental calcium may increase this risk. This apparent difference may be associated with the timing of calcium ingestion relative to the amount of oxalate consumed. However, other factors in dairy products, the main source of dietary calcium, could be responsible for the reduction in risk associated with dietary calcium.

▶ This is another helpful report from the Nurses' Health Study. As in men, a high intake of dietary calcium is associated with fewer kidney stones, possibly because of the reduction in absorption of oxalate. However, the intake of supplemental calcium was associated with no decrease in the rate of stones and, possibly, an increase (in the multivariate analysis). Thus, the adage that cautious avoidance of calcium supplements when one has a history of renal stones may be appropriate (depending on whether you think kidney stones or osteoporosis is worse). The authors' suggestion that the large unit doses of supplements be spread out over the day—particularly at the time of ingestion of oxalate—might also work. As expected, increased fluids and increased dietary potassium were also associated with fewer kidney stones.

M.A. Bowman, M.D., M.P.A.

9 Musculoskeletal Conditions

Introduction

A fascinating study following patients with whiplash long term and a rare randomized controlled trial of treatment open this chapter. Miscellaneous articles cover a proposed guideline for use of X-rays in the diagnosis of low back pain, a randomized trial of treatment of ulnar shaft fractures, and a useful empirical study of orthopedic implants that set off airport metal detectors.

Randomized controlled trials: Abstracts 9–2, 9–4, and 9–5.

Alfred O. Berg, M.D., M.P.H.

Whiplash

A Prospective Study of 39 Patients With Whiplash Injury
Karlsborg M, Smed A, Jespersen A, et al (Univ Hosp of Hvidovre, Copenhagen)
Acta Neurol Scand 95:65–72, 1997   9–1

Background.—Whiplash trauma is reported to affect more than 1 million individuals in the United States each year. The highest incidence occurs in the 20- to 24-year age group, a cohort that costs insurance companies more than $18 million (U.S.) annually. Most of these injuries result from rear-end collisions. Although the acute symptoms are caused by neck sprain, it is uncertain why symptoms persist and why some patients experience "late whiplash syndrome." A prospective study of 39 patients with whiplash injury sought to determine whether any common clinical signs might predict clinical outcome.

Methods.—Eligible patients were aged 18–65 years, had no direct head trauma or fracture of the neck, did not abuse drug or alcohol, and were seen within 2 weeks after the whiplash injury. Included in the study were 23 women and 16 men with a median age of 33 years. All but 1 had been involved in traffic accidents; of these, all but 1 used seat belts and headrests. Patients were evaluated within 14 days of the injury, after 1 month, and at 7 months. At 1 month postinjury, all were examined with MRI of the brain and cervical spine, neuropsychological tests, and motor evoked potentials (MEP). These tests were repeated at 6 months if abnormalities were present.

Results.—None of the patients had fractures, dislocations, or posture abnormalities at admission radiography. The most common initial symptoms were neck pain (100%), headache (94%), and limited motion of the cervical spine (91%); at 7 months, the percentage of patients with these symptoms had fallen to 47%, 44%, and 32%, respectively. Ten patients (29%) reported complete recovery after 7 months and 2 (6%) had more symptoms at the final examination. None of the variables examined, including sex, age, and number of symptoms at first visit, were predictive of outcome, and the correlation between MRI and clinical findings was poor. Results of all MEP examinations were normal and no patient exhibited cognitive dysfunction. There was a relationship, however, between stress unrelated to whiplash injury and persistence of symptoms.

Conclusion.—Although most of these patients with whiplash injury improved considerably during the following 6 months and 29% became completely symptom-free, the symptoms associated with the injury tended to persist among those who had experienced other stressing life events close to the accident.

▶ How well people recover from injuries is often related to their psychosocial situation. This study from Denmark shows that patients with persistent cervical symptoms of whiplash 6 months after a traffic accident have findings similar to those that we see in the United States. There is a high frequency of stressful life events. It is not mentioned whether secondary gain—such as litigation from the injury or long-term disability payments—played a role in the persistent symptoms. I usually tell patients that their body wants to heal, but sometimes they simply won't let that happen.

J.E. Scherger, M.D., M.P.H.

The Effect of Soft Cervical Collars on Persistent Neck Pain in Patients With Whiplash Injury

Gennis P, Miller L, Gallagher EJ, et al (Bronx Municipal Hosp, NY; Albert Einstein College, Bronx, NY)
Acad Emerg Med 3:568–573, 1996   9–2

Introduction.—In emergency medicine, whiplash injuries are a common problem, with more than 1 million occurrences in the United States each year. A whiplash is a soft tissue cervical injury resulting from hyperextension or sudden flexion of the neck. The most common mechanism of injury is motor vehicle crashes. The traditional management of whiplash injury in the emergency department is rest, analgesia, and a soft cervical collar. The use of the collar has been controversial, and no study has compared rest, analgesia, and a soft cervical collar with rest and analgesia alone.

Methods.—There were 250 patients with neck pain after an automobile crash who were asked to indicate their initial degree of pain on a visual analog scale in an emergency department. Based on their medical record, patients were randomized to receive a soft cervical collar or no collar. At 6 weeks, patients were asked to record their level of pain as none, better, same, or worse. They were considered recovered if there was no pain, improved if the pain was none or better, and deteriorated if the pain was worse.

Results.—Follow-up was conducted with 196 of the 250 patients (78%). The soft cervical collar group was composed of 104 (53%) patients, and the control group was composed of 92 (47%) patients. These groups had similarities in initial pain score, seat belt use, seat position in the car, gender, and age. There were 122 (62%) patients who had pain persisting 6 weeks or more. The groups showed no difference in follow-up pain category, complete recovery, improvement, or deterioration.

Conclusion.—Pain persists for at least 6 weeks for most patients with whiplash injuries. However, the duration or degree of persistent pain is not influenced by a soft cervical collar. Future studies should determine the potential value of complete and constant soft cervical collar immobilization for the prevention of prolonged pain.

▶ It has become much more unusual to see patients in soft cervical collars than it was 10 years ago. Studies such as this reinforce their lack of utility and potential harm. This study is helpful in that a substantial number of patients were monitored, and the natural history of whiplash is described. When patients have symptoms for 6 weeks, they often wish that something more could be done. Physical therapy and strengthening exercises may be appropriate, but soft cervical collars are not.

J.E. Scherger, M.D., M.P.H.

Miscellaneous

Use of Lumbar Radiographs for the Early Diagnosis of Low Back Pain: Proposed Guidelines Would Increase Utilization
Suarez-Almazor ME, Belseck E, Russell AS, et al (Univ of Alberta, Edmonton, Canada)
JAMA 277:1782–1786, 1997

9–3

Objective.—The Agency for Health Care Policy and Research (AHCPR) practice guidelines recommend lumbar radiographs for patients with low back pain. Because diagnostic tests increase utilization and health care costs, the potential impact of these guidelines in patients with new episodes of low back pain was assessed.

Methods.—In a retrospective cohort study in 4 family clinics in Edmonton, Canada, records of 963 patients, seen in 1992 and 1993 for a new episode of back pain were reviewed. Physicians were paid on a fee-for-service basis. Lumbar radiograph utilization and incidences of spinal tumor, infection, or fractures were recorded.

Results.—Lumbar radiographs were done on 127 patients at the initial visit; 68 were oblique views. Radiographs were normal in 44 patients (35%). If all 426 patients who met AHCPR criteria for lumbar radiographs had received them, utilization would have increased by 238%. Only 4 of 8 patients with a subsequent diagnosis of spinal tumors or fractures did not have an initial lumbar radiograph. The sensitivity and specificity of physician utilization patterns were 50% and 84%, respectively. The sensitivity and specificity of AHCPR guidelines were 93% and 56%, respectively.

Conclusion.—The AHCPR recommendations for lumbar radiographs for patients with low back pain would increase utilization and health care costs without contributing significantly to the diagnosis.

▶ Almost weekly in our heavily managed care community, a new clinical guideline is proposed for the management of some condition. Although the stated purpose of these guidelines is to standardize care among all physicians and to improve care given to patients with the particular condition, the clear underlying message is to reduce the use of diagnostic tests that may be unnecessary. The relentless pressure to reduce overutilization, and thereby costs, seems to be the motivating factor.

On the federal level, the AHCPR has been developing a series of practice guidelines and disseminating them widely. Among these were practice guidelines for the management of patients with acute low back pain. The authors of this study did a retrospective review of patients seen in primary care offices with low back pain and analyzed what would have been the effect of applying these AHCPR guidelines. Surprisingly, if the AHCPR guidelines had been implemented, there would have been over a 300% increase in the use of radiographs of the low back. Of the 963 patients included in this retrospective study, only 4 not given an X-ray study were found to have a condition that would have been diagnosed by X-ray.

I predict that we will be in for several years of arguing over proposed guidelines. Through this process, we may well come out with some generally accepted guidelines that most people can agree upon. However, expect that the first recommended guidelines, regardless of the condition, will be scrutinized and argued about in the literature.

R.C. Davidson, M.D., M.P.H.

Treatment of Ulnar Shaft Fractures: A Prospective, Randomized Study
Atkin DM, Bohay DR, Slabaugh P, et al (Univ of California, San Francisco; Kaiser Hosp, Santa Rosa, Calif)
Orthopedics 18:543–547, 1995   9–4

Objective.—There is no general agreement on the duration of casting and the need for elbow immobilization in isolated fractures of the ulna. Which form of immobilization is optimal in treating forearm fractures was examined in a prospective, randomized study.

Methods.—Between May 1989 and November 1991, 31 patients (9 women), aged 19–50 years, with closed midshaft or distal ulnar fractures were randomly allocated to treatment with long arm plaster immobilization (9 patients), short arm plaster immobilization (14 patients), or Ace Wrap bandages (8 patients). Patients were studied clinically and radiographically until union.

Results.—Fractures located at the middle and distal thirds took significantly longer to heal than fractures located at the midshaft. Fractures in long arm immobilization casts healed in an average of 7.2 weeks, with an average change in angulation of 2.7 degrees. One patient lost significant range of motion, and 2 patients were unable to return to their previous jobs. Fractures in the short cast healed in an average of 7.9 weeks, with an average change in angulation of 3.5 degrees. Two patients experienced significant loss of range of motion, and 2 were unable to return to work. Fractures treated with Ace Wrap healed in an average of 7.7 weeks, but 6 treatments were considered failures because of pain and were changed to another treatment. These patients had significantly more change in angulation than did patients in the long arm casts (4.0 degrees vs. 2.7 degrees). Three patients rated their results as poor because of pain.

Conclusion.—Long arm casting did not improve outcome and left 1 patient with significantly decreased elbow range of motion. Ace Wrap was unsuccessful because 6 patients had to be converted to another treatment as a result of pain. The short arm cast with immobilization for 8 weeks is recommended.

▶ Forearm fractures are commonly managed by family physicians. Most of us have been taught to immobilize the joint above and below the fracture which, in this case, would include the elbow and the wrist. Immobilization of the elbow is uncomfortable and results in considerable stiffness. This study confirms that isolated ulnar shaft fractures do well without immobilization of the elbow. A short arm cast should be the standard treatment for this condition.

J.E. Scherger, M.D., M.P.H.

Treatment of Early Rheumatoid Arthritis With Minocycline or Placebo
O'Dell JR, Haire CE, Palmer W, et al (Univ of Nebraska, Omaha; Omaha VA Hosp, Neb)
Arthritis Rheum 40:842–848, 1997   9–5

Background.—Rheumatologists currently emphasize the importance of early control of rheumatoid arthritis (RA). Evidence suggests that tetracyclines may have antiarthritic action. Thus, the efficacy of minocycline in the treatment of seropositive RA within the first year of diagnosis was investigated.

Methods.—Forty-six patients with RA were enrolled in the 6-month study. The patients received 100 mg of minocycline twice a day or placebo.

Findings.—Eighteen patients had met 50% improvement criteria at 3 months and maintained at least a 50% improvement for 6 months. No significant toxicity was documented. The responders included 65% of the patients receiving minocycline and only 13% of the patients receiving placebo.

Conclusions.—Minocycline is effective in the treatment of patients with seropositive RA in the first year of disease. Further research is needed to establish optimal treatment duration and to investigate the mechanism(s) of action.

▶ Recent rheumatology literature has a number of articles regarding the use of antibiotics in treatment of RA. Minocycline seems to be the antibiotic of choice. These studies have consistently found improvement in symptoms of RA in patients treated with antibiotics. This prospective study of a small group of 46 patients found similar findings with a 50% improvement in 6 months of patients with early RA who were given antibiotics vs. placebo.

Curiously enough, nobody has yet been able to find a reason that antibiotics should help in treating RA. The use of antibiotics would obviously lead one to think of an infectious agent. However, our current level of culture and detection has found no evidence of an infectious agent.

I included this study to remind us that there are therapies for RA beyond antiinflammatory drugs and pain medication. I have become much more likely to seek early consultation for patients who show clinical and laboratory evidence of RA.

R.C. Davidson, M.D., M.P.H.

Detection of Orthopaedic Implants by Airport Metal Detectors

Basu P, Packer GJ, Himstedt J (Southend Hosp, Prittlewell Chase, England)
J Bone Joint Surg Br 79B:388–389, 1997   9–6

Background.—Many patients with metallic implants express concern that these implants may activate alarms at airport security gates. Patients may ask their physicians for certificates to allow them to pass through airport security if the alarm goes off. The current study determined which implants, if any, activate metal detectors at airports so that patients can be forewarned and given a certificate.

Methods and Findings.—A volunteer with various metal implants strapped on and patients with implants in situ walked through airport security gates. Implants such as plates, screws, and nails used for internal fixation did not usually activate the detector. One exception was Richards cannulated screws, which set off the device at a higher setting of 7. In addition, patients with a single joint replacement were unlikely to activate the metal detector at the normal setting, but patients with 2 total replacements may set off the alarm at higher settings. Patients with 1 Austin-Moore prosthesis or 3 or 4 standard hip and knee replacements usually activated the alarm.

Conclusions.—Airport security alarms may be set off by Richards cannulated screws used for fixation, an Austin-Moore prosthesis, and 3 or 4 joint replacements. Patients with such implants should be warned of this and given an appropriate certificate.

▶ This is one of those small but interesting studies that say to me, "Gee, I never thought about that." The authors studied metal orthopedic implants of all varieties and whether they are likely to trigger an airport metal detector. They found that it took a significant amount of metal to set off the alarm. This generally meant 3 or more joint replacement prostheses or an Austin-Moore prosthesis. The authors used an alarm sensitivity setting of 5. They did note that some hip prostheses triggered the alarm when the setting was placed at a higher sensitivity level (7). I have no idea what most airports use. Apparently a setting of 10 is the highest sensitivity and activates minute metal objects such as rings and coins. I suspect that most airports do not use this high a setting.

The take-home message for me is that most patients with simple screws or fixation devices should not be worried about triggering airport security devices. Only multiple joint replacements or Austin-Moore prosthesis patients are likely to trigger such devices.

R.C. Davidson, M.D., M.P.H.

10 Mental Health and Psychiatry

Introduction

The opening section on depression contains a couple of sobering articles about the relative usefulness of the serotonin-specific reuptake inhibitors and older tricyclics and 2 rare randomized clinical trials on the treatment of depression in primary care settings. A thoughtful article on the treatment of depression in children closes the section.

Kindergarten behavior as a predictor of later substance abuse, screening for alcohol problems, and a randomized trial of a brief physician intervention for problem drinkers highlight the next section.

The miscellaneous section addresses long-term effects of sexual abuse, results from a large study of mental disorders in primary care settings, an interesting comparison of outpatient psychiatric services in the U.S. and Canada, and a thoughtful article on the evidence base for psychotherapy.

Randomized controlled trials: Abstracts 10–3, 10–5, 10–7, and 10–14.

Alfred O. Berg, M.D., M.P.H.

Depression and Dysthymia

Discontinuation Rates of SSRIs and Tricyclic Antidepressants: A Meta-analysis and Investigation of Heterogeneity
Hotopf M, Hardy R, Lewis G (King's College School of Medicine, London; Univ College London; Univ of Wales, Cardiff)
Br J Psychiatry 170:120–127, 1997   10–1

Purpose.—Despite the many randomized controlled trials (RCTs) comparing the serotonin-specific reuptake inhibitors (SSRIs) and tricyclic or heterocyclic antidepressants, it remains unclear which should be the first-line treatment for depression. Meta-analyses of RCT data have suggested that the discontinuation rate is lower for patients taking SSRIs than for those taking tricyclic antidepressants. However, many RCTs have used older tricyclic antidepressants, such as imipramine and amitriptyline, which may cause more problems with side effects than the newer drugs.

This meta-analysis compared the discontinuation rate with SSRIs vs. the newer tricyclic or heterocyclic antidepressants.

Methods.—The analysis included 92 RCTs comparing SSRIs with tricyclic or heterocyclic antidepressants. Of the latter, 51 evaluated old tricyclics; 24 evaluated new tricyclics, such as nortriptyline and desipramine; and 17 evaluated heterocyclics, such as bupropion and trazodone. Odds ratios for discontinuation were calculated for each of these 3 groups.

Results.—Odds ratios for treatment discontinuation were 0.82 for old tricyclics, 0.89 for the newer tricyclics, and 1.02 for the heterocyclics. The SSRIs had a significant advantage only over the older compounds. On pooled analysis, the SSRIs had a lower discontinuation rate whether the population studied was younger adults or the elderly. There were no differences in discontinuation rates between individual SSRIs.

Conclusions.—Meta-analyses suggesting that tricyclic/heterocyclic antidepressants have a higher discontinuation rate than SSRIs may reflect the use of older tricyclics as reference drugs. Discontinuation rates are similar for SSRIs and the newer tricyclics or heterocyclics. The results support the use of tricyclic antidepressants as first-line therapy for depression.

Which Antidepressant? A Commentary From General Practice on Evidence-based Medicine and Health Economics
Kernick DP (St Thomas Med Group, Exeter)
Br J Gen Pract 47:95–98, 1997   10–2

Background.—Evidence-based medicine, coupled with health economics, can aid in making decisions about the allocation of limited health care resources. In evidence-based medicine, needs are stated in a specific question, and critically appraised evidence is applied. Depression is a very common and important illness that is usually treated in general practice. An evidence-based approach was applied to the decision of whether to treat depression with a tricyclic antidepressant (TCA) or a selective serotonin reuptake inhibitor (SSRI).

Methods.—The question posed was, "Should depression be treated in primary care, and by which drug?" The 2 competing treatments were compared according to the criteria of appropriateness, efficacy, effectiveness, and value for money, using evidence from the literature.

Results.—Given the frequency of depression and the costs of treatment, general practice treatment of depression seemed clearly appropriate. Both SSRIs and TCAs were deemed efficacious treatments for depression, although the dropout rate was somewhat higher for TCAs. In terms of effectiveness, there was no clear evidence regarding the relative efficacy of SSRIs and TCAs in the general practice setting. The issue of value for money included analysis of direct and indirect costs, the latter including loss of productivity, suicide and parasuicide, and behavioral toxicity. Taking all these factors into consideration, the economic implications of treatment with SSRIs vs. TCAs were unclear.

Conclusions.—An evidence-based approach shows that SSRIs and TCAs are both efficacious treatments for depression. However, their relative effectiveness and value for money remain unclear. Future studies should be relevant to the setting in which care is delivered, i.e., general practice. Primary care research should seek answers to questions that will complement and support a pragmatic system of health delivery, rather than trying to direct it.

▶ The first study (Abstract 10–1) is one of a series of articles in the British medical literature publishing annoying evidence that the SSRIs are not as great as generally accepted when compared with older drugs. The evidence summarized here (from both sides of the Atlantic) is quite convincing that discontinuation rates for SSRIs and tricyclics/heterocyclics are very much the same.

The second study (Abstract 10–2), also British, systematically reviews earlier literature on the choice of antidepressants using evidence-based criteria of appropriateness, efficacy, effectiveness, and value for the money. The authors conclude that there is insufficient evidence to make a recommendation for typical general practice settings between SSRIs and other agents. Certainly in this country most physicians use SSRIs as drugs of first choice. Exactly why the American and British experiences with SSRIs are so different is a mystery, because the data we are looking at are the same. The British seem to be a more critical lot in attempting to rely on evidence; the Americans seem to be driven more by individual clinical experience and have more faith in new drugs.

I have read enough of the literature to make me skeptical of some of the extraordinary claims made in this country about SSRIs. On this subject our British colleagues have good advice: don't forget about the tricyclics and heterocyclics.

A.O. Berg, M.D., M.P.H.

Double-blind Comparison of Sertraline, Imipramine, and Placebo in the Treatment of Dysthymia: Psychosocial Outcomes
Kocsis JH, Zisook S, Davidson J, et al (New York Hosp/Cornell Med Ctr; Univ of California, San Diego; Duke Univ, Durham, NC; et al)
Am J Psychiatry 154:390–395, 1997   10–3

Background.—Dysthymia is a chronic depressive disorder that may greatly impair social and occupational function and lead to poor general medical health. Recent studies suggest that most patients with this condition are undertreated. A double-blind trial was conducted to determine the effects of treatment with sertraline, imipramine, and placebo on mood symptoms and psychosocial outcomes in patients with primary dysthymia.

Methods.—The multicenter study comprised 416 patients with a DSM-III-R diagnosis of early-onset primary dysthymia without concurrent major depression. The inclusion criterion was a current episode of dysthymia that had lasted at least 5 years without a depression-free period of more than 2 consecutive months. Patients were randomized to receive 12 weeks of acute-phase therapy with sertraline, imipramine, or placebo. Both clinician-rated and self-rated depression and psychosocial rating instruments were administered at baseline and during the course of therapy.

Results.—Patients ranged in age from 25 to 65 years; most were white, female, and middle-aged. The mean baseline 17–item Hamilton Depression Rating Scale score was 12.9, indicating mild depression. Patients had a mean duration of dysthymia of 30 years and an average age at onset of 12 years. Half reported a history of episodes of major depression. The 12-week treatment was completed by 84.3% of the sertraline group, 66.9% of the imipramine group, and 75.7% of the placebo group. Both active treatments were significantly superior to placebo in bringing about improvement and in achieving full remission. The proportions of patients classified as demonstrating a full remission were 49.5% for sertraline, 43.5% for imipramine, and 27.8% for placebo. Both active agents improved overall psychosocial function as measured with the Global Assessment of Functioning Scale, significantly more than placebo.

Conclusions.—Both sertraline and imipramine were effective treatments for dysthymia, improving depressive symptoms and psychosocial function in patients with a long history of the condition. The responses to these agents support the view that mild chronic depression is a mood disorder rather than an underlying character trait.

▶ The treatment of dysthymia (chronic, low-level depression) has not been studied as well as major depression, although most primary care physicians probably end up treating it much the same, with antidepressants. In this well-designed study, a serotonin-specific reuptake inhibitor, a tricyclic antidepressant, and a placebo were compared directly, with focus placed on psychosocial function in addition to the usual measures of depressive symptoms. The positive results are good news, even though the study was not large enough to determine which of the drug treatments was more effective (the serotonin-specific reuptake inhibitor was better tolerated than the tricyclic antidepressant). These findings give physicians a reasonable basis on which to prescribe antidepressants to patients with dysthymia. Although the study period was short, I think we know enough about the safety of long-term medication to extend the recommendation for the long term if symptoms warrant, as they usually do with this difficult diagnosis.

A.O. Berg, M.D., M.P.H.

Exercise and Depression in Midlife: A Prospective Study
Cooper-Patrick L, Ford DE, Mead LA, et al (Johns Hopkins Univ, Baltimore, Md)
Am J Public Health 87:670–673, 1997   10–4

Background.—Previous reports have suggested that exercise is related to better mental health. However, this link has been difficult to prove, with prospective observational studies giving conflicting results. The possible protective effect of physical activity against depression and psychiatric stress was assessed, with an emphasis on vulnerable individuals.

Methods.—The prospective observational study included 973 formal medical students from 1 medical school. The subjects were asked about their level of physical activity—defined as the frequency of exercising to a sweat during an average week—on 2 occasions. On later occasions, their incidence of self-reported clinical depression and psychiatric distress was assessed on the General Health Questionnaire. The protective effect of exercise was assessed, particularly in respondents with an "unstable" temperament or a parental history of depression.

Results.—At 15 years' follow-up, the cumulative incidence of depression was about 6% and the prevalence of psychiatric distress was 15%. Risk of depression was not affected by frequency of exercise in any analysis. Neither was there any link between physical activity level and subsequent psychiatric distress.

Conclusions.—This observational study does not show a protective effect of exercise against depression or psychiatric distress. If there is any such effect, it is probably a small one that will require a larger sample size to measure.

▶ To rely on this study you need to assume that medical students at Johns Hopkins are representative of the population in general (at least with respect to physical and mental health) and that you can believe uncontrolled cohort studies. I don't find those 2 beliefs too much of a stretch, and in any case doubt that the outcome of midlife depression would be biased, so I find the results intriguing. Regular exercise has many benefits, but less depression and better psychiatric health are not yet proven to be among them.

A.O. Berg, M.D., M.P.H.

Treating Major Depression in Primary Care Practice: Eight-Month Clinical Outcomes
Schulberg HC, Block MR, Madonia MJ, et al (Univ of Pittsburgh, Pa; Western Pennsylvania Hosp, Pittsburgh, Pa; State Univ of New York at Stony Brook)
Arch Gen Psychiatry 53:913–919, 1996   10–5

Background.—Major depression can lead to serious disability and generate significant health care costs. The manifestations of affective illness are often minimized, however, by both physicians and patients in the primary care setting. To advise primary care physicians about beneficial treatments for major depression, investigators designed a randomized, controlled trial of depression-specific therapies.

Methods.—The study was conducted at 4 ambulatory health centers. Potential participants were aged 18 to 64 years and scored at or above the positivity criterion on the Center for Epidemiologic Studies–Depression Scale. After a second assessment, 678 patients were identified who met

Diagnostic and Statistical Manual of Mental Disorders, 3rd Edition criteria for current major depression. Of these 678 referred patients, 403 agreed to complete a third assessment, 283 were judged clinically eligible for the study, and 276 were assigned to treatment. Randomization was to nortriptyline (NT), interpersonal psychotherapy (IPT), or a physician's usual care (UC). Patients were followed for 8 months for symptomatic improvement and rates of recovery.

Results.—Only 33% of patients in the NT group and 42% of the IPT group completed the full drug regimen or recommended psychotherapy protocol. In the UC group, 63% were provided some mental health treatment within 2 months of randomization. An antidepressant had been prescribed to 45% of UC patients within 2 months of study entry, and 41% of individual prescriptions were for nortriptyline. Both NT and IPT were more clinically and rapidly effective than UC in reducing severity of depression. The 3 treatment groups were comparable in baseline characteristics, but at 8 months only 20% of UC patients who completed treatment were judged to have recovered. In contrast, approximately 70% of treatment completers in the NT and IPT groups had recovered.

Discussion.—Both standardized pharmacotherapy and psychotherapy were found to be more effective than a primary physician's usual care in treating episodes of major depression. The treatment principles followed in the NT and IPT treatment groups were those recommended by the Depression Guidelines Panel for the Agency for Health Care Policy and Research. These findings are important because of the large number of depressed patients who seek help from generalist physicians.

A Multifaceted Intervention to Improve Treatment of Depression in Primary Care

Katon W, Robinson P, Von Korff M, et al (Univ of Washington, Seattle; Group Health Cooperative of Puget Sound, Seattle)
Arch Gen Psychiatry 53:924–932, 1996   10–6

Introduction.—Almost half of the patients treated for major or minor depression are seen in the primary care setting. Many of these patients do not receive an accurate diagnosis, however, and the most efficacious treatments for depression may not be prescribed or continued for an adequate period. A randomized, controlled trial was designed to evaluate the benefits of collaborative care for management of depression in primary care.

Methods.—The trial included 153 primary care patients who had received a diagnosis of major or minor depression by a primary care physician. Exclusion criteria included current alcohol abuse, psychotic symptoms, and dementia. All patients agreed to initiate antidepressant therapy. Randomization was to usual care (UC) or to a multifaceted intervention based on a collaborative model of care. With UC, patients commonly received a prescription for an antidepressant, were seen 2 or 3 times over the first month of treatment, and had the option of being referred to the HMO's mental health services. Intervention patients were enrolled in a structured depression treatment program that included medication, behavioral treatment, and counseling.

Results.—Sixty-five patients with major depression and 88 with minor depression were treated: 77 in the intervention group and 76 in the UC group. All 3 follow-up evaluations (at 1, 4, and 7 months) were completed by 73.8% of patients. Significantly more patients in the intervention group than in the UC group adhered to antidepressant medication and rated the quality of care received for depression as good or excellent. On all 4 outcome analyses, intervention patients with major depression experienced a significantly greater decrease in depression severity over time than UC patients with major depression. Among patients with minor depression, the multifaceted intervention yielded significant benefits vs. UC in only 1 of 4 study outcome analyses.

Conclusion.—Primary care patients with major and minor depression had better adherence to antidepressant regimens and greater satisfaction with care when they entered a treatment intervention that included behavioral strategies and counseling than when "usual" care by the primary care physician was offered. Depression outcomes were clearly more favorable for patients with major depression randomized to intervention, whereas those with minor depression tended to have similar outcomes whether assigned to UC or intervention.

▶ Randomized, controlled trials for mental health interventions that are conducted in primary care settings are rare birds, but here we have 2, and regarding the most common mental health problem seen in primary care—depression—to boot. The interventions in the 2 studies were different, but the results were remarkably similar, indicating a 2- to 4–times greater likelihood of the patient being symptom free at 8 months compared with UC controls. Although the Schulberg study (Abstract 10–5) found that psychotherapy was roughly equivalent to medication in producing a favorable outcome, the IPT that was used might prove a challenge for the average family physician to implement.

The multifaceted therapy used in the Katon study (Abstract 10–6) would also require resources that most family physicians would find difficult to replicate. Nonetheless, these 2 studies provide a standard against which our routine treatment might be measured. These 2 studies provide a strong argument for a multifaceted and interdisciplinary approach using both medications and psychotherapy. Family physicians in large group practices should be able to work toward establishing just such a system. Family physicians practicing alone or in resource-poor areas are going to find implementing these findings a challenge.

A.O. Berg, M.D., M.P.H.

Randomised Controlled Trial of Effect of Intervention by Psychogeriatric Team on Depression in Frail Elderly People at Home

Banerjee S, Shamash K, Macdonald AJD, et al (Inst of Psychiatry, London; St Thomas's Hosps, London)
Br Med J 313:1058–1061, 1996

Objective.—Home care enables the disabled elderly to be maintained in their own households. Unfortunately, the prevalence of depression in these patients is estimated to range from 26% to 44%. Results of a randomized controlled trial of intervention by a psychogeriatric team in southeast London are presented.

Methods.—A multidisciplinary team, consisting of community psychiatric nurses, occupational therapists, senior and junior medical staff, a social worker, and a psychologist, evaluated 69 depressed home care patients (12 men), 65 or older, and randomly allocated them to intervention (n = 33) or to the control group (n = 36), which received medical care only. Six months later, the patients were interviewed by an observer unaware of the group assignments. Recovery from depression was based on the AGECAT (automated geriatric examination for computer-assisted taxonomy) rating system. Results were compared statistically.

Results.—At follow-up, 4 patients in the intervention group and 3 in the control group had died. At baseline, 3 control patients and 4 intervention patients were taking antidepressant drugs. At follow-up, 5 control patients and 20 intervention patients were taking antidepressant drugs. During the study, 2 control patients were referred to the psychiatric team. Three intervention patients and 1 control patient were admitted to a psychiatric facility. Nineteen intervention patients and 9 control patients recovered. Use of antidepressant drugs did not produce a significant treatment effect. Increasingly severe depression and first episode of depression were predictive of a worse outcome at 6 months.

Conclusion.—Only 9 of the control group recovered in 6 months, indicating that the natural course of this disease is grim. The poor prognosis after a first episode of depression is probably the result of a combination of factors including many irreversible physical or social factors that limit recovery. Additional investigations need to be conducted to determine the degree to which these depressed patients can be managed and the cost associated with that management.

▶ Although from a British site, the results from this study should be generalizable to the U.S. setting. Professionals caring for the homebound elderly should be alert for signs of depression and ensure that resources are used. As pointed out by the authors, "therapeutic nihilism" regarding depression in the elderly is not appropriate.

A.O. Berg, M.D., M.P.H.

Major Depressive Disorder in the 6 Months After Miscarriage

Neugebauer R, Kline J, Shrout P, et al (New York State Psychiatric Inst, New York; Columbia Univ, New York; New York Univ, New York; et al)
JAMA 277:383–388, 1997   10–8

Background.—Miscarriage occurs in up to 20% of clinically recognized pregnancies. Miscarriage is an unanticipated, traumatic event and as such may have important mental health consequences. Few studies have examined the possible psychiatric effects of miscarriage. One previous study found that women who miscarry have elevated depressive symptoms. The miscarriage-associated risk of an initial or recurrent episode of major depressive disorder was analyzed.

Methods.—The study included 229 women who had had a miscarriage, defined as involuntary termination of a non-viable pregnancy, and a population-based cohort of 230 women without recent pregnancy. Half the women were 25 to 34 years old, most with more than a high school education. Forty percent were white and 35% Hispanic. The Diagnostic Interview Schedule, customized to detect recent episodes, was used to assess the presence of major depressive disorder. The a priori hypothesis was that the miscarriage group would be at higher risk for an episode of major depressive disorder. Risk for the miscarriage group in the first 6 months after the pregnancy loss was compared with risk in the previous 6 months for the community group. Risk was predicted to be higher for childless women, those who had lost previous pregnancies, and those aged 34 years or older.

Results.—The incidence of major depressive disorder was 11% in the miscarriage group versus 4% in the community group. Relative risk (RR) was 2.5 for the miscarriage group overall. Within the miscarriage group, risk was higher for childless women than for those with children, RR 5.0 versus 1.3. Nearly three fourths of the depressive episodes in miscarrying women occurred within the first month after the pregnancy loss. The risk of recurrence for miscarrying women with a history of major depressive disorder was 54%. Risk was unaffected by previous pregnancy loss, maternal age, time of gestation, or attitude toward pregnancy.

Conclusions.—Miscarriage appears to raise the risk of new or recurrent major depressive disorder. Women who miscarry should be evaluated for signs of depression in the first few weeks after the event, especially childless women and those with previous depressive episodes. Such high-risk women may benefit from referral to a mental health professional.

▶ The linkage between pregnancy and postpartum depression has been well studied empirically. Most physicians are pretty good at detecting it, I would guess because the association is well known and because the women are coming in often in conjunction with well-child visits, so there are plenty of opportunities for the physician to make the connection. This article documents a problem of similar scope, but in women who miscarry. Detection might be more of a problem because the woman might not be making regular office visits. This suggests several possible interventions, including discussing the risk of depression with the woman at the time of the miscarriage, scheduling 1 or more brief visits 3 to 6 months later, and arranging for nurse or physician follow-up at a reasonable interval.

A.O. Berg, M.D., M.P.H.

Antidepressants for Children: Is Scientific Support Necessary?
Fisher RL, Fisher S (State Univ of New York, Syracuse, NY)
J Nerv Ment Dis 184:99–102, 1996   10–9

Background.—Although it is generally accepted that treatment should be based on a scientific rationale, the application of this concept is complex, overlaid with ambiguity and even defensive rationalization. The nature of this dilemma was explored in an analysis of antidepressant use in depressed children and adolescents.

The Role of Scientific Support in Antidepressant Prescription for Children.—A review of the relevant scientific literature demonstrated unanimous evidence that antidepressants are no more effective than placebo in treating children with symptoms of depression. However, the prescription of antidepressants for such patients is widely practiced. Some child psychiatrists have tried to find other rationales for this practice. In one editorial, reasons as to why clinicians may actually "know better" than the published research about the efficacy of antidepressants in children were given. In a recently published *Handbook of Depression in Children and Adolescents*, the authors state that clinicians would be unlikely to continue to give antidepressants to children if there were no clinical benefit. In essence, these authors say that if the scientific data do not come out as expected, another set of criteria can be used to justify a certain practice. Other authors argue that using a treatment of questionable efficacy or safety is unethical.

Conclusions.—The continued prescription of antidepressants for children clearly shows how a significant group of clinicians can persist in and justify the use of a treatment contradicted by research data. Just how far practitioners are at liberty to deviate from scientific findings needs to be better defined.

▶ For those physicians who are interested in evidence-based practice, the topic of antidepressants for children is a fascinating debate. Although they are in wide use based on clinical and anecdotal experience, no randomized trials (of which there have been several quite good ones) have shown antidepressants to be effective in children and adolescents. This paper thoughtfully considers some of the arguments on both sides of the decision to prescribe. My own view is that the issue is important; that we are ethically bound to conduct appropriate studies to settle the question; and that, in the interim, these agents should be prescribed rarely, if at all, especially by primary care physicians.

A.O. Berg, M.D., M.P.H.

Drug and Alcohol Use

Behavior of Boys in Kindergarten and the Onset of Substance Use During Adolescence

Mâsse LC, Tremblay RE (Univ of Texas, Houston; Univ of Montreal)
Arch Gen Psychiatry 54:62–68, 1997   10–10

Introduction.—Recent longitudinal studies indicate that certain childhood behaviors and family characteristics are predictive of substance abuse among adolescents. Some authors hypothesize that basic personality dimensions may be the link between disruptive behavior and substance abuse. A sample of high-risk young boys was tested to determine whether a relationship exists between high novelty-seeking, low harm avoidance, and low reward dependence and subsequent cigarette use, alcohol abuse, and other drug use.

Methods.—The initial study sample included 1,034 white boys who attended French-speaking schools in Montreal. All lived in poor areas of the city, and 67% lived in a home with both parents when they attended kindergarten. The boys were evaluated at ages 6 and 10. Teachers' ratings of behaviors were used to assess childhood personalities. Measurement of substance use was obtained by self-reports at ages 11 to 15. Questionnaires were used to gather information on cigarette smoking, getting drunk, and drug use.

Results.—The proportion of substances used increased with age. By age 15, nearly half of the boys (47.5%) reported being drunk in the preceding year, and almost one third (30.5%) said they had used other drugs in the preceding 12 months. Whereas high novelty-seeking and low harm avoidance at age 6 or 10 significantly predicted the early onset of substance use, reward dependence was unrelated to smoking, getting drunk, or using drugs. Children usually experimented with alcohol first, at age 13, then tried other drugs about 1 year later. Cigarette smoking probably started before age 13, but earlier data on this variable were not available.

Conclusions.—The presence of the personality dimensions of high novelty-seeking and low harm avoidance at ages 6, 10, or both significantly predicts the onset of cigarette smoking, getting drunk, and using drugs in adolescent boys. Assessments of such behavior in early childhood, even in the preschool years, may help identify those at risk for early onset of substance use.

▶ The observation reported in this article is of the sort that has plenty of methodologic limitations and is difficult (impossible?) to act on but is fascinating nonetheless. The methodologic limitations include the unusually homogeneous population (lower socioeconomic class but intact families, French-Canadian setting) and the substantial dropout rate. These findings join a mountain of data showing that personality characteristics, including the extremes, are well developed early in life, suggesting a strong genetic component. Although we don't have reliable tools to protect children at risk, recognition of the increased risk is the first step. These investigators expect to follow the cohort into adulthood, so more information will come.

A.O. Berg, M.D., M.P.H.

Prevalence of Alcohol-impaired Driving: Results From a National Self-reported Survey of Health Behaviors
Liu S, Siegel PZ, Brewer RD, et al (Natl Ctr for Chronic Disease Prevention and Health Promotion, Atlanta, Ga; Ctrs for Disease Control and Prevention, Atlanta, Ga)
JAMA 277:122–125, 1997   10–11

Introduction.—Alcohol-related motor vehicle crashes are a major cause of death in the United States. Physicians can play an important role in advising their patients not to drive while under the influence of alcohol. There are no data on the actual number of episodes of alcohol-impaired driving that occur. Data from a national health survey were used to estimate and analyze the prevalence of alcohol-impaired driving in the United States.

Methods.—The analysis used data from the 1993 Behavioral Risk Factor Surveillance System, a nationwide survey of self-reported health behaviors. The responses of more than 100,000 non-institutionalized adults were analyzed. The study looked at the percentage of respondents who reported driving while under the influence of alcohol, the number of episodes of alcohol-impaired driving per 1,000 population, and the overall number of such episodes. The results were analyzed by age, sex, race, education, and state.

Results.—The results suggested that 123 million episodes of alcohol-impaired driving occurred in 1993. The percentage of respondents who reported driving while under the influence was 2.5%. The rate of alcohol-impaired driving was 655 episodes per 1,000 adult population. This rate varied considerably among states, from 165/1,000 in Maine to 1,550/1,000 in Alaska. Young men aged 21 to 34 years had the highest rate of impaired driving, 1,739 episodes per 1,000 population. The rate was similar for men aged 18 to 20 years, 1,623/1,000, even though all states had laws prohibiting the sale of alcohol to people younger than 21 years. People who reported 2 or more drinks per day and "binge drinkers" who recently had had 5 or more drinks on 1 occasion, were more likely to drive while under the influence.

Conclusions.—Data from a nationwide survey suggest that rates of driving while under the influence of alcohol are very high in the United States. Efforts are needed to combat this problem, including strict enforcement of laws against driving under the influence of alcohol and community and patient education. The Behavioral Risk Factor Surveillance System provides a valuable source of specific data for monitoring of trends and for evaluating the effectiveness of interventions to reduce alcohol-impaired driving.

▶ The fact that this article is based on more than 100,000 individual interviews should not make us too complacent about the fact that it is all self-report. We can never be absolutely sure that the findings are "true" because there is no way to validate the interview responses. Self-report in this case, though, makes the findings even more alarming, because it almost certainly means that the estimates of driving while under the influence of alcohol are underestimates (at least it is hard to imagine that individuals would overstate the number of events reported). This line of research then points to a problem of such size that only substantial interventions in several areas are likely to address it. Certainly, individual physicians have a role here, but most of the interventions will be carried out at the community level or higher.

A.O. Berg, M.D., M.P.H.

A Two-item Screening Test for Alcohol and Other Drug Problems
Brown RL, Leonard T, Saunders LA, et al (Univ of Wisconsin, Madison)
J Fam Pract 44:151–160, 1997   10–12

Introduction.—A brief, accurate screening tool is needed to assess substance use disorders (SUDs) in health care settings. Direct questions may not yield reliable results. The current screening protocols recommended for health care settings assess only alcohol use. The criterion validity of a two-item conjoint screening (TICS) test for alcohol and other drug abuse or dependence was evaluated in a random sample of 434 patients receiving primary care.

Methods.—A focus group process was used to develop 9 screening items. The criterion standard was the DSM-IIIR criteria for SUDs. An exhaustive analysis of combinations of items revealed that the best 2–item screening strategy was a positive response to 2 items: "In the last year, have you ever drank or used drugs more than you meant to?" and "Have you felt you wanted to cut down on your drinking or drug use in the past year?" Research subjects were interviewed, then completed a brief questionnaire with the TICS items and questions regarding their comfort level with the interviewer. Urine tests were collected for drug screening in participants who blindly drew 1 particular marble from a pouch of 4 marbles.

Results.—Of 494 patients recruited, 434 participated (response rate of 87.9%). More than half the participants had lifetime SUDs, greater than one third had a lifetime history of substance abuse, more than one fourth had a current SUD, and one fifth were currently dependent on at least 1 substance. Compared with other age groups, the TICS was less specific for patients aged 40–49 years and significantly less specific for patients aged 30–39 years. The sensitivity and specificity was about 81% with at least 1 positive response to the TICS. The TICS was especially sensitive to polysubstance use disorders. The chance of a positive SUD was 7.4%,

45%, and 75%, respectively, for respondents with zero, 1, and 2 positive responses.

Conclusions.—Two screening questions on TICS can identify more than 80% of young and middle-aged adults with SUDs and can classify severity of risk for drug and alcohol disorders.

▶ Last year, Dr. Berg reviewed an article that seriously questioned the utility of a 2–item screening test for alcohol abuse (see 1997 YEAR BOOK OF FAMILY PRACTICE, p 410). (This effectively halted one of my interview shortcuts, and I went back to the CAGE [*C*ut down, *A*nnoyed by criticism, *G*uilty about drinking, *E*ye-opener drinks] technique.) Here is a potential "replacement" 2–item test that shows more promise. I was intrigued by the use of conjoint questions—probably harder to evade (but possibly harder for the interviewer to remember, too!)—and by the fact that the questions used screen for drugs and alcohol. Comparisons here are difficult—very different demographics and different design. Nevertheless, this appears to be an easily administered, quick test which reliably screens for substance abuse.

W.W. Dexter, M.D.

Screening for Problem Drinking in Older Primary Care Patients
Adams WL, Barry KL, Fleming MF (Univ of Wisconsin, Madison)
JAMA 276:1964–1967, 1996   10–13

Background.—Heavy use of alcohol contributes to morbidity and mortality among the elderly. In the general population older than 65 years, the incidence of alcohol abuse is 2% to 4%, and the incidence of less severe alcohol-related problems is as high as 10%. In the United States, even if the current incidence remains the same, the number of elderly individuals with alcohol problems will increase because the population is aging. Alcohol consumption can exacerbate or increase the risk of other health problems. Screeing tools for problem drinking in the elderly should be able to identify those who may be at risk for medical problems related to alcohol abuse. The ability of the CAGE (Cut down, Annoyed by criticism, Guilty about drinking, Eye-opener drinks) questionnaire to identify heavy and binge drinking in elderly individuals was evaluated in a cross-sectional study.

Methods.—A survey was conducted of 5,065 individuals older than 60 years who were enrolled from the offices of 88 primary care physicians. The Health Screening Survey, which asks about drinking, smoking, exercise, and diet, was distributed to patients on arrival at their physician's office. The CAGE questionnaire was also completed by patients. Demographic data were obtained.

Results.—Of the 5,065 individuals who completed the questionnaire, 56% were women, 84% were aged 60–75 years, 16% were older than 75 years, and 23% lived alone. Regular drinking exceeding the limits recommended by the National Institute of Alcohol Abuse and Alcoholism was reported by 15% of men and 12% of women (more than 7 drinks per week for women and more than 14 drinks per week for men). Also, 9% of men and 2% of women reported consuming more than 21 drinks per week on a regular basis. The CAGE questionnaire identified 9% of men and 3% of women positive for alcohol abuse within 3 months. The CAGE questionnaire was poor at detecting individuals who drank heavily or who were binge drinkers.

Discussion.—These findings indicate that the CAGE questionnaire cannot adequately identify problem drinking in an elderly, primary care population. It is recommended that various screening tools be combined when screening for problem drinking. This and other studies have shown that men, college graduates, and married individuals are more likely to drink heavily. Consuming 2–3 alcoholic drinks per day raises the risk of hypertension and possibly diabetes, breast cancer, head and neck cancers, and hip fracture.

▶ This large and well-conducted questionnaire study defines a problem but does not provide a satisfying answer. I think the authors have shown persuasively that the CAGE questions have inadequate sensitivity in older patients—they miss detecting individuals with problem drinking. It is not clear, though, exactly how the CAGE should be supplemented, that is, what questions should be added? What this article says to me is that older patients merit a bit more careful questioning on their alcohol habits than the CAGE provides. I hope these researchers will give us specific tools to use both to improve the validity of the assessment and to keep the complexity of the assessment at a minimum.

A.O. Berg, M.D., M.P.H.

Brief Physician Advice for Problem Alcohol Drinkers: A Randomized Controlled Trial in Community-based Primary Care Practices
Fleming MF, Barry KL, Manwell LB, et al (Univ of Wisconsin, Madison; Univ of Michigan, Ann Arbor; Family Health Plan Cooperative, Milwaukee, Wis)
JAMA 277:1039–1045, 1997
10–14

Background.—Alcohol use disorders are associated with adverse health and economic effects. A randomized controlled clinical trial was designed to determine whether brief physician advice delivered in community-based primary care practices could reduce alcohol use in problem drinkers.

Methods.—Project TrEAT (Trial for Early Alcohol Treatment) was conducted in 17 primary care practices located in 10 counties in Wisconsin. Sixty-four family physicians and general internists were recruited for the project; 34 had received training in alcohol use disorders during medical school and residency. Patients aged 18 to 65 years were asked to complete a health screening survey at regularly scheduled appointments. Problem drinking was defined as more than 14 drinks per week (168 g alcohol) for men and more than 11 drinks per week (132 g alcohol) for women. Individuals who had attended an alcohol treatment program in the preceding year had been advised by a physician in the preceding 3 months to change their alcohol use, drank more than 50 drinks per week, or reported symptoms of suicide were excluded. The intervention consisted of 2 15-minute counseling visits delivered 1 month apart by physicians. A workbook containing information on the adverse effects of alcohol, a drinking agreement, and drinking diary cards was used. Patients were monitored for 12 months for alcohol use measures, emergency department visits, and hospital days.

Results.—The study group comprised 482 men and 292 women; 392 were randomized to the intervention and 382 to a control group. Controls were given a booklet on general health issues. The 2 groups were similar at baseline in alcohol use and other potentially confounding variables. At 12-month follow-up, patients in the intervention group showed significant reductions compared with the control group in 7-day alcohol use (mean number of drinks in the preceding 7 days), in episodes of binge drinking during the preceding 30 days, and in frequency of excessive drinking in the preceding 7 days. Men in the control group had substantially longer hospitalizations during the study period than men in the intervention group. The 2 groups did not differ in number of emergency department visits or other health status measures.

Conclusion.—Brief advice protocols in the primary care setting can be effective in changing drinking behavior and improving health outcomes for at-risk and problem drinkers. Alcohol use was also reduced among controls, perhaps because of an intervention effect of the research procedures.

▶ One of the things that the U.S. Preventive Services Task Force struggled with in producing its 1996 report is how to evaluate evidence for primary preventive services—often, office-based physician counseling. For many primary preventive interventions we know that a change in behavior changes health outcomes (e.g., exercise, smoking cessation, safe-sex practices), but the evidence showing that physicians in practice can persuade patients to change is often thin indeed. This article provides the first evidence in primary care practices that such counseling is effective for problem drinkers. The intervention is too briefly described to be used immediately in practice, but with support from a federal grant the investigators expect to make the materials widely available within a short time. The basic components of the intervention have already been published and are available from National Institute of Alcohol Abuse and Alcoholism (NIH publication 95–3769, U.S. Government Printing Office).

A.O. Berg, M.D., M.P.H.

Miscellaneous

Clinical Characteristics of Women With a History of Childhood Abuse: Unhealed Wounds

McCauley J, Kern DE, Kolodner K, et al (The Johns Hopkins Univ, Baltimore, Md; Montgomery County Health Department, Montgomery, Ala; Hahnemann Univ, Philadelphia)
JAMA 277:1362–1368, 1997
10–15

Background.—A variety of psychosocial problems are associated with previous childhood abuse, such as poor self-esteem, depression, and anxiety disorders. Prevalence estimates of childhood sexual and physical abuse vary among settings. The prevalence of such abuse in primary care practices was determined, and the physical and psychologic effects in victims of different types of abuse were compared.

Methods.—The cross-sectional study included 1,931 women seen at 4 community-based, primary care internal medicine practices. The women, of various ages and marital, educational, and economic status, completed a self-administered, anonymous survey.

Findings.—Twenty-two percent reported childhood or adolescent physical or sexual abuse. Compared with the 1,257 women who reported no abuse, the 204 women who reported abuse in childhood but not in adulthood had more physical symptoms and higher scores for depression, anxiety, somatization, and interpersonal sensitivity. These women were also more likely to be abusing drugs or to have a history of alcohol abuse, to have attempted suicide, and to have a psychiatric admission. Number of physical symptoms, emotional distress, substance abuse, and suicide attempts did not differ significantly between women abused only as children and those abused only as adults. Women experiencing both childhood and adult abuse had greater levels of psychological problems and physical symptoms than those with childhood or adulthood abuse alone.

Conclusions.—In this large, socioeconomically diverse, community-based population of primary care patients, 1 in 5 women was the victim of sexual or physical abuse. Physical and psychological problems are associated with such abuse, even in women abused in childhood only. Recognizing this may alter health care providers' diagnostic and treatment plans for such patients.

▶ This article was published in an issue of JAMA (May 1997) with two other articles dealing with the issues of violence and abuse. This article makes it clear that the consequences of abuse fade very little with time. A table in the article documents the toll, showing that 20 of 23 chronic symptoms and maladies are more common in those with a positive history of abuse. Family physicians who ask their patients about abuse are likely to find it more often than expected. But once identified, effective "treatment" or "management" is usually elusive. Patients often carry the scars for years, regardless of treatment plan.

An accompanying editorial attempts to bring some perspective to a series of issues and paradoxes that seem to have no rational explanation.[1] The writer of the editorial comments that definitions are changing, that the relevant disciplines do not share definitions and measures of success, and that researchers and practitioners are widely separated by experience, authority, and goals. It is little wonder that patients and physicians find this area so frustrating.

A.O. Berg, M.D., M.P.H.

Reference

1. Flitcraft A: Learning from the paradoxes of domestic violence. *JAMA* 277:1400–1401, 1997.

Gender, Quality of Life, and Mental Disorders in Primary Care: Results From the PRIME-MD 1000 Study
Linzer M, Spitzer R, Kroenke K, et al (Columbia Univ, New York; Uniformed Services Univ, Bethesda, Md; Albert Einstein College of Medicine, Bronx, NY; et al)
Am J Med 101:526–533, 1996

10–16

Introduction.—Many studies indicate that women in primary care have an excess of certain mental disorders, particularly mood disorders, and that physicians often fail to diagnose these disorders. Data from a large primary care study (PRIME-MD 1000) were analyzed for differences between the sexes in the frequency of mental disorders in the primary care setting and the potential impact of these differences on health-related quality of life (HRQL).

Methods.—One thousand patients were examined at 4 primary care sites using PRIME-MD, a questionnaire that helps to diagnose mood, anxiety, somatoform, alcohol, and binge-eating disorders. The instrument contains 2 parts: a 1–page patient questionnaire and a clinician's evaluation guide. The clinician's evaluation guide is a structured clinical interview designed to follow up on positive responses to the patient questionnaire. Health-related quality of life was assessed with the Medical Outcomes Study SF-20 General Health Survey. Patients in the study had a mean age of 55 years; 56% were women and 58% were white. Sixty-one percent of physicians were men. The most common physical disorders in the group were hypertension (48%) and arthritis (23%); 39% had 1 or more mental disorders.

Results.—Men and women differed significantly in certain baseline demographic characteristics. Women were less likely to have a college degree and to be married and more likely to be nonwhite. Half of the women were obese, but only one third of the men were. Women were significantly more likely than men to have any mental disorder (43% vs. 33%) and to have psychiatric co-morbidity (26% vs. 15%). Particularly prominent among the women patients were mood disorders, anxiety disorders, somatoform disorders, and binge eating. Women had significantly worse HRQL than men, scoring lower in all 6 domains of the SF-20. After controlling for the number of mental disorders, however, differences in HRQL were eliminated in 5 of 6 domains. Female physicians were more sensitive than male physicians to PRIME-MD diagnosed psychiatric caseness, but women patients were not less satisfied with care from male physicians.

Discussion.—Women in this sample of primary care patients were significantly more likely than men to have mood, anxiety, and somatoform disorders and psychiatric co-morbidity. Largely as a result of these mental disorders, women scored significantly lower on HRQL. It is important for primary care physicians to screen for and treat common mental disorders in their female patients.

▶ The conclusions here are not surprising, but I include the article because it confirms countless smaller regional studies of less rigorous design showing much the same thing. The PRIME-MD instrument is fast becoming one of the best-tested tools to assess mental health because it is short, easy to use, and valid. (The instrument was initially published in *JAMA*[1] and is available from Pfizer Pharmaceuticals.) These authors and others have shown persuasively that common mental disorders are especially common in women, but we still have too few data showing that screening the general population is beneficial. We need better quality data showing that HRQL actually improves with routine screening and treatment for the disorders here studied: mood, anxiety, and somatoform disorders.

A.O. Berg, M.D., M.P.H.

Reference

1. Spitzer RL, Williams JBW, Kroenke K, et al: Utility of a new procedure for diagnosing mental disorders in primary care: The PRIME-MD 1000 study. *JAMA* 272:1749–1756, 1994.

Differences in the Use of Psychiatric Outpatient Services Between the United States and Ontario
Kessler RC, Frank RG, Edlund M, et al (Harvard Med School, Boston; Univ of Michigan, Ann Arbor; Univ of Toronto; et al)
N Engl J Med 336:551–557, 1997   10–17

Introduction.—Although the mental health care system in the United States has been criticized for restricting access to care for the uninsured, some believe that expanded coverage will lead to more resources being devoted to individuals with low levels of need. Canada and the United States are similar in many ways, but Canada has universal health coverage and spends relatively less on health care. To clarify the relation between health insurance and mental health care, 2 general population surveys were done separately in the United States and Ontario.

Methods.—Ontario was selected for comparison because it is the largest Canadian province and similar to the United States in key sociodemographic variables. Canada places no limits, however, on visits to a physician for mental health problems, whereas mental health coverage often is limited in the United States, even for the insured. The household surveys on use of psychiatric outpatient services were conducted in 1990 and aimed at young and middle-aged adults (15 to 54 years). Analyses were from self-reports of disorders listed in *Diagnostic and Statistical Manual of Mental Disorders*, ed 3, revised and other indicators of need for mental health services.

Results.—Compared with respondents in Ontario, those in the United States were significantly more likely to report having had psychiatric disorders, poor mental health, or workdays lost or cut short because of psychiatric problems. The probability of use of services for psychiatric problems was significantly higher in the United States (13.3%) than in Ontario (8.0%). When subgroups were analyzed, however, the higher probability of use in the United States was confined to individuals with less severe mental illness and low levels of need. The rates of use of the human-services and self-help sectors, as opposed to the health care sector, was significantly higher in the United States at several levels of illness severity. In patients who had similar numbers of psychiatric disorders over the same time periods, the average number of visits did not differ significantly between the 2 survey areas.

Conclusions.—A higher prevalence of psychiatric problems was found in the general household population in the United States than in Ontario. Nevertheless, the greater use of the health care sector for psychiatric problems in the United States is confined to individuals with less severe illness. This mismatch between measures of need and treatment must be addressed in any plan to expand access to mental health services in the United States.

▶ I find studies comparing the United States and Canadian health care experiences endlessly fascinating because our populations are so alike in most ways but so divergent in others. Here is an area of divergence. The United States has more individuals with psychiatric visits, but the visits are concentrated among those with the lowest level of "need" if need is defined by severity of the condition. It is not hard to speculate on why need does not match utilization: with the low levels of third-party reimbursement for mental health services, only the well-off can afford them, and the well-off are not as likely to be afflicted with the most serious mental diseases. The explanation for why psychiatric conditions are so much more common in the United States than in Canada is not clear. One can invoke the usual comments about the differences between the 2 countries in personal health behaviors and expectations regarding medical care, but the truth is that no one knows.

A.O. Berg, M.D., M.P.H.

Is Psychotherapy Ever Medically Necessary?

Bennett MJ (Harvard Med School, Boston)
Psychiatric Serv 47:966–970, 1996   10–18

Background.—Mental health care has become controversial, as the needs of patients and the allocation of resources are rethought by managed care providers. The usefulness of psychotherapy is no longer taken for granted. A framework for providing mental health care to populations rather than individuals was presented and a role for psychotherapy was suggested.

Psychotherapy Prior to Managed Care.—Studies performed on the mental health care system that existed before the advent of managed health care have revealed that mental disorder was common, whereas treatment was not common. Among those who did receive mental health treatment, most did not have a diagnosable mental disorder at the time of treatment. Mental health care specialists frequently practiced long-term psychotherapy, which accounted for most mental health expenditures. There does not appear to have been a strong relationship between need for treatment and receipt of treatment under the system that existed before managed care. At least some mental health care appeared to be discretionary.

Medically Necessary Psychotherapy.—Most managed care organizations consider treatments to be medically necessary if they establish or re-establish normality or limit disability associated with a diagnosable disorder. Because mental health treatment is heterogeneous and large, long-term controlled clinical trials are often unavailable, it is difficult for exact treatment paradigms to be created. Managed care systems determine a need for mental health services based on the presence of a mental disorder and either a state of clinical instability or impaired function resulting from the specific disorder. Within this context, psychotherapy will be viewed as medically necessary if it is effective in treating defined mental disorders by itself, as short-term adjunctive therapy, or as the best therapy when effective therapy has not been defined. Treatment is most controversial for patients who have complex disorders that are refractory to treatment. These patients function poorly on a chronic basis and require long-term treatment. For these complex cases, brief periods of psychotherapy to achieve stabilization or remediation could be interspersed with longer periods of case management and support for rehabilitation.

Conclusion.—Despite its limitations, the *Diagnostic and Statistical Manual of Mental Disorders* system has value in setting thresholds beyond which need for treatment can be defined. These thresholds are important in rational resource application by managed care entities. Psychotherapy is a treatment tool and will continue to be considered useful as long as it can be shown to be effective in treating mental disorder.

▶ This provocative title introduces a controversial subject, thoughtfully presented. The key to the author's 3 scenarios in which he defines medical necessity is the issue of efficacy. Efficacy in psychotherapy should be evaluated just as it is in any other condition, with rigorous controlled trials demonstrating that the treatment works when compared with placebo and is cost effective when compared with other proven therapies. As I read the literature on psychotherapy (and my wife is a psychiatrist, so I see a lot of it), we are just beginning to see the quality of research improve so that the value of psychotherapy can be objectively assessed. The author of this article sets high standards. I agree with them.

A.O. Berg, M.D., M.P.H.

11 Preventive Medicine

Introduction

The chapter begins with a section of 3 articles on exercise, including a systematic review of what works in practice settings and a welcome plea for moderation. The miscellaneous section opens with a study of centenarians, followed by quite a few provocative studies on attendance at religious services and mortality, dangers of driving while talking (on cell phones), screening for lung cancer, maternal smoking as a risk for attention deficit–hyperactivity disorder and the difficulties of providing high quality prevention services to adolescents.

Alfred O. Berg, M.D., M.P.H.

Fitness and Physical Activity

A Systematic Review of Physical Activity Promotion Strategies
Hillsdon M, Thorogood M (London School of Hygiene and Tropical Med)
Br J Sports Med 30:84–89, 1996   11–1

Background.—There is considerable evidence showing the health benefits of physical activity. However, there are few data on the effectiveness of strategies designed to increase physical activity sufficiently to achieve these benefits. This study reviewed recent studies on the effectiveness of physical activity promotion strategies.

Methods and Findings.—A literature search identified 11 randomized, controlled trials of physical activity promotion strategies. The exercise was home-based in 7 interventions and facility-based in 5. In the exercise interventions, the subjects were to exercise between 3 and 5 times per week for 20–60 minutes. The outcome was positive in 5 of the 7 home-based interventions and in 2 of the 5 facility-based interventions. In a study comparing home- and facility-based interventions, subjects assigned to the home-based arm completed significantly more prescribed exercise sessions. Walking was the prescribed mode of exercise in half of the studies, and all studies of walking showed a significant increase in exercise compared with controls. For subjects who achieved an initial increase in exercise, regular follow-up improved the proportion of subjects able to maintain their improvement. All home-based studies using telephone follow-up showed positive outcomes.

Conclusions.—Exercise promotion strategies that encourage walking and do not require traveling to a facility appear to give the best chance of sustainable increases in physical activity. The form of exercise with the greatest potential for increasing activity levels in the population and meeting public health recommendations is brisk walking. It also is most likely to be adopted by diverse age, socioeconomic, and ethnic groups. More studies of exercise promotion strategies are needed.

▶ For such an important public health issue, we know strikingly little about how to achieve exercise and fitness goals. I was surprised by how few studies had been done; at their size (small); follow-up, or lack of it; and lack of consistency. The good news is that there is some evidence indicating that some exercise interventions (notably home-based walking programs) might promote positive, long-term change. Although disheartening for the authors, it was heartening for me to learn that nearly all the interventions were taking place here in the United States. We are far too sedentary, too heavy, and too unfit. How do we change this? It is not at all clear, but walking programs are a place to start—after you have assessed your patient's readiness to change (see Abstract 11–2).

W.W. Dexter, M.D.

Reasons for Not Exercising and Exercise Intentions: A Study of Middle-aged Sedentary Adults

Auweele YV, Rzewnicki R, van Mele V (Catholic Univ of Leuven, Belgium)
J Sports Sci 15:151–165, 1997   11–2

Introduction.—A low percentage of the population engages in vigorous and frequent physical activity. Many people have continued to be sedentary despite encouragement to increase their physical activity. A questionnaire study was done to identify the reasons why people do not exercise and to find out what might lead them to become more active.

Methods.—Based on interviews with sedentary people, the investigators developed a questionnaire addressing why people do not participate in leisure-time physical activities and what steps might be taken to change the situation. The questionnaire consisted of lists of reasons for not exercising and lists of conditions to promote exercise. The subjects were to indicate the extent to which each statement applied to them. Responses from 265 middle-age Belgian adults were analyzed .

Results.—Factor analysis of the results suggested that reasons for inactivity were related to the subjects' self-concept and the irrelevance of exercise; the perception that exercise was "unnecessary"; anticipated negative feelings related to exercise; the perception that exercise was risky; and the perception that exercise was too much effort. Factors related to the conditions needed to start exercising related to an unacceptable perceived decrease in health and to the appropriateness of the activity. Discriminant analysis identified significant differences between subjects who never exercised and those who had stopped exercising, and between those who had stopped exercising a long time ago and those who stopped recently. A typology of sedentariness was created by cluster analysis, identifying the following 3 groups of sedentary adults: the "unconcerned," the "opposed," and the "approachable."

Conclusions.—Among sedentary middle-age adults, reasons for not exercising are related to the person's self-concept, cognitive cost-benefit processes, and negative emotions associated with exercise. Some people might be convinced to exercise if they perceived a decrease in their health or if the proposed exercise was seen as appropriate. Simple indifference to exercise may be the greatest barrier. These kinds of beliefs, attitudes, and interests must be considered in any health promotion policy attempting to change behavior and adjust priorities in adults.

▶ Overcoming barriers to exercise is a windmill I tilt at nearly every day. I have heard the most outlandish excuses, from the standard "I've only got so many heartbeats, and I don't want to waste them, Doc" to "I'd have to go upstairs from the TV room, and I'd miss my shows." The latter patient, by the way, eventually agreed to exercise, but only during commercials. This allowed him to accumulate nearly 1 hour a day of physical activity! The point is that my approach, perhaps yours, has been haphazard at best. This study, at the least, provides a base for adding structure to the process. I like the groupings and the types identified. This allows us, with a few simple questions, to stratify patients and apply "change contemplation" techniques, which are time-efficient and can be effective. Just don't spend too much time on the precontemplators (the opposed).

W.W. Dexter, M.D.

How Much Physical Activity Should We Do? The Case for Moderate Amounts and Intensities of Physical Activity
Blair SN, Connelly JC (Cooper Inst for Aerobics Research, Dallas)
Res Q Exerc Sport 67:193–205, 1996   11–3

Background.—Over the past half century, numerous epidemiologic studies have documented an association between a sedentary way of life and various health problems, most notably, coronary artery disease. Research on the role of exercise, usually carried out by physiologists, has centered on physical fitness as measured as maximal oxygen uptake (VO_2max). More recent investigations have combined some elements of the 2 research themes of physical activity and health and exercise training experiments on VO_2max. Yet to be determined are the appropriate dose of activity and the recommended intensity of exercise for health and fitness outcomes.

Methods.—Several recent representative studies and a few classic investigations from past years were reviewed and summarized in an attempt to produce a cogent recommendation for the type and amount of physical activity required for health and function. Of particular interest was evidence relating to the benefits of moderate amounts and intensities of physical activity. Other issues considered were the relation of physical fitness to mortality and the effect of exercise on health outcomes.

Moderate Exercise.—A number of recent population-based studies indicate that moderate and moderately vigorous activity can significantly reduce fatal and nonfatal coronary heart events, compared with a sedentary way of life. Exercise test heart rate is a significant independent predictor for both coronary heart disease and all-cause mortality, even after adjustment for age, smoking, blood pressure, and serum cholesterol concentration. A trend was noted for dose response, and substantial benefits were obtained when individuals changed from low to moderate physical fitness. Among women, a walk of only about 1 mile per day increased bone density, compared with sedentary women.

Exercise Intensity.—Early exercise training studies were limited in number of subjects and duration of the exercise regimen. In addition, most participants were young men who were relatively fit at baseline. Training intensity was found, however, to have a direct effect on the amount of improvement in aerobic power. Increases in overall fitness are accompanied by reductions in weight, lipid levels, and blood pressure.

Discussion.—In terms of risk of clinical disease, some activity is clearly better than none, and low to moderately intense activity is better than remaining sedentary. The least active 20% to 30% of the adult population has an increased mortality of at least 2-fold, but their risk can be substantially reduced with even moderate activity.

▶ I have hope that the release of the Surgeon General's report on physical activity and health will have the same impact on our thinking and behavior that the report on smoking has had. It is unrealistic, though, to expect the general population to become vigorously active. In this article by Blair (a major architect of the Surgeon General's report) and Connelly, they quite effectively make the case for moderate levels of activity and suggest focusing attention on the least fit quartile as a way to reap the greatest public health gains. This article succinctly reviews the evidence supporting the benefits of exercise and its inverse relationship to risk of disease. It also supports the concept of "accumulated" exercise over the course of a day.

There is no dispute that the most sedentary 25% of the population would benefit the most from an exercise program. How to get these "hard-core sedentaries" moving is the question. I am convinced that lack of physical activity, while clearly a risk factor for various diseases, is probably a part of a complex, ingrained behavior pattern. It has, for instance, been linked to a variety of adolescent risk behaviors.[1]

An intriguing construct for this problem is the transtheoretical model of behavioral change. Using the percentages in a recent survey from Canada, precontemplators and contemplators (no intention of changing and just thinking about it) constitute over 20% of the population.[2] This, I suspect, corresponds pretty closely to the most sedentary quartile of our society. This is a tough one, folks. The ones who need it and would benefit the most desire it the least, and it is pretty well ingrained.

So, how do we get our patients moving and then keep them moving? No good answers, as yet. There have been multiple studies of various stripes showing some success with a broad range of approaches. This is fairly well reviewed in a recent article by Dunn.[3] It is discussed in Abstract 11–1. In the office, work with patients one at a time, find out where they are in their readiness to change, recommend modest activity levels, perhaps accumulated over a day, and don't get discouraged. To paraphrase the commercial, "Measure success one exerciser at a time!"

W.W. Dexter, M.D.

References

1. Pate RR, Heath GW, Dowda M, et al: Associations between physical activity and other health behaviors in a representative sample of U.S. adolescents. *Am J Public Health* 86:1577–1582, 1996.
2. Potvin L, Gauvin L, Nguyen NM: Prevalence of stages of change for physical activity in rural, suburban, and inner-city communities. *J Commun Health* 22:1–13, 1997.
3. Dunn AL: Getting started—A review of physical activity adoption studies. *Br J Sports Med* 30:193–199, 1996.

Miscellaneous

Centenarians: Human Longevity Outliers
Smith DWE (Northwestern Univ, Chicago)
Gerontologist 37:200–207, 1997

11–4

Objective.—A few individuals live to be very old. The characteristics that allow them to survive for so long are examined.

Centenarians as Longevity Outliers.—Although mortality rates of most animals increase exponentially with age, mortality rates of the very old are lower than predicted. The increase in mortality rates results from multi-hit mechanisms caused by exogenous and endogenous risks that increase and accumulate with time.

Causes of Human Death and Resistance to Them.—Diseases of the circulatory system are the most common causes of death in the United States. Voluntary behavioral risk factors such as smoking can increase the risk. Mortality rates for all types of cancers also increase with age, family history, smoking, and occupational exposure to carcinogens. Individuals who are very old have a lower mortality rate from cancer because they may have more resistance.

Resistance to Other Causes of Death.—There are fewer hits contributing to mortality today than in the past. Maximum life spans are inherited.

The Condition of Human Longevity Outliers.—Whereas centenarians are a heterogeneous group, most are in poor health and many have dementia.

Causes of Death of Longevity Outliers.—Most very old individuals (63%) are said to die of diseases of the circulatory system, 10% of cerebrovascular disease, 4% of cancer, and 10% of pneumonia. The few studies that have compared causes of death on certificates with results of autopsies find significant disagreement. A cause of death could not be found in 26% of autopsies.

The Future.—The number of centenarians will increase. Their physical and mental condition and their survival rate are unknown.

▶ This is a wonderful review, full of interesting data and references to other interesting articles about the very, very old. Despite everyone's wish that it were otherwise, there is no compelling evidence that long life is predictable. Although there is strong evidence for "shortivity" (e.g., families who live short lives), there is little evidence for the inheritance of long life in humans. Centenarians are a heterogeneous group, and most have major health problems, not the least of which is dementia, as it appears that "normal aging" and dementia converge in the very old. It is clear that the absolute and relative numbers of the very old are increasing in this country, so we can expect to see more about this rare group. If you want to learn about the limits of human existence and the problems that the very old (and their physicians!) face, track this one down.

A.O. Berg, M.D., M.P.H.

Frequent Attendance at Religious Services and Mortality Over 28 Years
Strawbridge WJ, Cohen RD, Shema SJ, et al (California Public Health Found, Berkeley; California Dept of Health Services, Berkeley)
Am J Public Health 87:957–961, 1997   11–5

Objective.—Studies of religious groups have found that members of strict religious groups live longer because they subscribe to moderation in behavior and are more likely to have good health practices. Because social and psychological factors may be important in any study of longevity, the long-term correlation between religious attendance and mortality was examined to determine if the association is explained by improvements in health practices and social connections for frequent attenders.

Methods.—A longitudinal health and mortality study in Alameda County, California, measured religious service attendance of 6,928 individuals, aged 16 to 94, in 1965, 1974, 1983, and 1994, and assessed sociodemographic variables, religious affiliation, health variables, health practices and conditions, and social connections. The study also assessed improved health practices, increased social contacts, and stable marriages during the study period. Multiple logistic regression was used to relate attendance and other variables during the study period.

Results.—Females, blacks, the mobility impaired, and the overweight were frequent attenders. Frequent attendance was also associated with the number of close social contacts and group memberships but not with marriage. Smokers and heavy drinkers were less likely to attend. There was a weak but significant correlation between frequent attendance and lower mortality rates when health conditions, social connections, health practices, and body mass index were included (relative hazard=0.77). The relationship was stronger for females than for males (RH=0.66 vs. 0.90). Compared with infrequent attenders, frequent attenders who smoked in 1965 were almost twice as likely to quit, frequent attenders who never or rarely exercised in 1965 were almost 33% more likely to increase their exercise frequency. There was a tendency for reducing drinking and for losing excess weight among frequent attenders. Frequent attenders were more socially adept, stayed married, increased memberships, and increased social contacts.

Conclusion.—Frequent attendance at religious services results in improved health practices and social skills or contacts.

▶ The authors are academically circumspect about positing a direct link between religious service attendance and mortality. But whether it is attendance per se that makes the difference (which I doubt), or the intervening variables of improved health practices and social connections that does it (which seems more plausible), the bottom line is the same: quite an astonishingly large effect. Using number needed to treat, only about four would need to attend religious services to prevent one death in 28 years. If this were a public health intervention, it would rank right up there with smoking cessation in effectiveness!

A.O. Berg, M.D., M.P.H.

Association Between Cellular-Telephone Calls and Motor Vehicle Collisions

Redelmeier DA, Tibshirani RJ (Univ of Toronto; Sunnybrook Health Science Centre, North York, Ont, Canada)
N Engl J Med 336:453–458, 1997   11–6

Background.—The use of cellular telephones while driving seems to many observers to be distracting to the driver, and it seems likely that such use would increase the risk of motor vehicle collisions. However, 2 industry-sponsored surveys have found no increased risk. This study investigated the risk by using a case-crossover design, a technique that assesses the brief change in risk associated with a transient exposure and in which research subjects serve as their own controls.

Methods.—Consenting subjects were enrolled if they came to a collision reporting center in Toronto during peak hours between July 1, 1994, and August 31, 1995; their collision had involved substantial property damage as judged by the police (collisions involving injuries are not reported to the center); they reported owning a cellular phone; and their cellular phone bills could be obtained. Subjects answered a brief questionnaire about themselves and the collision, and the time of the collision was estimated from subject reports, police records, and telephone records of calls to emergency services. Telephone bills were examined to determine telephone use during the 10 minutes before the collision and during the comparable time on the day preceding the collision. If more calls were made immediately before the collision than would be expected as a result of chance, that was interpreted as an increase in risk. Supplemental analyses were made to evaluate alternative comparison days and shorter and longer times before the collision. In addition, the data were adjusted to account for intermittent driving (i.e., not all participants had driven on the previous day).

Results.—Of 5,890 eligible drivers, 1,064 acknowledged owning a cellular phone, 742 agreed to participate, and billing records were obtained for 699. After adjusting for intermittent driving, analysis indicated that cellular telephone activity in the 10 minutes immediately before the collision was associated with a 4.3 relative risk of a motor vehicle collision (95% confidence interval, 3.0–6.5). The results were not significantly different for drivers using hands-free telephones.

Conclusions.—In this population, use of a cellular telephone while driving was associated with a risk of motor vehicle collision 4 times higher than that for the same drivers when they did not use their cellular telephones. This association does not prove a causal relationship. However, individual drivers who use cellular telephones are at greater risk and should act accordingly (e.g., abstain from alcohol use, avoid speeding, minimize other distractions, place and receive only important calls, interrupt conversations if necessary, and keep calls brief). Physicians have a responsibility to identify patients who may be at risk and counsel them about safety precautions.

▶ The cellular telephone has truly been a boon to this family doctor's family life. A longer electronic leash has allowed me to be a coach-dad on Saturdays, take bicycle rides, etc. It has been a boon on the sidelines, too, providing quick access to 911, arranging x-rays, and calling parents. There is a "dark side to this force," though (with apologies to the *Star Wars* screenwriter!). The convenience is seductive, and I am sure we have all seen drivers chatting on their phones, oblivious to the traffic around them and sometimes, probably unintentionally, breaking traffic laws. I have been that oblivious driver, I am sorry to say. In their conclusion, the authors correctly state that the use of cellular phones is associated with an increased risk for accidents. They do not claim causality. Anyone believe that one does not lead to the other here? Some suggestions are made to reduce the risk of collisions. Let me add another: Pull over and park while you are making the call. I agree that we should include this as another item in our health screening questionnaires. We are, of course, asking about seat belt use. Ask about cellular phone use, too.

W.W. Dexter, M.D.

Don't Ask, They Won't Tell: The Quality of Adolescent Health Screening in Five Practice Settings
Blum RW, Beuhring T, Wunderlich M, et al (Univ of Minnesota, Minneapolis)
Am J Public Health 86:1767–1772, 1996   11–7

Introduction.—The American Medical Association issued The Guidelines for Adolescent Preventive Screening, a comprehensive set of guidelines created to provide a framework for adolescent preventive services within the clinical setting. The medical records of 788 adolescents aged 13–17 years were randomly chosen from 5 practice settings to determine the extent to which comprehensive, age-appropriate adolescent health screening was accomplished.

Methods.—Medical records were examined for the number of biomedical and sociobehavioral health risks screened. Data were obtained from 2 pediatric private practices, 2 community family practices, 1 private family practice, 1 school teen clinic, and 1 community teen clinic.

Results.—No setting met recommended guidelines for adolescent health screening. The most comprehensive assessment of behavioral, psychosocial, substance use, and sexual behavioral risks were performed in the 2 teen clinics, followed by the community family practice setting, then the private family practice or private pediatric practice settings (which were similar in health risk screening). Although expected to be opposite of what was observed, adolescents aged 13–14 years were screened for the most

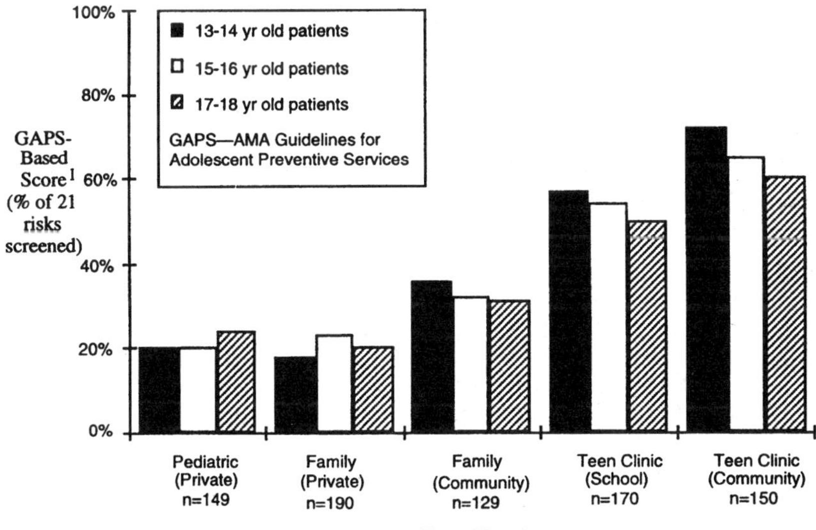

FIGURE 1.—Percentage of adolescent preventive health screening questions asked, by age and practice setting. *Abbreviation: GAPS,* Guidelines for Adolescent Preventive Screening. (Courtesy of Blum RW, Beuhring T, Wunderlich M, et al: Don't ask, they won't tell: The quality of adolescent health screening in five practice settings. *Am J Public Health* 86:1767–1772, 1996. Copyright 1996, American Public Health Association.)

risks and adolescents aged 17–18 years were screened for the least risks in the community family practices, school teen clinic, and community teen clinic (Fig 1).

Conclusions.—It cannot be assumed that high-risk behaviors are limited to certain adolescent populations. If the right questions are not asked, appropriate services cannot be offered to adolescent health care consumers.

▶ The title of this article says it all. As family doctors, we are in exactly the right position to offer comprehensive care for our adolescent patients. As this study indicates, we are probably falling short on our responsibilities in this regard.

I have been intrigued, and bothered, by the move to specialty training in adolescent health care. It seems to me that the underlying difference is really in communicating with this particular age group—no question, it can be difficult. There are many barriers, not the least of which is that this age group does not frequent the doctor's office regularly. One of the exceptions to this is the preparticipation evaluation (PPE). One of the drawbacks of mass PPEs is lack of time, rapport, and privacy, all diminishing the chances of solid communication with the patient. It was especially troubling to learn that the physicians in private practice, those ostensibly with the most and best opportunities to establish this rapport, had the worst track record in this regard.

It is a fact that adolescents wish to discuss a variety of health and behavior topics with their health care providers. We simply are not giving them a chance. One study, for instance, found that a significant percentage of primary care physicians did not provide privacy for interviewing adolescents.[1] It would seem it is time to change the paradigm under which we approach our adolescent patients. A place to start might be with some privacy, and perhaps, a structured format for the interview. An excellent example of this is the West Virginia University Adolescent Health Risk Score—a comprehensive biopsychosocial interview—described in a recent article in *Clinical Pediatrics*.[2]

W.W. Dexter, M.D.

References

1. Purcell JS, Hergenroeder AC, Kozinetz C, et al: Interviewing techniques with adolescents in primary care. *J Adoles Health* 20:300–305, 1997.
2. Perkins K, Ferrari N, Rosas A, et al: You won't know unless you ask: The biopsychosocial interview for adolescents. *Clin Pediatr* 36:79–86, 1997.

Screening for Lung Cancer: Another Look; A Different View
Strauss GM, Gleason RE, Sugarbaker DJ (Harvard Med School, Boston; McGill Univ, Montreal; Caro Research, Boston)
Chest 111:754–768, 1997   11–8

Background.—Because no randomized trials have shown that lung cancer screening results in decreased mortality rates, such screening is generally thought unnecessary. Prospective studies on lung cancer screening were reviewed to determine the effects of known biases.

Methods.—The analysis included 4 randomized, controlled studies. Research at Memorial–Sloan Kettering and Johns Hopkins compared annual chest radiography (CXR) in a control group with CXR plus sputum cytologic findings. In the Mayo Lung Project and Czechoslovakian study, regular and frequent rescreening CXR was compared with sporadic or infrequent rescreening in a control group.

Findings.—In the Memorial Sloan–Kettering and Johns Hopkins studies, the addition of cytologic assessment to CXR did not affect outcomes. However, long-term survivals in both studies were about 3 times those predicted by other data. The Mayo and Czech studies showed a striking advantage for regular screening in stage distribution and in resectability, survival, and fatality rates. In both studies, however, mortality rate was somewhat greater in the screened groups. Survival and fatality comparisons may be confounded by overdiagnosis bias, lead-time bias, and length bias, whereas mortality rate is not subject to these biases.

Conclusions.—Periodic CXR results in clinically meaningful improvements in stage distribution and in resectability, survival, and fatality rates among patients with lung cancer. Though mortality rate reductions have not been shown, mortality rate did not accurately reflect lung-cancer-related death rates in the Mayo and Czech studies. Thus, periodic CXR screening may be reconsidered for persons at high risk for lung cancer.

▶ I am often attracted to investigations that challenge dogma. One dogma that is well ingrained is the lack of utility of screening for lung cancer with CXR. I suspect that many of us hedge a bit here—perhaps leaning toward CXR for our patients who smoke, particularly when symptoms such as cough are present. This dogma is widely adhered to, and probably correctly so, because the evidence does not support use of CXR as a screening tool for lung cancer. Still, these authors make a case that the evidence is perhaps not as compelling as we have held and should be revisited.

W.W. Dexter, M.D.

Serum Potassium, Cigarette Smoking, and Mortality in Middle-aged Men

Wannamethee SG, Lever AF, Shaper AG, et al (Royal Free Hosp School of Medicine, London; Gardiner Inst, Glasgow, Scotland)
Am J Epidemiol 145:598–606, 1997   11–9

Purpose.—Previous studies have suggested that elevated serum potassium levels (6.0 mmol/L or higher) may be related to increased mortality. However, there have been no studies of the long-term relationship between potassium and morality in the general population. This longitudinal study evaluted the assocation between serum potassium and all-cause mortality in middle-aged men.

Methods.—The analysis included 7,636 Brititsh men aged 40 to 59 years from the British Regional Heart Study. At baseline, the men completed a standard questionnaire and series of physical assessments, including blood sampling for biochemical measurements. They were then followed for 11.5 years. Associations between potassium level and all-cause mortality were evaluated in normotensive vs. hypertensive subjects, in subjects who were and were not receiving antihypertensive treatment, and in subjects with and without evidence of ischemic heart disease.

Results.—Excluding 374 men who were receiving antihypertensive therapy, there were 771 deaths among 7,262 subjects. Mortality was not increased for men with a low serum potassium level, defined as less than 3.7 mmol/L. Mortality was significantly increased for men with serum potassium levels of 5.2 mmol/L or greater. The increase was especially great for noncardiovascular deaths and was present even after adjustment for potential confounders. However, serum potassium level was strongly linked to smoking, and the potassium-related increase in mortality was seen only in smokers. The relative risk of all-cause mortality was 1.7 for current smokers with high serum potassium values. This group had a 1.8 relative risk for overall cancer mortality and a 2.5 relative risk for lung cancer mortality. For subjects receiving antihypertensive therapy, high serum potassium values carried an excess risk of cardiovascular and noncardiovascular mortality. Low serum potassium levels were not associated with excess mortality in this group.

Conclusion.—These epidemiologic data suggest that smoking-related increases in serum potassium level may increase the risk of death from noncardiovascular disease, especially lung cancer. Alternatively, high serum potassium levels could reflect some other smoking-related risk factor. More study is needed to clarify the prognostic and treatment implications of increased mortality related to high serum potassium values. Mortality is not increased for men with low serum potassium values, whether or not they are receiving antihypertensive treatment.

▶ The window of safety for serum potassium levels is notoriously narrow. Because many of the medications we use for hypertension and other cardiovascular diseases, as well as diabetes, significantly affect the serum potassium levels, we are forced to routinely monitor these levels and attempt to compensate if they are out of the therapeutic window.

In this very interesting study of more than 7,000 middle-aged British men, the authors studied the relationship between serum potassium level and all-cause mortality, as well as cardiovascular mortality. There was a somewhat surprising and reassuring finding that low serum potassium levels—even those of men treated for hypertension—did not increase overall mortality or cardiovascular mortality. However, there was a significant increase in all-cause mortality for high serum potassium levels, particularly related to smoking.

This study found several variables associated with high potassium levels. Certainly, 2 of the most glaring were smoking and alcohol use. It may be that an elevated serum potassium level is simply a marker for risky habits that contribute to an increased all-cause mortality. My take-home message from this study is to be comforted somewhat by a serum potassium level between 3.5 and 4 and to more vigorously pursue causes for potassium levels greater than 5.

R.C. Davidson, M.D., M.P.H.

Is Maternal Smoking During Pregnancy a Risk Factor for Attention Deficit Hyperactivity Disorder in Children?
Milberger S, Biederman J, Faraone SV, et al (Massachusetts Gen Hosp, Boston; Harvard Med School, Boston; Massachusetts Mental Health Ctr, Boston; et al)
Am J Psychiatry 153:1138–1142, 1996   11–10

Background.—Attention-deficit hyperactivity disorder (ADHD) begins in early childhood and is characterized by difficulties with attention, motor activity, and impulsiveness. It affects from 6% to 9% of school-age children. Genetic and environmental factors are involved in the cause of this disorder. Maternal smoking during pregnancy may be an important environmental risk factor. Nicotinic receptors modulate dopaminergic activity, and it is believed that dopaminergic dysregulation is involved in the underlying pathophysiology of ADHD.

Methods.—The following 2 groups of children were studied: 140 children with ADHD and 120 control subjects. All subjects were male and were between 6 and 17 years old. Information on maternal smoking was obtained by an interviewer.

Results.—A maternal history of smoking during pregnancy was found in 22% of the children with ADHD and in 8% of the control subjects. This association was still significant after adjusting for socioeconomic status, parental IQ, and parental ADHD status. There were significant differences in IQ between the children whose mothers smoked and the children whose mothers did not smoke during pregnancy.

Discussion.—These results suggest that there is a correlation between maternal smoking during pregnancy and ADHD in children. They are consistent with a nicotinic-receptor hypothesis of ADHD. These findings are consistent with a growing body of evidence of the long-term medical, behavioral, and cognitive problems in children associated with smoking during pregnancy.

▶ Raising a child with ADHD can be a long and arduous process. I always look for the most distressing conditions to convince women not to smoke during pregnancy, such as the greatly increased risk of sudden infant death syndrome. The increased risk of ADHD would follow as a serious warning. Frightening patients is generally not good practice, but it is appropriate for avoiding maternal smoking during pregnancy. I give such warnings with care and compassion.

J.E. Scherger, M.D., M.P.H.

Immunization of Adolescents
Averhoff FM, Williams WW, Hadler SC (Ctrs for Disease Control and Prevention, Atlanta, Ga)
Am Fam Physician 55:159–167, 1997   11–11

Introduction.—Many adolescents and young adults in the United States continue to be affected by diseases that are preventable by vaccine. Current immunization programs have not focused on improving the rate of vaccination in adolescents. Recommendations for immunization of adolescents were developed to improve vaccination coverage in this age group and to establish a routine visit to a health care provider. It is important to ensure that adolescents receive hepatitis B and varicella virus (if indicated) vaccines and that they receive the second dose or booster for measles, mumps, rubella, tetanus, and diphtheria toxoid, as well as other vaccines, such as influenza, which may be recommended for certain adolescents.

Administration of Vaccines.—Although all indicated vaccines should be administered to adolescents who are 11 or 12 years of age, multiple vaccinations may be required in some individuals. Factors that affect the decision not to administer all vaccines during a single visit and to schedule the adolescent for return visits include vaccines requiring multiple doses and diseases that may be an immediate threat to the individual.

Documentation.—The clinician should attempt to obtain documentation of previous vaccines from the parent, previous physicians, or school. If documentation is unavailable at the time of the first visit, it is recommended that the clinician assume that the individual has received the vaccinations required by law or regulation and administer the vaccines not so required.

Discussion.—The recommendations for each vaccine discussed are consistent with current Advisory Committee on Immunization Practices, American Academy of Pediatrics, American Academy of Family Physicians, and American Medical Association documents. However, recommendations for the first diphtheria toxoid booster have recently been

TABLE 1.—Recommended Schedule of Vaccinations for Adolescents Aged 11 to 12 Years

Immunobiologic	Indications	Name	Dose	Frequency	Route
Hepatitis A vaccine	Adolescents who are at increased risk of hepatitis A infection or its complications	Havrix	720 EL.U. per 0.5 mL*	A total of two doses at 0,† 6 to 12 months	Intramuscular injection
		Vaqta	25 U per 0.5 mL	A total of two doses at 0, 6 to 18 months	Intramuscular injection
Hepatitis B vaccine	Adolescents not vaccinated previously for hepatitis B	Recombivax HB	5 µg per 0.5 mL	A total of three doses at 0, 1 to 2, 4 to 6 months	Intramuscular injection
		Engerix-B	10 µg per 0.5 mL	A total of three doses at 0, 1 to 2, 4 to 6 months	Intramuscular injection
Influenza vaccine	Adolescents who are at increased risk for complications caused by influenza or who have contact with persons at increased risk for these complications	Generic— influenza virus	0.5 mL	Annually (September-December)	Intramuscular injection
Measles, mumps and rubella	Adolescents not vaccinated previously with 2 doses of measles vaccine at 12 months of age or more	MMR II	0.5 mL	One dose	Subcutaneous injection
Pneumococcal polysaccharide vaccine	Adolescents who are at increased risk for pneumococcal disease or its complications	Generic— pneumococcal vacine polyvalent	0.5 mL	One dose	Intramuscular or subcutaneous injection
Tetanus and diphtheria toxoids (Td)	Adolescents not vaccinated within the previous five years	Generic—tetanus and diphtheria toxoids, adsorbed (for adult use)	0.5 mL	Every 10 years	Intramuscular injection
Varicella virus vaccine	Adolescents not vaccinated previously and who have no reliable history of chickenpox	Varivax	0.5 mL	One dose‡	Subcutaneous injection

*Alternative dosage and schedule of 360 enzyme-linked immunosorbent assay units per 0.5 mL and a total of 3 doses administered at 0, 1, and 6 to 12 months.
†Ten months represents timing of the initial dose, and subsequent numbers represent months after the initial dose.
‡Adolescents aged 13 years or older should be given a total of 2 doses (0.5 mL/dose) subcutaneously at 0 and 4 to 8 weeks.
Abbreviation: EL.U, enzyme-linked immunosorbent assay unit.
(Reprint from the January 1997 volume 55 issue of *American Family Physician*, courtesy of Averhoff FM, Williams WW, Hadler SC: Immunization of adolescents. *Am Fam Physician* 55:159–167, 1997, published by the American Academy of Family Physicians.)

changed; the first booster may now be given at 11 to 12 years. Recommendations for hepatitis B, measles, mumps, rubella, diphtheria toxoid, varicella virus, influenza, pneumococcal polysaccharide, and hepatitis A vaccines are included, as well as general immunization recommendations and a suggested schedule of vaccinations for this age group (Table 1).

▶ Usually, the *American Family Physician* presents practical and useful articles. The Advisory Committee on Immunization Practices is the recognized authority for immunization recommendations for all ages. In this review of immunizations of adolescents, the American Medical Association, American Academy of Family Physicians, and the American Academy of Pediatrics have all agreed that adolescence is an important time for reviewing and updating immunizations. The recommendation for a second measles, mumps, and rubella vaccine, if necessary, is probably the most important recommendation of all. However, the recommended schedule in Table 1 may not be realistic. Vaccinations for hepatitis A (2 doses) and hepatitis B (3 doses) are very expensive, and few adolescents have received them as infants. Because tetanus and diphtheria toxoids are effective for 10 years and adolescents would have received 5 doses in childhood, I do not understand why a booster would be necessary within 5 years of the previous vaccination. Either a new series of "well child care" visits for adolescents must be developed, or these recommendations are going to have to be reconsidered to make them more practical.

J.E. Scherger, M.D., M.P.H.

Determination of Deltoid Fat Pad Thickness: Implications for Needle Length in Adult Immunization

Poland GA, Borrud A, Jacobson RM, et al (Mayo Clinic, Rochester, Minn)
JAMA 277:1709–1711, 1997   11–12

Introduction.—The Advisory Committee on Immunization Practices stated in 1994 that needles should be long enough for all intramuscular injections to reach the muscle mass and prevent vaccine from leaking into subcutaneous tissue. The range of deltoid fat pad thickness was evaluated in healthy adult males and females to help guide the selection of a needle length adequate for intramuscular injection into the deltoid muscle.

Methods.—Two hundred twenty consecutive health care workers undergoing hepatitis B immunization underwent high-resolution ultrasound scanning, and measurement of weight, height, and middeltoid arm circumference to determine deltoid fat pad thickness. There were 126 females and 94 males.

Results.—There was a highly significant difference in deltoid fat pad thickness between males and females. Females had a thicker deltoid fat pad (11.7 mm vs. 8.3 mm) and deltoid skin-fold thickness (34.7 mm vs. 17.2 mm) than males. The body mass index was similar for both sexes. Ultrasound findings indicated that a standard 16-mm (⅝–inch) needle would not have reached 5 mm into the muscle in 17% of males or 48.4% of females.

Recommendations and Conclusions.—In the healthy adults evaluated, the appropriate needle lengths for true deltoid intramuscular immunization is 25-mm (1 inch) for males weighing between 59 and 118 kg. For females, recommended needle lengths are 16 mm (⅝-inch needle) for females weighing less than 60 kg; 25 mm (1-inch needle) for women 60–90 kg; and 38 mm (1.5-inch needle) for females greater than 90 kg. These findings demonstrate the importance of choosing an adequate needle length, particularly in females, to ensure deltoid intramuscular immunization.

▶ Are you sure that your immunizations are going where they are supposed to? I was reassured by our head nurse that our staff makes allowances for size and weight in choosing the needles to use when administering immunizations. Taking at face value the assumption that the Mayo Clinic employees are representative of U.S. healthy adults, these results are useful guidelines for the office. The data presented here allow us to take some of the guesswork out of choosing needle size. Prevention of disease via immunization is one of the greatest services we provide. An important step in this process is proper technique—size them up.

W.W. Dexter, M.D.

12 Neurologic Conditions

Introduction

The first section on stroke contains important articles on general stroke risk, the specific effect of "statins" on stroke risk, treatment with thrombolysis, secondary prevention, and quite an interesting observation of a handful of individuals whose stroke sequelae include a new passion for good food. Two randomized trials of intranasal lidocaine and sumatriptan comprise the section on migraine headache, followed by articles on diagnosis and management (with midodrine) of syncope, and a final (and very useful) article on the alcohol sniff test as a screen for function of the first cranial nerve.

Randomized controlled trials: Abstracts 12–2, 12–4, 12–7, 12–8, and 12–11.

Alfred O. Berg, M.D., M.P.H.

Stroke and Stroke Prevention

A Population-based Model of Risk Factors for Ischemic Stroke: Rochester, Minnesota

Whisnant JP, Wiebers DO, O'Fallon WM, et al (Mayo Clinic and Mayo Found, Rochester, Minn)
Neurology 47:1420–1428, 1996
12–1

Background.—Previous epidemiologic studies have linked stroke with hypertension, diabetes mellitus, ischemic heart disease, transient ischemic attack (TIA), and perhaps atrial fibrillation. There is conflicting evidence as to whether stroke is related to alcohol consumption and smoking. A population-based cohort of patients with ischemic stroke was used to assess the relevant risk factors and the interactions between them.

Methods.—The study was based on 1,444 incidence cases of ischemic stroke identified in the Rochester Epidemiology Project from 1960 to 1984. They were matched 1:1 for age and sex to control subjects from the same population. Risk factors for ischemic stroke were evaluated by multiple logistic regression, with adjustment for confounding variables. The final model included age, date of stroke, TIAs, hypertension, smoking, atrial fibrillation, ischemic heart disease, mitral valve disease other than

TABLE 2.—Transient Ischemic Attack, Smoking, Mitral Valve Diseases, Ischemic Heart Disease, and Diabetes Mellitus

Risk factor	Odds ratio* (95% confidence interval)				
	50 yr	60 yr	70 yr	80 yr	90 yr
Transient ischemic attack					
Female	31 (6.1–158)	20 (5.8–68.5)	13 (5.1–32)	8 (3.8–17.8)	5 (2.2–12.8)
Male	11 (3.0–41.6)	7 (2.9–18.2)	5 (2.4–8.9)	3 (1.5–5.8)	2 (0.7–5.0)
Current smoking	3.6 (1.7–7.6)	2.7 (1.6–4.3)	1.9 (1.4–2.8)	1.4 (0.9–2.3)	1.0 (0.5–2.1)
Mitral valve disease	2.1 at all ages (1.1–3.8)				
Ischemic heart disease	1.9 at all ages (1.4–2.5)				
Diabetes mellitus	1.7 at all ages (1.2–2.4)				

*From the final multivariable model adjusted for age, stroke, or reference date, and an interaction between age and time period.

(Courtesy of Whisnant JP, Wiebers DO, O'Fallon WM, et al: A population-based model of risk factors for ischemic stroke: Rochester, Minnesota. *Neurology* 47:1420–1428, 1996. Copyright American Academy of Neurology. Used with permission of Lippincott-Raven.)

prolapse, and diabetes mellitus. The model also was designed to assess interactions between risk factors.

Results.—Of all the risk factors studied, the only ones that were not significant were mitral valve prolapse and aortic valve disease. The incidence of stroke associated with TIAs was greater for women than men and declined with advancing age. The stroke risk associated with hypertension and with current smoking also decreased with age (Table 2). Intermittent and persistent hypertension had comparable effects on stroke risk in patients with hypertension. However, when hypertension was absent, the risk was 7 times greater with persistent than with intermittent atrial fibrillation. There were no significant differences in the odds ratios encountered over the various periods studied. Anti-hypertensive treatment had no apparent effect on stroke risk.

Conclusions.—Risk factors for ischemic stroke include ischemic heart disease, mitral valve disease, diabetes mellitus, hypertension, TIA, smoking, and atrial fibrillation. Many stroke risk factors interact with each other; for some of these factors, the associated stroke risk gets lower with age. The risk factors were stable over the 25-year period studied. The study was conducted in a predominantly white population, so the results cannot be extrapolated to other ethnic groups.

▶ The strengths of this article are its population base and the quality of the statistical analysis. The table contains the most useful summary, with the odds ratios representing the approximate relative risks for each factor in each age group. For example, an odds ratio of 3.6 in a current smoker aged 50 means that such a patient is 3.6 times more likely to have a stroke than his or her non-smoking control subject. Importantly, the mostly white population of Rochester makes it impossible to use these findings in a more ethnically diverse practice, except for the whites. I like the article, though, because it summarizes important risk factors in 1 place and gives a sense of the relative importance of the risk factors studied.

A.O. Berg, M.D., M.P.H.

Stroke, Statins, and Cholesterol: A Meta-analysis of Randomized, Placebo-controlled, Double-blind Trials With HMG-CoA Reductase Inhibitors

Blauw GJ, Lagaay AM, Smelt AHM, et al (Leiden Univ, The Netherlands)
Stroke 28:946–950, 1997   12–2

Objective.—The 3-hydroxy-3-methylglutaryl-coenzyme A (HMG-CoA) reductase inhibitors, or "statins," have proven effective in the prevention of coronary heart disease. However, their effects on stroke and other manifestations of atherosclerotic disease are unclear. To answer this question, all data on stroke occurrence from published randomized, placebo-controlled, double-blind trials of HMG-CoA reductase inhibitor treatment were combined.

Methods.—Thirteen trials published between 1980 and 1996 met criteria for inclusion in the analysis. Design aspects considered included placebo control, monotherapy, and double-blinding. When there were incomplete data on the type of stroke or the rates of clinical events or adverse effects, the study authors were contacted. For each study, the number of strokes occurring in patents receiving active statin treatment was compared with the number of strokes expected.

Results.—In 20,438 study participants, there were 462 evaluable strokes. One hundred eighty-one strokes occurred in patients receiving HMG-CoA reductase inhibitor treatment, and 261 in patients receiving placebo. Twelve of the 13 trials showed a smaller-than-expected number of strokes with statin treatment. The overall odds ratio of stroke with HMG-CoA reductase inhibitor treatment was 0.69, with a 95% confidence interval of 0.57–0.83.

Conclusions.—Meta-analysis of randomized trial data suggests that treatment with HMG-CoA reductase inhibitor reduces the risk of stroke in middle-aged patients. The 31% reduction shown in this study is comparable to the effects of statins in preventing coronary heart disease. The findings underscore the need to test the ability of statins to prevent stroke in the elderly.

▶ This is an especially interesting application of meta-analysis in that the studies included in the analysis primarily focused on coronary heart disease rather than stroke. The studies also reported on stroke, but because stroke was a secondary end point, the individual studies were too small to reach conclusions. Despite the novelty of the method, however, I would approach the conclusion of net benefit with caution. First, trials (mostly small) that did not include at least 1 stroke were excluded from the analysis, possibly biasing the meta-analysis in favor of treatment. Second, the quality screen used to decide whether to include studies was fairly crude, allowing in some marginal studies. I would conclude that there is fair evidence of a beneficial effect of the statins on stroke, but that 1 or more properly designed studies with stroke as a primary end point need to be conducted before we can be sure.

A.O. Berg, M.D., M.P.H.

When Is Thrombolysis Justified in Patients With Acute Ischemic Stroke?: A Bioethical Perspective

Furlan AJ, Kanoti G (Cleveland Clinic Found, Ohio)
Stroke 28:214–218, 1997   12–3

Introduction.—The use of IV thrombolysis in acute ischemic stroke is known to increase the risk of clinically significant intracerebral hemorrhage. With the exception of the National Institutes of Neurological Disorders and Stroke recombinant tissue plasminogen activator trial, which showed a net benefit in certain subgroups, other studies indicate a 44% increase in the odds of death among fibrinolysis-treated patients. The bioethical issues involved in offering thrombolysis to patients with acute ischemic stroke were studied.

Justification of Thrombolysis.—The justification of a treatment involves scientific, ethical, and economic standards. One author (JS Schwartz, 1995) has suggested criteria for evaluation of medical therapies (Table 1). Randomized clinical trials can show a net benefit under ideal circumstances ("safety and efficacy"), but in the current health care environment more is required. The benefit must justify the cost, there must be a benefit in routine conditions, and benefits must be proportional to the risk accepted with informed consent.

Clinical Trials.—A rigorous new standard for assessing benefit was set with the National Institutes of Neurological Disorders and Stroke trial, in which the primary end point was full neurologic recovery at 90 days. There is likely to be variation, however, among physicians and patient subgroups in setting the relative risk-to-benefit ratio and cost-effectiveness of thrombolysis. Because stroke outcome end points are not standardized, comparisons between studies are difficult, and it is not yet possible to predict response to treatment in individual patients. Some selection factors proposed are early CT changes, National Institutes of Health Stroke Scale score greater than 22, and age older than 77 years. It is important to remember that there may be major discrepancies between patients' and providers' perceptions of functional capabilities and preferences.

TABLE 1.—Criteria for Justification of Medical Interventions

Criterion	Question
Safety	Risks acceptable?
Efficacy	Can it work? (net benefit in ideal conditions)
Effectiveness	Will it work? (net benefit in routine conditions)
Efficiency	Is it worth it? (net benefit versus net cost)
Outcome	Are benefits proportional to risk?
	Informed consent

Note: Modified from Schwartz JS: Clinical economics and noncoronary vascular disease. *J Vasc Interv Radiol* 6:1165–1245, 1995.

(Courtesy of Furlan AJ, Kanoti G: When is thrombolysis justified in patients with acute ischemic stroke?: A bioethical perspective. *Stroke* 28:214–218, 1997. Reproduced with permission [*Stroke*]. Copyright 1997, American Heart Association.)

Conclusions.—No stroke thrombolysis regimen has met all proposed criteria for justification of medical interventions. Without data from trials that have precisely identified important subgroups and contain cost-efficiency analyses, there is no clear answer to the question of when the increased risk of hemorrhage and death justifies thrombolysis treatment for patients with acute ischemic stroke.

▶ This article should make those enthusiastic about thrombolysis in the context of stroke pause in their enthusiasm. I reproduce the table here because it is a handy summary of the criteria that any therapy should meet. Thrombolysis in acute stroke is a good example of an area in which too much of the evidence is disease-oriented rather than patient-oriented. There are no data showing that the treatment works and is safe and effective in typical practice settings in typical patients. Further, there are no data at all on patients' preferences—a key variable. These factors add up to a recommendation not to use the treatment until more data are available and patient preferences can be determined.

A.O. Berg, M.D., M.P.H.

European Stroke Prevention Study 2. Dipyridamole and Acetylsalicylic Acid in the Secondary Prevention of Stroke
Diener HC, Cunha L, Forbes C, et al (Univ of Essen, Germany; Hospitais da Universidade de Coimbra, Portugal; Ninewells Hosp, Dundee, Scotland; et al)
J Neurol Sci 143:1–13, 1996   12–4

Background.—The European Stroke Prevention Study, first published in 1987, showed that combined treatment with dipyridamole and acetylsalicylic acid (ASA) reduced secondary stroke by 38% compared with placebo in patients with prior stroke or transient ischemic attack (TIA). This was a markedly greater reduction than achieved with ASA alone. The second European Stroke Prevention Study determined the efficacy of dipyridamole and ASA alone for preventing secondary stroke, whether combined treatment is better than each agent alone, and whether low-dose ASA (50 mg/day) eliminates the propensity to induce bleeding.

Methods.—Data were obtained from 6,602 patients. The primary end points were stroke, death, and the combination of stroke and death. Secondary end points were TIA and other vascular events. Treatment and follow-up was continued for 2 years.

Findings.—In a factorial analysis, ASA and dipyridamole alone significantly reduced the risk of stroke and stroke or death combined. Compared with placebo, stroke risk was reduced by 18% with ASA alone, 16% with dipyridamole alone, and 37% with combined treatment. The risk of stroke or death was decreased by 13%, 15%, and 24% with ASA alone, dipyridamole alone, and combined treatment, respectively. Treatment did not significantly affect death rate alone. Dipyridamole and ASA also signifi-

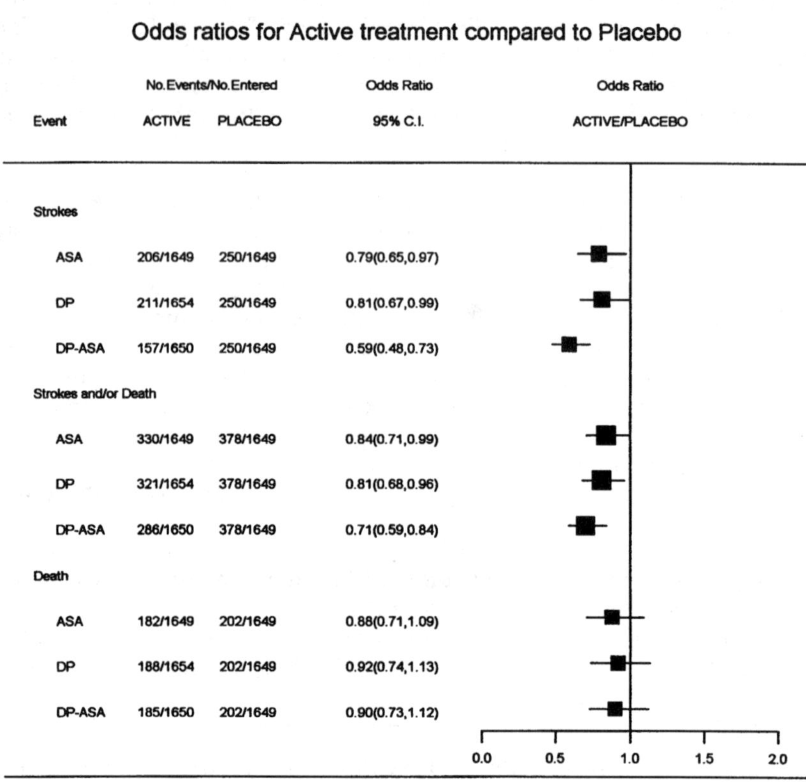

FIGURE 2.—Odds ratios and 95% confidence intervals for the effect of active treatment vs. placebo on the principal endpoints: stroke, stroke or death, and death. (Courtesy of Diener HC, Cunha L, Forbes C, et al: European Stroke Prevention Study 2: Dipyridamole and acetylsalicylic acid in the secondary prevention of stroke. *J Neurol Sci* 143:1–13, 1996.)

cantly prevented TIA. Compared with placebo, combined treatment reduced the risk by 36%. The most common adverse event was headache, occurring more often in patients receiving dipyridamole. Patients receiving ASA had significantly more common instances of all-site bleeding and GI bleeding (Fig 2).

Conclusions.—The efficacy of ASA, 25 mg twice daily, and modified-release dipyridamole, 200 mg twice daily, is equal in the secondary prevention of ischemic stroke and TIA. When prescribed together, the protective effects are additive. Combined treatment is significantly more effective than treatment with either agent alone. Low-dose ASA does not eliminate the propensity for induced bleeding.

▶ This is an excellent study with several clinically useful messages, all graphically summarized in Figure 2. First, aspirin in low dosage works well in secondary prevention. Second, for those who cannot tolerate aspirin, dipyridamole works equally well. Third, the combination works best of all. Keep the relative risk reductions in perspective, though. A 13% reduction in risk for stroke or death in the aspirin-treated group translates into an absolute risk reduction of about 3%, or number needed to treat of about 34. In other words, you would need to treat 34 patients with aspirin alone to prevent 1 stroke or death. Numbers needed to treat for dipyridamole alone and for the combination are 25 and 18, respectively. I think the main clinical question is whether this study provides sufficient evidence to make prescribing the combination routine. I would say it certainly makes it clinically acceptable, although the cost will be very high compared to that with aspirin alone.

A.O. Berg, M.D., M.P.H.

Reductase Inhibitor Monotherapy and Stroke Prevention
Crouse JR III, Byington RP, Hoen HM, et al (Bowman Gray School of Medicine, Winston-Salem, NC)
Arch Intern Med 157:1305–1310, 1997   12–5

Objective.—Although epidemiologic studies have not established a link between hypercholesterolemia and stroke, these investigations have not examined the effect of using reductase inhibitors. Results of a meta-analysis of the effect of reducing cholesterol levels on stroke in all reported clinical trials (4 primary and 8 secondary) using reductase inhibitor monotherapy were presented.

Methods.—Eight studies used pravastatin, 3 used lovastatin, and 1 used simvastatin monotherapy. The effect of reductase inhibitor therapy on stroke incidence was estimated using the Mantel-Haenszel test. The logical regression models used gave similar results. Event rate and risk reduction estimates were calculated.

Results.—During the 88,647 person-years of follow up in these trials, there were 430 strokes. The use of reductase inhibitors significantly decreased stroke in both primary and secondary trials by 27%. An analysis of the secondary trials only, showed a 31% reduction in stroke with the use of reductase inhibitors. A similar analysis of the primary trials showed a 15% reduction.

Conclusion.—Reducing cholesterol levels with reductase inhibitor monotherapy in patients with hypercholesterolemia and coronary artery disease reduces the incidence of stroke.

▶ The relationship of stroke to cholesterol has been enigmatic. First, we know strokes are related to atherosclerosis, often in the carotid arteries. Given this, it seems that stroke should be associated with hypercholesterolemia. However, most major trials have found little relationship between the occurrence of stroke and high cholesterol values but have found a strong relationship of stroke to blood pressure. This study is a meta-analysis of all studies using monotherapy with a statin and presenting data on stroke incidence. Statins generally lower low-density lipoprotein (LDL) cholesterol more than other treatments do, and if there is some benefit to lowering LDL cholesterol, it may be more obvious in this type of study.

The results indicate a substantial reduction in rate of strokes, more so in the secondary than in the primary prevention trials. Of note, these trials were not designed specifically for strokes but were for coronary artery disease. However, lowering the rate of strokes is 1 more reason to treat hypercholesterolemia aggressively.

M.A. Bowman, M.D., M.P.A.

"Gourmand Syndrome": Eating Passion Associated With Right Anterior Lesions

Regard M, Landis T (Univ Hosp, Zurich, Switzerland; Hôpital Cantonal Universitaire de Genève, Switzerland)
Neurology 48:1185–1190, 1997

12–6

Objective.—Eating disorders can arise from a variety of causes. The "gourmand syndrome," a consequence of focal lesions of the right anterior cerebral hemisphere, is described.

Case 1.—A right-handed man, 48, with high blood pressure, non-insulin dependent diabetes mellitus, and chronic smoker's bronchitis, had left hemiparesis resulting from a hemorrhagic infarction of the right middle cerebral artery including the basal ganglia. Before injury, although slightly overweight, the patient was an average eater with no food preferences. His writings in the hospital were filled with thoughts of food. After his release, he was interested only in conversations about food, often left home to eat in restaurants, and gained 3 kg in 1 year.

Case 2.—An ambidextrous man, 55, was hospitalized for headache, which was caused by a hemorrhage in the right anterior basal ganglia. After his left hemiplegia recovered, he made sexual advances to the nurses, ate goodies constantly, and had impaired figural memory and fluency. Before injury, he was an active, fit businessman. After injury he wrote almost solely of food. Although he resumed his normal activities after his release, he was less engaged in them. He talked about food often and dined out frequently.

Methods.—A prospective study found that the characteristics of the "gourmand syndrome" were normal hunger and satisfaction signals with distinctive food preferences, preoccupation with food and eating, a single cerebral lesion, syndrome onset with lesion, absence of the medical or social triggers, and no previous history of eating disorders.

Results.—Thirty-six of 723 patients with known or suspected single cerebral lesions had "gourmand syndrome." Fourteen were women, 35 were right-handed. Ages ranged from 15 to 77. All had focal right-sided damage, and most had left-sided hemisyndromes. Twelve had abnormal mental status. Most had visual-spatial dysfunctions, 26 had impaired memory, 24 had impaired learning and recall of figures. Lesions were caused by tumors in 14 patients, strokes in 12, focal seizures in 8, and head trauma in 2. The eating disorder was strongly associated with damage in the right anterior part of the brain involving the basal and limbic areas.

Conclusion.—Lesion localization is the primary cause of the "gourmand syndrome," a preoccupation with food and eating.

▶ This article caused quite a stir among immediate acquaintances, with concern that some might have had subclinical cerebrovascular events leading to their perfectly obvious obsession with good food. Actually, the message for me in this article is not so much about poststroke interest in food, but rather that this documents a subtle behavioral change with an organic/structural substrate in the poststroke patient. All of us have had patients with strokes who develop odd behavioral characteristics in the post-stroke interval. I also have had patients with transient ischemic attacks (who I did not think had completed strokes) who experienced subtle behavioral or personality change. Is it possible that subclinical cerebrovascular events might cause more behavioral or personality change than we have recognized?

A.O. Berg, M.D., M.P.H.

Migraine Headache

Intranasal Lidocaine for Treatment of Migraine: A Randomized, Double-blind, Controlled Trial
Maizels M, Scott B, Cohen W, et al (Southern California Permanente Med Group, Woodland Hills, Calif)
JAMA 276:319–321, 1996   12–7

Introduction.—Current therapies for migraine have a slow onset and unpredictable absorption, and may cause adverse effects. A recent open-label study reported that intranasal lidocaine provided rapid and complete pain relief in 52% of patients. The efficacy of intranasal lidocaine in the treatment of acute migraine was evaluated in a prospective, double-blind study.

Methods.—Eligible patients were older than 18 years, met the criteria of the International Headache Society for migraine with or without aura, and sought outpatient therapy for a headache of at least moderate intensity. Patients rated the baseline level of their headache, nausea, and photophobia on a scale of 0 to 10. A similar rating was completed immediately after treatment and 2, 5, 10, and 15 minutes later. Clinical disability also was rated by the patients, using a scale of 0 (normal function) to 3 (bed rest required). Patients were randomly assigned in a 2:1 ratio to receive intranasal lidocaine (a 4% solution of topical lidocaine) or placebo (normal saline).

Results.—Ninety-one patients completed the protocol—57 in the lidocaine group and 34 in the placebo group. Study criteria were fully met by 53 patients randomly assigned to receive lidocaine and 28 assigned to receive placebo. The 2 groups were comparable in all pre-treatment characteristics. Within 5 minutes of instilling the lidocaine drops, patients in the active treatment group experienced significant relief of headache pain, nausea, and photophobia. Complete or nearly complete headache relief was achieved in 21% of the lidocaine group versus 7% of the placebo group. Rescue medication was required by 28% of the lidocaine group versus 71% of the control group. No headache characteristic predicted a response to intranasal lidocaine. Adverse local effects, observed almost exclusively in the lidocaine group, included burning or numbness in the nose, eye, and/or throat and an unpleasant taste.

Discussion.—Intranasal lidocaine was effective in providing rapid relief of pain in about 55% of patients seeking therapy for migraine at an urgent care department. Nausea and photophobia also were relieved, usually within 5 minutes. Intranasal lidocaine appears to have an effect on the sphenopalatine ganglion, a possible causative site of cluster headache and link with the trigeminal system.

▶ This article reports a rare placebo-controlled trial; most such trials compare 1 drug of more-or-less known effectiveness to a new drug. The percentage of patients who benefited from the intranasal lidocaine (55%) is comparable to the percentage who benefit from other standard treatments, although one would need a direct comparison trial to determine whether lidocaine was more or less effective. The quick onset of action is a real advantage, but the short duration of action is a just-as-important disadvantage. Still, the rapid relief experienced by some patients might be worth a try while the longer-acting and more established treatments take effect. Until specific sequential regimens are actually tested, however, I would file this one away for the future.

A.O. Berg, M.D., M.P.H.

A Double-blind Study of Subcutaneous Dihydroergotamine vs Subcutaneous Sumatriptan in the Treatment of Acute Migraine

Winner P, Ricalde O, Le Force B, et al (Palm Beach Headache Ctr, West Palm Beach, Fla; Keesler Med Ctr, Keesler Air Force Base, Miss; Lackland Med Ctr, Lackland Air Force Base, Tex; et al)
Arch Neurol 53:180–184, 1996   12–8

Background.—Serotonin receptor binding is believed to be the main mechanism in migraine relief. Dihydroergotamine mesylate (DHE-45) and sumatriptan succinate both work in this way. However, there have been no published studies comparing these 2 agents. The effects of subcutaneous DHE-45 and sumatriptan on initial and persistent pain relief in patients with migraine were compared in a multicenter, double-blind trial.

Methods.—By random assignment, patients with moderate or severe head pain received 1 mg of subcutaneous DHE-45 or 6 mg of subcutaneous sumatriptan. The patients rated head pain, functional ability, nausea, and vomiting at baseline and at 0.5, 1, 2, 4, and 24 hours after administration. A second injection of the same medication was administered if pain persisted after 2 hours, and self-ratings were obtained 0.5 and 1 hour later.

Findings.—Two hundred ninety-five patients were evaluable. Pain relief at 2 hours was documented in 73.1% of the patients given DHE-45 and in 85.3% of those given sumatriptan. Headache relief at 3 and 4 hours did not differ significantly between groups. At 24 hours, 89.7% of those given DHE-45 and 76.7% of those given sumatriptan had relief. Headache recurred within 24 hours after treatment in 45% of the sumatriptan group and in 17.7% of the DHE-45 group. No serious adverse effects occurred with either drug.

Conclusions.—Both DHE-45 and sumatriptan effectively alleviate the initial pain of migraine headache. Although sumatriptan had a faster onset of relief, by 3 hours the 2 agents were equally effective. The relief attained with DHE-45 was more sustained, with significantly less headache recurrence. With both agents, efficacy did not require concomitant anti-emetic administration.

▶ This was a fair head-to-head contest between a relatively new drug (sumatriptan) and an old one administered in a new way (DHE). The randomized, controlled design is everything one would wish to see, although I am always nervous when the drug that comes out ahead happens to be the one made by the company that put up the money for the study (Sandoz). The fact that the 2 treatments were roughly equivalent (DHE was a little slower) in the first few hours was surprising because all one hears nowadays is about the "superiority" of sumatriptan. The DHE group also had slightly more nausea requiring treatment. But the second surprise was the significant difference in recurrence in 24 hours, with the sumatriptan-treated group experiencing 2.5 times the recurrences in the DHE group (see Fig 2 in the original article). This study gives the family physician and the patient more to work with in managing migraines—2 efficacious treatments with slightly different effectiveness profiles initially and at 24 hours, and slightly different side effects. Cost also might be a factor. Patient preference should be strongly supported on all counts.

A.O. Berg, M.D., M.P.H.

Hypotension and Syncope

Syncope: The Diagnostic Value of Head-up Tilt Testing
Oribe E, Caro S, Perera R, et al (City Univ of New York)
PACE 20:874–879, 1997
12–9

Background.—Neurally mediated syncope (NMS), a common cause of unexplained syncope, is characterized by a sudden decrease in sympathetic vasoconstrictor outflow along with an increase in parasympathetic activity, resulting in vasodilation and relative bradycardia. Accurately diagnosing NMS by history alone is often difficult. The value of the passive head-up tilt test in the diagnosis of NMS was investigated.

Methods and Findings.—Two hundred one patients with a history of syncope of unknown cause and 102 control subjects matched by age and sex underwent a 40-minute 60-degree head-up tilt test. Head-up tilt elicited syncope in 37% of the patients with a history of unexplained syncope, compared to 6% of the control subjects. In patients 60 years of age and older, the test had a 100% specificity. The patients said that the symptoms experienced during tilt-induced syncope were similar to those experienced during spontaneous episodes. All 80 subjects with tilt-induced syncope recovered without complication. A positive response to head-up tilt had a positive predictive value of 93% and a negative predictive value of 43%.

Conclusions.—The prolonged head-up tilt test is very specific and highly diagnostic in patients with a history of unexplained syncope. This test is especially useful in elderly patients with a high incidence of syncope.

▶ The workup of a patient with new onset syncope frequently provides no initial demonstrable cause. These authors took 201 patients with a history of syncope of unknown cause and matched them with 100 age- and gender-matched healthy controls. They studied the prognostic value of a simple head-up tilt test. The patient was placed supine for 20 minutes, and once blood pressure and heart rate had stabilized, the patients were passively tilted to a 60-degree head-up position in 15 seconds. A positive test result was defined as hypotension, slowing of heart rate, and/or symptoms of decreased cerebral perfusion. The authors described these as positive signs for NMS.

It certainly is not surprising that you would find a higher number of positive head-up tilt tests in a patient population with known syncope when compared to controls without syncope. However, the authors found a specificity greater than 90% for a positive tilt test with a lower sensitivity of approximately 37%. Because the test has little risk to the patient in a controlled situation, it can be very helpful in diagnosing an autonomic nervous system dysfunction leading to syncope.

R.C. Davidson, M.D., M.P.H.

Syncope in Children and Adolescents

Driscoll DJ, Jacobsen SJ, Porter C-BJ, et al (Mayo Clinic and Found, Rochester, Minn)

J Am Coll Cardiol 29:1039–1045, 1997

12–10

Background.—Syncope is a common and usually benign problem in adolescence. However, sometimes it signals a dangerous problem. There have been no population-based studies of syncope in children and adolescents. The incidence and outcomes of syncope in children and adolescents

TABLE 3.—Attending Physicians' Diagnoses After Initial Evaluation of Incident Syncopal Events

	1950 to 1954 (n = 43)		1987 to 1991 (n = 151)		Total (n = 194)		p Value*
	No.	%	No.	%	No.	%	
Simple faint	21	49	44	29	65	34	0.016
Vasodepressor/vasovagal	6	14	61	40	67	35	0.001
Hysteria psychogenic	1	2	3	2	4	2	1.00
Breathholding	0	0	6	4	6	3	0.34
Concurrent infectious disease	1	2	3	2	4	2	0.89
Possible epilepsy	6	14	3	2	9	5	0.001
Syncope	3	7	6	4	9	5	0.41
Orthostatic	1	2	2	1	3	2	0.64
Hyperventilation	1	2	1	1	2	1	0.34
Hypoglycemia	0	0	3	2	3	2	0.35
Unknown	6	14	6	4	12	6	0.017
Other†	4	9	22	15	28	13	0.37

Note: Incident event was the first syncopal episode brought to medical attention.

*P value for test of difference between time periods.

†Includes, among other diagnoses, chest pain, sunburn, exhaustion, dysmenorrhea, medication-related condition, vertigo, trauma, dehydration, stress, alcohol-related condition.

(Reprinted with permission from the American College of Cardiology, courtesy of Driscoll DJ, Jacobsen SJ, Porter C-BJ, et al: Syncope in children and adolescents. *J Am Coll Cardiol* 29:1039–1045, 1997.)

from 1 to 22 years of age was evaluated. Changes over time in the evaluation of pediatric syncope and the charges for such evaluation were studied as well.

Methods.—Children and adolescents with syncope were identified by data from the Rochester Epidemiology Project. This population-based data base supplied information to evaluate the incidence and outcomes of the problem of pediatric syncope. Two groups of patients—1 seeking medical attention for syncope in the 1950s and another seen in the late 1980s and early 1990s—were studied. Changes in the patterns of evaluation and charges for evaluation between these 2 periods were assessed.

Findings.—In the initial cohort, the incidence of syncope leading to medical attention was 71.9/100,000 population. In the later cohort, the incidence rose to 125.8/100,000. Females were more likely to have syncope than males. The incidence peaked at 15 to 19 years of age. The most frequent diagnoses were simple fainting and vasodepressor or vasovagal syncope (Table 3).

The syncope was related to acute illness in about one fourth of cases and to noxious stimuli in one fourth. The long-term survival of patients with syncope was similar to that of the general population. However, in 1 child with syncope, sudden death resulted, and another had hereditary prolonged QT interval syndrome. These and 4 other patients had syncope related to exertion. Although evaluation charges were comparable for the 2 cohorts, related charges were greater in the latter cohort ($289/patient vs. $77/patient) (Table 4).

TABLE 4.—Laboratory and Clinical Tests Performed During Initial Evaluation of Incident Syncopal Events

| | 1950 to 1954 (n = 43) | | | 1987 to 1991 (n = 151) | | | |
| | Patients Tested | | Tests Performed | Patients Tested | | Test Performed | p Value* |
	No.	%	No.	No.	%	No.	
CBC	13	30	13	63	42	76	0.22
Glucose	4	9	4	48	32	67	0.003
Electrolytes	0	0	0	48	32	67	0.000001
Urinalysis	15	35	15	31	21	40	0.07
ECG	1	2	1	35	23	37	0.001
24-h ECG	0	0	0	10	7	10	0.12
Echocardiogram	0	0	0	4	3	4	0.58
Tilt table	0	0	0	1	1	1	1.00
Electrophysiologic study	0	0	0	1	1	1	1.00
Exercise test	0	0	0	1	1	1	1.00
Electroencephalogram	6	14	6	27	18	28	0.65
CT scan	0	0	0	22	15	26	0.005
Skull radiograph	8	19	8	15	10	17	0.18
Other	24	56	24	79	52	104	0.73
Total tests			71			479	

Note: Initial evaluation included all tests performed within the first 6 months after the initial medical visit for syncope. Incident event was the first syncopal episode brought to medical attention.

*P value for test of difference in proportion of patients tested between time periods.

Abbreviation: CBC, complete blood count.

(Reprinted with permission from the American College of Cardiology, courtesy of Driscoll DJ, Jacobsen SJ, Porter C-BJ, et al: Syncope in children and adolescents. *J Am Coll Cardiol* 29:1039–1045, 1997.)

Conclusion.—Syncope is a common problem in children and adolescents and does not usually herald a serious problem. Patients with exercise-related syncope are more likely to have a potentially life-threatening condition. Certain factors should prompt a detailed evaluation: exercise-related syncope or a family history of syncope, sudden death, myocardial disease, or arrhythmias. An ECG may be considered for all patients with syncope.

▶ This is one of the more interesting articles I have reviewed for the YEAR BOOK OF FAMILY PRACTICE. Its purpose was to evaluate the incidence and etiology of syncope in children and adolescents. This it did by comparing 2 populations separated by more than 30 years. The causes of syncope in these 2 populations were remarkably similar. About 70% of incidences of both populations were attributed to either a simple faint or a vasovagal reaction. Both of these conditions are considered benign.

What was more interesting to me were the results displayed in Table 4. Even though the outcomes and causes in the 2 populations were very similar, the number of tests performed to evaluate these patients varied significantly. Studying these data reminds us why the cost of medicine continues to go up and why, with managed care, we are faced with prior authorization and other utilization management techniques designed to reduce our use of tests.

R.C. Davidson, M.D., M.P.H.

Efficacy of Midodrine Vs Placebo in Neurogenic Orthostatic Hypotension: A Randomized, Double-blind Multicenter Study

Low PA, for the Midodrine Study Group (Mayo Clinic, Rochester, Minn)
JAMA 277:1046–1051, 1997   12–11

Introduction.—Autonomic neuropathies, such as those of diabetes and amyloidosis, can cause neurogenic orthostatic hypotension, probably the most devastating of the manifestations of generalized autonomic failure. The United States Food and Drug Administration recently approved midodrine hydrochloride for use in treating orthostatic hypotension. An α-agonist, midodrine activates α-1 receptors on arterioles and veins to increase total peripheral resistance and to reduce orthostatic hypotension. A double-blind, randomized multicenter study compared placebo with midodrine for neurogenic orthostatic hypotension.

Methods.—In a 6-week study, 171 patients were randomized to placebo or a 10-mg dose of midodrine 3 times per day. At week 1, there was a single-blind run-in, and there was a washout at weeks 5 and 6. During weeks 2 to 4, there was an intervening double-blind period. Measurements were taken of standing systolic blood pressure, global symptom relief score, and symptoms of lightheadedness.

Results.—During all time points, midodrine resulted in improvements in standing systolic blood pressure. There was an improvement in reported symptoms by the end of the second week of treatment with midodrine. During the entire period, there was a major improvement in lightheadedness over baseline. There was also improvement in the global symptom relief score with midodrine as rated by the investigator and the patient. No effect was seen by use of fludrocortisone or compression garments, diagnosis, or severity of orthostatic hypotension. Supine hypertension, urinary retention, and pilomotor reactions were the main adverse effects.

Conclusion.—Midodrine is efficacious and safe in the treatment of neurogenic orthostatic hypotension. Nocturnal hypertension was avoided by avoiding midodrine after 6 p.m.

▶ The definition of neurogenic hypotension used here does not give the reader a lot to work with, but I expect it would cover many patients for whom another organic cause is not identified. Midodrine is now United States Food and Drug Administration–approved for orthostatic hypotension. This carefully designed study shows that it works and is reasonably well tolerated, although the midodrine group did have side effects. Interestingly, a number of the midodrine-treated patients elected to continue the drug after the trial was completed, despite the side effects, indicating that the benefits were worth it. The benefits were statistically and clinically apparent (see Fig 3 in the original article). This is a treatment worth trying in symptomatic patients.

A.O. Berg, M.D., M.P.H.

Miscellaneous

Rapid Clinical Evaluation of Anosmia: The Alcohol Sniff Test

Davidson TM, Murphy C (Univ of California, San Diego; San Diego State Univ, Calif)

Arch Otolaryngol Head Neck Surg 123:591–594, 1997   12–12

Objective.—Loss of smell affects 1% to 2% of Americans. The alcohol sniff test (AST) is a simple test of olfactory function. The ability of AST to discriminate between patients with anosmia or hyposmia and persons with normal function, estimating the correlation of AST results with results of other tests, and estimating the reliability of the AST are discussed.

Methods.—The AST was administered to 64 patients (32 males), average age 47, and 36 controls (19 males), average age 47. The patient, with mouth and eyes closed, is asked to breathe normally and indicate when the odor from a standard 70% isopropyl alcohol on a preparation pad is detected. The pad is held 30 cm below the nose and moved 1 cm closer with each expiration until the odor is detected. The test is repeated 4 times. Results were compared with the standard butanol olfactory threshold test.

Results.—The AST threshold values (in cm) were significantly lower for patients than for controls. Repeated tests showed no significant variation. Because neurodegenerative diseases can impair olfactory sensation, olfactory testing may be useful in detecting Alzheimer's disease, Parkinson's disease, Huntington's disease, and HIV. The test may also prove useful in discovering nutritional problems in the elderly that result from lack of aroma-based appetite stimulation.

Conclusion.—The AST is an effective screening test for anosmia and hyposmia.

▶ This article fills an important gap in neurological testing of cranial nerves in a way that is useful to primary care physicians. The test is simple and reproducible. It looks to me like the test will be best at discriminating between the anosmic and normosmic, and that a score of 10 would be a pretty good cut-off (a lower score indicates trouble). In order to reduce time needed for the test, the authors suggest a single presentation as a screen: if patients detect the odor at 10 cm, they are unlikely to have a serious olfactory deficiency.

A.O. Berg, M.D., M.P.H.

13 Eye Conditions

Introduction

Three articles comprise this short chapter, providing near–population-based data on contact lens complications, a comprehensive study of visual impairment in older adults, and the slightly increased risk of ocular hypertension in open-angle glaucoma in individuals taking high-dose inhaled glucocorticoids.

Alfred O. Berg, M.D., M.P.H.

A Prospective Study of Contact Lens Complications in a Managed Care Setting
Keech PM, Ichikawa L, Barlow W (Group Health Cooperative of Puget Sound, Seattle; Univ of Washington, Seattle)
Optom Vis Sci 73:653–658, 1996

13–1

Introduction.—Contact lens complications are fairly common, particularly among users of extended wear soft lenses. Even minor complications can be a significant factor in long-range eye health and represent a major cost and inconvenience to the wearer. In the managed care setting, knowledge of factors contributing to contact lens–related complications could aid in prescribing decisions. A prospective study measured the prevalence of complications in a large group of primary care patients.

Methods.—Over 1 month, 11 optometrists at 8 locations reported the prevalence of anterior segment conditions associated with contact lens wear. Only a small minority (less than 5%) of patients seen in these practices require specialty lens services. Demographic and clinical data were collected for patients wearing contact lenses at the time of the visit. A total of 1,496 patient visits were evaluated.

Results.—Most of the patients wore rigid gas permeable (RGP) or conventional soft lenses (38% and 32%, respectively). Approximately 40% of patients had 1 or more anterior segment complications. One fourth of these patients, or 10% of the entire group of contact lens wearers, had complications classified as serious. Such complications required refitting or discontinuation of contact lens use, with follow-up visits to resolve the problem. Complications most frequently encountered were superficial punctate staining (17.3%) and neovascularization (11.4%).

The prevalence of complications was lower with RGP lens wear and disposable soft lens wear. Factors associated with a higher prevalence of complications included an extended wearing time beyond 3 days, greater lens age, and use of inappropriate care systems. Serious complications were reduced when a 1–step care system was used.

Conclusion.—In a prepaid managed care system, the deliverer of services shares in the cost of contact lens complications. Thus, the prescriber's recommendations for lens type, wearing schedule, and care system can improve patient outcomes and reduce overall costs.

▶ Debates about the safety of contact lenses (including all the various types) have raged for years, but most studies are fundamentally uninformative because the methods used to select patients have tended to bias the results 1 way or the other. That is why this study is interesting: it comes closer to providing a population-based (and, thus, less biased) estimate of contact lens problems in patients typical of those seen in primary care. The half-full crowd will find the 61% prevalence of normality reassuring, whereas the half-empty group will find the 39% abnormal prevalence alarming. By any standard, this study shows that objective findings are very common among contact lens wearers, especially in the relatively small subset of extended-wear users. These numbers should be helpful both in counseling patients about likely problems and—for those in large managed care organizations such as the one in this study—helping the organization figure out which patients are at risk and how best to manage them.

A.O. Berg, M.D., M.P.H.

Function and Visual Impairment in a Population-based Study of Older Adults: The SEE Project
West SK, and the SEE Project Team (Wilmer Inst, Baltimore, Md; Johns Hopkins Univ, Baltimore, Md)
Invest Ophthalmol Vis Sci 38:72–82, 1997   13–2

Introduction.—A priority for research on aging is discovering the links between age-related diseases and the various domains of function. Visual impairment has been associated with functional dependence and progression of disabilities. Little is known about how different components of visual function relate specifically to various tasks associated with independent living. The impact of vision on functional status in a population-based sample of elderly people was assessed in the Salisbury Eye Evaluation (SEE) project.

Methods.—A random sample of 2,520 elderly people between the ages of 65 and 84 years underwent home interviews and SEE clinic examinations. During SEE clinical examination, binocular visual acuity was measured using Early Treatment Diabetic Retinopathy Study charts and protocols. The questionnaire included questions regarding activities of daily living, instrumental activities of daily living, physical function, social interaction, and activities of daily vision. Presenting visual acuity worse than 20/40, not best-corrected visual acuity, was used to reflect the acuity participants actually had while trying to accomplish activities.

Results.—A decline was observed with age in all measures of functional status. Females and blacks were the most likely groups to report problems. The age-adjusted proportions of research subjects with visual impairment were similar in males and females. Blacks had almost twice the rate of visual impairment as whites (10.4% vs. 5.6%). Declines in functional status were all significantly related to age, race, and gender.

Conclusions.—Data from the SEE project was similar to earlier findings in the United States population, based on the sample selected for the National Health Interview Survey 1986 Functional Limitations Supplement. Binocular visual acuity worse than 20/40 seemed to have an impact on all self-report measures of functional status. Further investigations regarding the interaction of vision with other comorbid conditions on functional status are needed.

▶ Function, function, function. The cornerstone of caring for the elderly. Sometimes the questions we should be asking are quite basic: "Are you having any difficulty with your vision?" The results of this study do not surprise me. On reflection, though, I am chagrined to admit that I probably have been remiss in giving only cursory attention to screening for this. A decline in visual acuity as we age is common and somewhat taken for granted. The authors convincingly demonstrate that this decline is strongly associated with declining functional status. Their results echo findings from other sizeable studies that have reported a significant impact on functional status and well-being from decreased visual acuity.[1] Once again, causality is not proven, and the authors suggest future studies look at outcomes of interventions to address vision loss in the elderly. No argument here, however—more aggressive screening and intervention make a lot of sense. The future for this, I think, is now.

W.W. Dexter, M.D.

Reference

1. Lee PP, Spritzer K, Hays RD: The impact of blurred vision on functioning and well-being. *Ophthalmology* 104:390–396, 1997.

Inhaled and Nasal Glucocorticoids and the Risks of Ocular Hypertension or Open-angle Glaucoma
Garbe E, LeLorier J, Boivin JF, et al (McGill Univ, Montreal; Royal Victoria Hosp, Montreal; Université de Montreal)
JAMA 277:722–727, 1997   13–3

Purpose.—Topical corticosteroids permit the therapeutic benefits of corticosteroids while reducing the adverse effects. However, as higher doses of inhaled and nasal steroids are prescribed, there is growing concern about the possibility of systemic adverse effects. Two recent case reports have suggested that ocular hypertension and open-angle glaucoma may occur in patients taking inhaled and nasal glucocorticoids. A case-control study was performed to evaluate this risk.

Methods.—The study used data on elderly patients from a Canadian universal health insurance data base. The case patients were 9,793 ophthalmology patients who had newly diagnosed borderline or open-angle glaucoma or started a new course of treatment for ocular hypertension or glaucoma between 1988 and 1994. The control patients were a random sample of 38,325 patients making ophthalmologist visits in the same month and year as the case patients. Conditional logistic regression analysis was used to evaluate the odds ratio (OR) of ocular hypertension or open-angle glaucoma among users vs. nonusers of inhaled or nasal glucocorticoids. Adjustments were made for other factors, such as age, sex, diabetes mellitus, systemic hypertension, use of ophthalmic and oral glucocorticoids, and pattern of health system utilization.

Results.—In general, users of inhaled and nasal glucocorticoids were not at increased risk for ocular hypertension or open-angle glaucoma. However, patients who had used high doses of inhaled corticosteroids for 3 months or longer ($n = 21$) were at significantly increased risk (OR 1.44). Risk was not increased for continuous users of low- to medium-dose inhaled steroids.

Conclusions.—The risk for ocular hypertension or open-angle glaucoma is increased in patients taking high doses of inhaled corticosteroids for an extended period. These patients may be candidates for intraocular pressure monitoring. Patients with newly diagnosed ocular hypertension and open-angle glaucoma should be asked about their use of inhaled steroids.

▶ Like many others, I embrace the recommendation that inhaled steroids be utilized as the cornerstone anti-inflammatory in asthma therapy. I have concomitantly increased my utilization of nasal steroids. This large-scale, epidemiologic study has some limitations but is, on balance, quite believable. It leads us to a good news–bad news situation. These drugs are quite beneficial but with potential flaws, one of which is a risk of ocular hypertension or open-angle glaucoma, but only with prolonged high-dose utilization. Fortunately, we can screen for this disorder. You should probably find a place for monitoring of ocular pressures in your flow sheets on your patients using these drugs regularly, particularly in high doses.

W.W. Dexter, M.D.

14 Pediatrics

Introduction

Two articles on infant colic open the chapter, including a politically incorrect (but possibly effective) suggestion to use sucrose, and a study showing that family problems persist after the symptoms subside. Sudden infant death syndrome is addressed in the 2 articles that follow on its relationship to smoking and an international comparison study discussing risk. A rare (and successful) randomized trial of a violence-prevention curriculum and a study of the effects of spending time with kids on family structure close the chapter.

Randomized controlled trial: Abstract 14–5.

Alfred O. Berg, M.D., M.P.H.

Infant Colic

Use of Sucrose as a Treatment for Infant Colic
Markestad T (Univ of Bergen, Norway)
Arch Dis Child 76:356–358, 1997   14–1

Introduction.—Uncertainty about the causes of infant colic has led to a wide range of treatment approaches. Previous studies have demonstrated an analgesic effect of sucrose in newborns. Sucrose was tested for its effects on infant colic.

Methods.—The study included 19 infants with typical colic, defined as at least 3 hours per day of crying for 3 days a week for the previous 3 weeks. All infants were 3 weeks to 3 months old. In a double-blind, crossover design, the infants received 2 mL of either 12% sucrose or distilled water when crying. The parents were to give the solutions by syringe while holding the infant in their arms. The effects were measured by parental scoring.

Results.—Twelve of the 19 infants had specific improvement with sucrose, that is, they had consistent improvements with sucrose and relapses with placebo. Most of the remaining infants also improved during the study, but had no consistent response to either solution. Five of the 12 infants who improved on sucrose stopped crying immediately, and 5 of the 12 showed a marked effect of sucrose.

Conclusions.—A 12% solution of sucrose appears to significantly reduce colic in infants. Sucrose seems likely to act through a pain-relieving effect. Sucrose may be tried as a treatment for infant colic; if there is no response within a day or two, the infant is unlikely to respond to future trials.

▶ I include this very small study of 19 infants because the therapeutic options for infant colic are quite limited. In Scandinavia (this study comes from Norway), simple and practical approaches to infant colic have been reported. Sucrose in water is easy to prepare, and it gives the distressed parents another option. Hopefully, a much larger study on this method will be done soon.

J.E. Scherger, M.D., M.P.H.

Family Life 1 Year After Infantile Colic
Räihä H, Lehtonen L, Korhonen T, et al (Turku Univ, Finland)
Arch Pediatr Adolesc Med 150:1032–1036, 1996   14–2

Background.—Infantile colic causes a crisis that may lead to parental depression, anxiety, stress, fatigue, and role ambivalence. The persistence of family psychological characteristics associated with infantile colic was investigated.

Methods.—Fifty-nine families with a colicky infant were surveyed. Data from these families were compared with data on 58 control families. Based on a structured diary of infant crying kept by the parents, 3 groups of families were identified: 36 had severely colicky infants; 23, moderately colic infants; and 58 (the control group), infants without colic. Interviews were conducted when the infants were 2 and 12 months old.

Findings.—The structural profiles of the families did not differ among the groups at 1 year. However, families with severely colicky infants had more problems with communication, more unresolved conflicts, more dissatisfaction, and less empathy than families in the other groups. Less flexibility was noted in both colic groups compared with the control group. During follow-up, coalition between the parents with moderately colicky infants became stronger than in the first assessment, and the atmosphere in all 3 groups improved significantly. However, the amount of empathy declined in families with severely colicky infants.

Conclusion.—Certain family characteristics associated with severe infantile colic persist for at least 1 year. In this study, families with moderately colicky infants coped almost as well as control group families. By the time the infant was 1 year old, the mood in all the families had improved a great deal.

▶ Yes, this is from Finland, so just maybe the situation is different from that in the United States. The authors believe that severe infantile colic continued to affect the family 1 year later. I suspect that the order is wrong. These families were not investigated before the colic and the lack of empathy and greater unresolved conflict may have predated the reporting of severe colic. What do you think?

M.A. Bowman, M.D., M.P.A.

Sudden Infant Death Syndrome

Sudden Infant Death Syndrome and Smoking in the United States and Sweden
MacDorman MF, Cnattingius S, Hoffman HJ, et al (Natl Ctr for Health Statistics, Hyattsville, Md; Univ Hosp, Uppsala, Sweden; NIH, Rockville, Md, et al)
Am J Epidemiol 146:249–257, 1997   14–3

Background.—Many predisposing factors have been reported for sudden infant death syndrome (SIDS), the leading cause of postneonatal death in both the United States and Sweden. Large variations in SIDS rates among U.S. ethnic groups continue to perplex researchers, as does the higher SIDS rate in the United States than in other developed nations, including Sweden.

Methods.—Associations between SIDS and such factors as ethnicity and maternal smoking were studied in the United States and Sweden. These countries differ in health care, social support, and sociocultural homogeneity.

Results.—The SIDS rates in 5 U.S. ethnic groups ranged from a low of 0.8 infant deaths per 1,000 live births among Hispanics, Asians, and Pacific Islanders to a high of 3.0 among Native Americans. In Sweden, the SIDS rate was 0.9. Risk factor prevalences in U.S. ethnic groups only partially explained differences in SIDS rates. The rate of SIDS increased with amount smoked in all U.S. ethnic groups and in Sweden. There was wide variation among groups with respect to percentage of mothers who smoked during pregnancy, with a range from 27% for Swedish mothers down to 5% to 6% for U.S. Asian, Pacific Islander, and Hispanic mothers. Amount smoked also varied considerably. Among U.S. non-Hispanic white women, more than 75% of smokers smoked 10 or more cigarettes per day, vs. less than 40% in Sweden. Independently, birth weight strongly correlated with SIDS rate, but its addition to risk models did little to lower maternal smoking odds ratios. Smoking probably does not increase SIDS risk through birth weight. The groups with the lowest SIDS rates showed the largest risk increases by amount smoked. Higher baseline SIDS rates may include factors not studied, lessening the relative effect of smoking.

Conclusions.—Smoking, a key preventable SIDS risk factor, apparently transcends ethnicity and nationality. Public health programs focusing on preventing and reducing smoking among pregnant women could substantially decrease SIDS rates in all populations.

► This study confirms that smoking is probably the most important risk factor for SIDS. It is also the most controllable risk factor. I found it interesting that the prevalence of smoking among pregnant women is substantially higher in Sweden than it is in the United States. After a legacy of exporting cigarettes, hopefully we will export methods of smoking cessation throughout the world.

J.E. Scherger, M.D., M.P.H.

Do Differences in the Prevalence of Risk Factors Explain the Higher Mortality From Sudden Infant Death Syndrome in New Zealand Compared With the UK?

Mitchell EA, Esmail A, Jones DR, et al (Univ of Auckland, New Zealand; St George's Hosp, England; Univ of Leicester, England)

N Z Med J 109:352–356, 1996　　　　　　　　　　　　　　　14–4

Introduction.—The mortality rate from sudden infant death syndrome (SIDS) is higher in New Zealand than in other comparable countries. Four risk factors for SIDS that are amenable to modification have been identified: prone sleeping position of infant, maternal smoking, lack of breast feeding, and infants' sharing a bed with another person. In 1989, the national mortality rate from SIDS in New Zealand was 4.1/1,000 live births, compared with 1.9/1,000 for the South West Thames (SWT) region of England. The prevalence of major risk factors for SIDS was compared in infants from New Zealand and SWT.

Methods.—Investigation methodologies were nearly identical in New Zealand and SWT. Research subjects were randomly selected from all births in selected study regions from 1987–1990. Parents of research subjects were interviewed and obstetrical records were reviewed.

Results.—Interviews were completed with parents or guardians of 1,592 infants in New Zealand and 511 infants in SWT. In New Zealand, the prevalence of maternal smoking, prone sleeping position, and infants' sharing of beds with another person was higher, compared with SWT. The rate and duration of breast feeding were higher in New Zealand than in SWT. The differences in the prevalence of the modifiable risk factors evaluated were of insufficient magnitudes to explain most of the difference between the SIDS mortality rates in New Zealand and England. The risk of SIDS was more than twice as high for infants in New Zealand, compared with infants in SWT.

Conclusion.—The high SIDS mortality rate in New Zealand cannot be simply explained by a high incidence of known and modifiable risk factors for SIDS.

▶ The causes of SIDS remain controversial. This article underscores the fact that maternal smoking in pregnancy may be the strongest risk factor. The prone sleeping position captures much attention. I have a suggestion as to why the prevalence of SIDS may be higher in New Zealand compared with England. The answer may be the sheep. Anecdotal evidence suggests that infants sleeping on sheepskins—especially in the prone position—are much more likely to have SIDS. Sheepskin and soft down comforters are not as safe as firm mattresses with thin sheets for sleeping infants. As I said, this evidence from New Zealand and Australia is anecdotal and needs confirmation in scientific studies.

J.E. Scherger, M.D., M.P.H.

Miscellaneous

Effectiveness of a Violence Prevention Curriculum Among Children in Elementary School: A Randomized Controlled Trial

Grossman DC, Neckerman HJ, Koepsell TD, et al (Univ of Washington, Seattle; Committee for Children, Seattle)
JAMA 277:1605–1611, 1997   14–5

Objective.—Violence is a growing social problem, and violence in adulthood has been linked to aggressive behavior in childhood. A number of school-based programs designed to teach social skills, conflict resolution, or violence prevention have appeared. However, there have been few studies to show whether these programs actually reduce aggressive or violent behavior. A randomized, controlled trial was done to test a commonly used violence-prevention curriculum for its ability to reduce aggressive behavior and increase prosocial behavior among children.

Methods.—The study was performed in second- and third-grade classrooms at 12 urban and suburban Washington state elementary schools. The sample was 79% white. The schools were randomly assigned in pairs to teach or not teach the popular "Second Step: A Violence Prevention Curriculum," which is designed to promote prosocial behavior and prevent aggressive behavior. Through 30 lessons, the curriculum seeks to teach social skills in several areas, including anger management, impulse control, and empathy. At 2 weeks and 6 months after the intervention, changes in aggressive and prosocial behavior were measured by parent and teacher reports made according to the Achenbach Child Behavior Checklist and Teacher Report Form, the School Social Behavior Scale, and the Parent-Child Rating Scale. In addition, behavioral observations were made of a random sample of 588 children in the classroom and in playground and cafeteria settings.

Results.—The parent and teacher reports showed no significant change in the children's behavior after participation in the "Second Step" curriculum after adjustment for sex, age, socioeconomic status, race, academic performance, household size, and class size. A reduction in physical aggression and an increase in neutral or prosocial behavior was noted at the 2-week observations in the intervention group. Most of the behavioral changes persisted at 6 months.

Conclusions.—Some reduction in physically aggressive behavior and some increase in neutral and prosocial school behavior is noted in grade-school children attending the "Second Step" violence-prevention curriculum. Though some of the improvements continue to be noted at 6 months of follow-up, their impact on behavior outside school is unknown. Violence prevention curricula may need to be supplemented by other interventions—through early childhood and adolescence—to be truly effective in reducing aggressive behavior.

▶ Thank goodness we are focusing some violence-prevention efforts on early education, and that at least someone is trying to evaluate the outcomes. Strengths of this study include the reasonable numbers of subjects and the 3 types of outcome evaluation. Overall, the classes were lengthy. The outcomes were modest and appeared only in the direct observation method, not on teacher or parent report. In general, I believe that only modest outcomes can be expected from any single course; behavior change takes time, repetition (frequently in different settings), and reinforcement. Improving the parents' skills would also allow more direct modeling of behavior. Multiple interventions through time are likely to be needed, but each small step helps and occasionally may result in magnified improvements years later.

M.A. Bowman, M.D., M.P.A.

Spending Time With His Kids: Effects of Family Structure on Fathers' and Children's Lives
Cooksey EC, Fondell MM (Ohio State Univ, Columbus)
J Marriage Fam 58:693–707, 1996   14–6

Background.—Fathers may be either more or less involved in the lives of their children, for a variety of reasons. The type of family structure is one important factor. The effects of family structure on fathers' and children's lives were investigated.

Methods.—The study was limited to men residing with children. A variety of family structures, including both biological fathers and stepfathers, were explored. Data from the National Survey of Families and Households were analyzed to determine how fathers spend time with the children, what encourages them to share activities, and how shared time affects children's welfare.

Findings.—Single fathers are very involved in their children's lives, being more likely to engage in a variety of activities (not related to sharing meals) compared with fathers in more traditional family settings. Fathers married to women who are not the children's biological mother also spend more time with their children than fathers married to the biological mother (although nonsignificantly so). In general, stepfathers are significantly less likely to engage in activities with their stepchildren than are biological fathers. Stepfathers with both biological children and stepchildren are more likely than stepfathers with only stepchildren to behave as other biological fathers do. However, stepfathers with no biological children are more likely than other stepfathers to read to their stepchildren or help them with homework. Family structure and father-child shared activity time were also correlated with children's grades.

Conclusion.—The type of family structure influences the activities that fathers engage in with their children. Family structure and shared activities between fathers and their children are associated with the children's academic achievement, although fathers' time apparently does not mediate the effects of family structure on grades.

▶ For me, the take-home message here is that there is a relationship between the time the father spends with the child and the child's grades in school. In the office, we can encourage father-children interaction. I also think it is interesting that the amount of time spent with the children is unrelated to the amount of time spent working, i.e., this is clearly a matter of priority setting.

M.A. Bowman, M.D., M.P.A.

15 Women's Health

Introduction

Breast cancer opens the chapter, with important articles on risk (physical activity, body mass, and education), a large, randomized clinical trial of breast self-examination (with disappointing results), strategies for mammography screening, what to do about genetic screening, and tantalizing data about the protective effects of tamoxifen therapy.

A substantial selection of articles on hormone replacement therapy and menopause includes both observational and intervention studies on body weight, menopausal symptoms, the effects of alcohol, and risks of venous thromboembolism, postural imbalance, and bone mineral density. Compliance (mediocre) with treatment is the subject of the final article.

The remainder of the chapter is divided into short sections on dysfunctional bleeding, spontaneous abortion (medical approaches to management, and long-term effects on fertility), androgen excess (a diagnostic aid and a treatment), and miscellaneous articles on normal vulvar anatomy, basal body temperature, and vaginal douching (a risk factor for ectopic pregnancy in black women).

Randomized controlled trials: Abstracts 15–4, 15–5, 15–11, 15–12, 15–13, 15–17, and 15–23.

Alfred O. Berg, M.D., M.P.H.

Breast Cancer

Physical Activity and the Risk of Breast Cancer
Thune I, Brenn T, Lund E, et al (Univ of Tromsø Norway; Cancer Registry of Norway, Oslo)
N Engl J Med 336:1269–1275, 1997   15–1

Background.—Physical activity may affect both hormonal concentrations and energy balance and therefore have an effect on risk of breast cancer in women. However, the relationship between energy balance, body-mass index, and energy expenditure on the risk for breast cancer is not well understood. To examine this issue, a cohort of 25,624 premenopausal and postmenopausal women were assessed for level of physical activity and breast cancer development.

Study Design.—From 1974 to 1978, the Norwegian National Health Screening Service invited people in 3 counties to participate in a survey of cardiovascular risk factors. A total of 31,556 women were invited to participate, and 28,621 women participated. These women, plus a random sampling of women aged 20 to 39 years, were invited to participate in a second study from 1977 to 1983. Of the 34,378 women invited, 31,209 women participated. Participants completed questionnaires pertaining to physical activity and food intake and underwent a clinical examination. The participants who completed the questionnaire, 25,624 women who had never been diagnosed with cancer, were followed up through their 11-digit national personal identification numbers to identify any cases of breast cancer reported to the Cancer Registry of Norway and Statistics Norway, through December 1994. There were 359,930 person-years of follow-up.

Results.—During the median follow-up period of 13.7 years, 351 cases of invasive breast cancer were detected among the 25,624 study participants. More physical activity during leisure time was associated with reduced breast cancer risk, after adjustments for age, body-mass index, height, parity, and county of residence. Among women who exercised regularly, the reduction in breast cancer risk was larger among premenopausal women than postmenopausal women, and larger in younger women than in older women. By stratified analysis, the risk of breast cancer was lowest in lean women who exercised at least 4 hours per week. Breast cancer risk was also reduced with increased levels of physical activity at work.

Conclusions.—In a large cohort of women, there was an association between increased levels of physical activity during work or leisure time and reduced risk of breast cancer. This association was stronger for younger, premenopausal women. The greatest protective effect occurred in lean women, which suggests that there may be an optimal energy balance that is inhibitory for mammary carcinogenesis.

▶ The association between increased levels of physical activity and reduced risk of breast cancer seems clear. What is not clear is causality. Should we be telling our patients that they will reduce their risk of breast cancer if they exercise more? I don't believe so. There are too many holes here to make that leap. Particularly striking is the association noted in younger (premenopausal) women, a group that, in my experience, often forgoes exercise as demands of family and career increase. I don't think we can draw any firm conclusions from this study, but I will share this information with my patients as I encourage them to begin or continue an exercise program.

W.W. Dexter, M.D.

Body Mass Index and Post-menopausal Breast Cancer: An Age-specific Analysis
La Vecchia C, Negri E, Franceschi S, et al (Istituto di Ricerche Farmacologiche, Milan, Italy; Università degli Studi di Milano, Milan, Italy; Centro di Riferimento Oncologico, Pordenone, Italy; et al)
Br J Cancer 75:441–444, 1997   15–2

Introduction.—Postmenopausal women who are overweight or obese have an increased risk for breast cancer, the result of elevated levels or availability of circulating estrogens. A pooled analysis of 3 Italian case-control studies was conducted. It examined the age-specific pattern of the relation between body mass index (BMI) and breast cancer risk in postmenopausal women.

Methods.—The 3 studies, published in 1985, 1986, and 1993, included 3,108 postmenopausal patients with breast cancer aged 50 years or older and 2,664 controls. Controls were women who had been hospitalized for conditions that were unrelated to risk factors for breast cancer and to long-term modification of diet. Multiple logistic regression was used to determine odds ratios (ORs) for breast cancer.

Results.—There was a moderate, but significant, association between BMI and postmenopausal breast cancer. The ORs were approximately 1.3 for the 3 intermediate quintiles of BMI, compared with the lowest quintile, and 1.4 for the highest quintile of BMI. The association between BMI and breast cancer was stronger among women 70 years or older (ORs of 1.6 for the fourth and 2.1 for the fifth quintiles) than among women aged 50 to 59 years and 60 to 69 years. The interaction with age proved significant. No relation was observed between height and breast cancer risk in postmenopausal women.

Discussion.—Postmenopausal women who are overweight or obese are at increased risk for breast cancer, and this association becomes stronger with advancing age. Because the incidence of breast cancer increases with age, the risk is even greater for women who are elderly and overweight. A similar age-related pattern of risk has been identified among postmenopausal women receiving hormone replacement therapy. For population-attributable risk, it is estimated that breast cancer in 19.6% of all postmenopausal patients with breast cancer and in 27.1% of those older than 70 years is attributed to excess weight. Controlling weight gain in elderly women can reduce breast cancer risk.

▶ The association between body mass and postmenopausal breast cancer has been observed many times before. This innovative research design pooling cases and controls from several large Italian studies expands our understanding of the relation by examining the effects of age. The findings are persuasive that increased body mass increases the risk of breast cancer the older you are. The findings are both statistically and biologically significant, because a relative risk of 1.6 in the oldest age group (already at high risk because of age alone) is very high indeed. As the authors point out, these findings have potentially important implications for prevention.

A.O. Berg, M.D., M.P.H.

Explaining the Relation Between Education and Postmenopausal Breast Cancer

Heck KE, Pamuk ER (Natl Ctr for Health Statistics, Hyattsville, Md)
Am J Epidemiol 145:366–372, 1997   15–3

Objective.—Studies have found that more highly educated and wealthier women have a higher incidence of breast cancer. The relation between socioeconomic status and development of breast cancer was studied using data from the National Health and Nutrition Examination Survey Epidemiologic Followup Survey.

Methods.—Of the 8,596 women who took part in the National Health and Nutrition Examination Survey, data were available on 229 individuals with breast cancer and 6,032 individuals without. Because of the limited number of premenopausal breast cancer cases, only postmenopausal cases were included in this analysis. Educational level, age at first birth, age at menarche, age at menopause, alcohol use, height, body mass index, family history, use of oral contraceptives, use of estrogen replacement therapy, and family income were compared.

Results.—There was an association between higher education and postmenopausal breast cancer. Women with more education had fewer births, were older at first birth, were more likely to have taken oral contraceptive and hormone replacement therapy, were more likely to have taken 1 drink of alcohol during the past year, and were significantly more likely to have breast cancer develop. Risk of breast cancer was increased for women with no children, women who were older at menopause, those who were taller, and those who had a history of breast cancer. Postmenopausal use of oral contraceptives or hormone replacement therapy did not affect breast cancer risk. Only women at the highest income levels were at increased risk for breast cancer. When these factors were adjusted for, the relation between breast cancer and socioeconomic level was no longer significant.

Conclusion.—The association between socioeconomic level and breast cancer appears to be spurious and can be explained by reproductive factors such as older age at first birth, no children, taller height, older age at menopause, and greater likelihood of having used oral contraceptives and hormone replacement therapy.

▶ I tend to forget that risk factors are not real things but indicators of real things. I am so accustomed to thinking of socioeconomic status (especially education) as a risk factor for breast cancer that I forget that socioeconomic status cannot be a primary biological factor but must stand as a surrogate for something else. This article provides convincing data that "something else" includes several common biological factors such as nulliparity, age at first birth, menarche, and menopause. Risk assessment for things that are not well understood can become an endless redux of social, biological, and environmental risk factors, none of which are the "real" cause. With breast cancer, discovery of specific associated genetic variants holds promise of eventually producing a more direct and robust predictor of breast cancer incidence.

A.O. Berg, M.D., M.P.H.

Randomized Trial of Breast Self-examination in Shanghai: Methodology and Preliminary Results

Thomas DB, Gao DL, Self SG, et al (Fred Hutchinson Cancer Research Ctr, Seattle; Shanghai Textile Industry Bureau, China)
J Natl Cancer Inst 89:355–365, 1997   15–4

Purpose.—Previous reports have suggested that women who regularly perform breast self-examination (BSE) have smaller breast cancers and are less likely to have axillary lymph node involvement at presentation. However, the effects of BSE on breast cancer mortality have never been clearly demonstrated. Initial results of a large, randomized trial of BSE were presented.

Methods.—The trial included 267,040 women who currently or previously worked in the Chinese textile industry. All participants were born between 1925 and 1958. They were assigned by factory to an intervention group, who were trained in BSE, or a control group. Women in the intervention group received intensive training in BSE, including the use of silicone models, personalized instruction, 2 reinforcement sessions, and frequent reminders to practice BSE. Women in the control group received an intervention on the prevention of low back pain. The 2 groups were compared for the development of breast disease and death from breast cancer.

Results.—Women in the intervention group showed a high level of BSE performance during the first 4–5 years of the trial. Compared with women in the control group, women trained in BSE were significantly more proficient in detecting lumps in breast models. The number of breast cancers detected during follow-up was 331 in the intervention group and 322 in the control group. Women from the BSE group did not have earlier-stage or smaller tumors at presentation than those from the control group. A total of 1,457 benign breast lesions were detected in the intervention group, compared with 623 in the control group. There was little difference in cumulative breast cancer mortality between groups through 5 years' follow-up (Fig 1).

Conclusions.—These preliminary results show no reduction in breast cancer mortality among women trained in BSE. Neither is there any evidence that the intervention is causing breast cancer to be diagnosed at an earlier stage. Final conclusions from this study will require longer

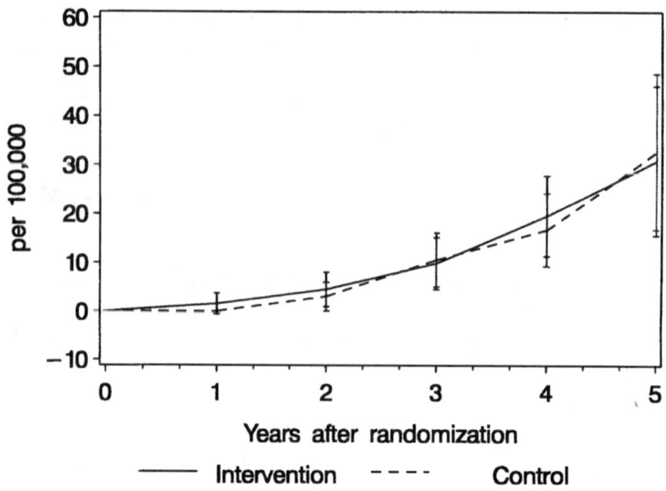

FIGURE 1.—Cumulative breast cancer mortality per 100,000 in women in the instruction and control groups. *Error bars* show 95% confidence intervals. (Courtesy of Thomas DB, Gao DL, Self SG, et al: Randomized trial of breast self-examination in Shanghai: Methodology and preliminary results. *J Natl Cancer Inst* 89:355–365, 1997. By permission of Oxford University Press.)

follow-up. The current data are insufficient to warrant recommendations for or against the teaching of BSE.

▶ We are not likely to see a randomized trial of BSE any bigger or better than this for quite some time. The results are disappointing (Fig 1) but not surprising given the large number of studies of lower-quality design that have shown the same thing. The U.S. Preventive Services Task Force reached the same conclusion in its 1996 report as do the authors of this study. Teaching BSE is of unproven benefit. Unless evidence of benefit emerges, if you are going to take time on breast cancer prevention, focus on groups (older women) and methods (mammography and clinical examination) that are known to work.

A.O. Berg, M.D., M.P.H.

A Test of Two Interventions to Improve Compliance With Scheduled Mammography Appointments

Margolis KL, Menart TC (Hennipin County Med Ctr, Minneapolis, Minn)
J Gen Intern Med 11:539–541, 1996   15–5

Background.—Screening mammography continues to be underutilized. Patient failure to keep scheduled mammography appointments is a problem. Two interventions designed to improve compliance with scheduled mammography appointments were tested.

Methods and Findings.—Consecutive women with mammography orders from October 1992 to November 1993 at 1 public teaching hospital were assigned to 1 of 3 groups. The 970 women, undergoing 1,072 mammograms, received usual care, a mailed reminder about the appointment, or a mailed reminder plus nurse counseling. In the usual care group, 25.5% of the patients missed their appointment. The failure rates in the mailed reminder group and the reminder-plus-counseling group were 20.3% and 19.7%, respectively.

Conclusion.—Mailed reminders modestly improve compliance with mammography appointments, lowering the failure rate by about 5%. The beneficial effects of adding nurse counseling to the reminder mailing are minimal.

▶ This study makes mailed reminders look worth the effort and nurse counseling a waste of money in improving mammogram completion rates. Bias may have been introduced because the patients were not individually randomized, but were randomized on the basis of the physician (and accompanying nurse). More important in my view, however, was that the mammogram scheduling was 1 to 3 weeks away. Same day appointments, when accepted, had no cancellations.

Perhaps mailed reminders would have had no effect if the mammogram appointment was within 2 to 3 days, as is possible at many mammogram screening centers. However, if your center has delayed appointment times, a mailed reminder system could be a reasonable practice-based intervention.

M.A. Bowman, M.D., M.P.A.

Breast-Cancer Screening With Mammography in Women Aged 40–49 Years
Tabar L, for the Organizing Committee and Collaborators, Falun Meeting, Falun, Sweden (Central Hosp, Falun, Sweden)
Int J Cancer 68:693–699, 1996   15–6

Introduction.—Considerable data are available regarding results of mammography screening of women ages 40–49 years. It may be that a more in-depth evaluation of mortality results could resolve some points of controversy. Reported are findings of a collaborative conference held in March 1996 in Falun, Sweden, on mammographic breast cancer screening in women aged 40–49 years.

Methods.—Data were gathered from Swedish randomized trials of breast cancer screening of women aged 40–49 years before a collaborative meeting of the Swedish Cancer Society and the Swedish National Board of Health and Welfare. The group objectives were to gather the most recent data on screening women in this age group and assess the qualities of the likely benefit in mortality rate, measures of screening performance and arrest of tumor progression through screening, costs and public-health implications, and prospects for future screening and research.

Findings.—The Swedish overview of results of mammographic screening trials indicated an estimated relative risk of breast cancer mortality

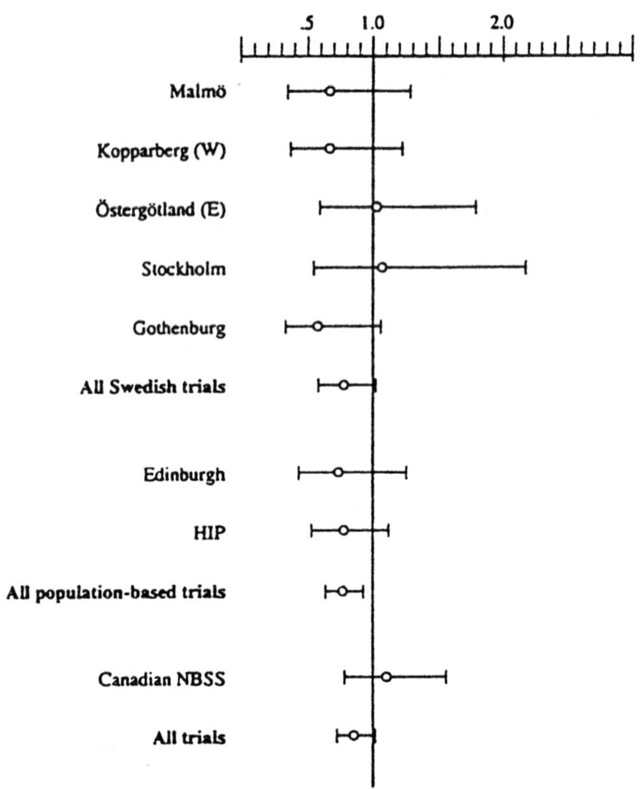

FIGURE 1.—Relative mortality in the age group of 40 to 49 from breast cancer in randomized trials of breast cancer screening (invitation vs. no invitation), with overall results from the Swedish trials, all population-based trials, and all trials. (Courtesy of Tabar L, for the Organizing Committee and Collaborators, Falun Meeting, Falun, Sweden: Breast-cancer screening with mammography in women aged 40–49 years. *Int J Cancer* 68:693–699, 1996. Reprinted by permission of Wiley-Liss, Inc., a subsidiary of John Wiley & Sons, Inc.)

associated with invitation to screening of 0.77 for women aged 40–49 years. Overall results indicate that there may be a 15% to 25% reduction in mortality associated with breast cancer screening by invitation (Fig 1). Detailed analysis suggested faster tumor progression in women aged 40–49 years, compared with women aged 50 or older. Optimal results are more likely with screening every 12–18 months and double reading of films.

Conclusion.—Findings of the Swedish overview show that women aged 40–49 years can benefit from mammographic breast screening in terms of reduced mortality. The timing and extent of reduced mortality needs further investigation and definition, but the existence of a reduction is no longer under question.

▶ Screening for breast cancer in women aged 40–49 years remains controversial. There are inherent risks in any screening program, such as false positive and false negative tests and the unintended consequences of these incorrect results. The current U.S. Preventive Services Task Force statement on breast cancer screening in this age group is that no recommendations are made either for or against, due to conflicting evidence.[1] This study, in a new look at (and meta-analysis of) old data, suggests that we should all reconsider recommending screening mammography for our patients in this age group. The data, all from studies outside the United States, when pooled, favored screening (see Fig 1) every 12–18 months. However, there were significant differences in screening parameters and techniques. The firm conclusion from this: Know how the test is done in the breast imaging facility you use (2 views and 2 readers is best). A softer conclusion: Consider screening mammography in this age group.

W.W. Dexter, M.D.

Reference

1. U.S. Preventive Services Task Force: *Guide to Clinical Preventive Services,* ed 2. Baltimore, Williams & Wilkins, 1996.

Recommendations for Follow-up Care of Individuals With an Inherited Predisposition to Cancer: II. *BRCA1* and *BRCA2*
Burke W, for the Cancer Genetics Studies Consortium (Univ of Washington, Seattle; et al)
JAMA 277:997–1003, 1997   15–7

Introduction.—Mutations in the *BRCA1* and *BRCA2* genes are associated with an inherited predisposition to breast and ovarian cancer. A task force with expertise in medical genetics, oncology, primary care, gastroenterology, and epidemiology was formed by the Cancer Genetics Studies Consortium, which is sponsored by the National Human Genome Research Institute. Their recommendations for the follow-up care of patients with an inherited predisposition to cancer were reported.

Data.—A MEDLINE search was conducted, as well as an evaluation of bibliographies of articles identified by MEDLINE, to find studies examining cancer risk, surveillance, and risk reduction in individuals genetically susceptible to breast and ovarian cancer. Quality of evidence was determined using criteria of the U.S. Prevention Service Task Force.

Provisional Recommendations.—Early screening for breast cancer and ovarian cancer are recommended for individuals with *BRCA1* mutations. For those with *BRCA2* mutations, early breast cancer screening is recommended. No recommendations were made by the task force for or against prophylactic mastectomy or oophorectomy. These surgeries are an option for mutation carriers, but there is no evidence of benefit. There have been documented case reports of cancer in patients who have undergone prophylactic surgery.

Conclusions.—Counseling regarding these recommendations should consider the uncertainties in risk estimates and in the efficacy of cancer surveillance for genetically susceptible individuals. It must be remembered that these recommendations are based upon potential, but unproven, benefits. These issues should be jointly evaluated by individuals at risk and their health care providers.

▶ Note that this is a consensus statement, not original research, and perhaps the take-home message here is "potential but unproven benefits." This is an exciting area of medicine. The mystery underlying genetic factors relating to the development of disease is slowly being unraveled. With this comes the opportunity to really target prevention strategies. These recommendations are of "low quality," based on expert opinion only, and identifying the individuals for whom we should target screening can be difficult. No practical take-home here but rather a "heads up" for what may be a future direction in cancer screening.

W.W. Dexter, M.D.

Diagnosis of Palpable Breast Lesions in Younger Women by the Modified Triple Test Is Accurate and Cost-effective

Vetto JT, Pommier RF, Schmidt WA, et al (Oregon Health Sciences Univ, Portland)
Arch Surg 131:967–974, 1996

15–8

Purpose.—The triple test (TT) refers to the use of physical examination, mammography, and fine-needle aspiration (FNA) for the diagnosis of palpable breast lesions. This approach is highly sensitive when all 3 elements are in agreement. However, most studies have used only selective confirmatory biopsy. The accuracy and cost of a modified TT (MTT)—using US instead of mammography—were evaluated in young women.

Methods.—The study included 55 women evaluated for unilateral, palpable breast lesions. Their mean age was 33 years, below the recommended age for screening mammography. In the MTT approach, all women underwent physical examination, US instead of mammography, and FNA. Each test element was classified as benign, suspicious, or malignant. When all 3 elements agreed that the lesion was benign, the patients were evaluated clinically for a mean of 11 months. Confirmatory open biopsy was obtained in women with suspicious or malignant FNA results.

Results.—Concordant benign results were obtained in 48 women, 14 of whom had breast cysts. None of these women had a cancer at that site during follow-up, for a negative predictive value and specificity of 100%. This included 5 patients who underwent biopsy at their request. The MTT showed non-concordant results in 7 patients; FNA and physical examination were more accurate than US in these cases. Compared with physical examination and open biopsy, MTT was able to avoid open biopsy in almost every patient. The average savings were as high as $623 per case.

Conclusions.—This MTT is a useful approach to the diagnosis of unilateral, palpable breast lesions in young women. It offers high accuracy while avoiding the need for open biopsy in most patients. The result is a significant reduction in patient charges. This approach is likely to become more popular as office-based US becomes more widely available.

▶ Evaluating young women with palpable breast masses can be a challenge. Most are going to be benign, but we want to find the malignant ones without too much difficulty. Mammograms are less useful in young women because of dense breast tissue, and biopsies can make future mammograms more difficult to read and are more expensive. This article suggests a combination of physical examination, US, and FNA, in that order. I do not think the number of patients (n = 55, 14 with cysts) and the length of follow-up (average, 11 months) is sufficient to be definitive, but I do think their method mostly makes sense and is likely to be sufficient when the 3 tests concur on a benign condition. However, I do not think even the 3 tests are necessary for obvious breast cysts, which I routinely aspirate and follow up without further definitive testing when no palpable lesion persists and the fluid is not bloody. The authors argue that imaging studies can be uninterpretable for weeks after an aspiration, but because the yield is so low in low-risk patients, I think the US should not always be required. Certainly, if the physical examination, US, and aspiration agree on a benign cyst, then an FNA for pathology review is not needed.

M.A. Bowman, M.D., M.P.A.

Coronary Heart Disease Mortality and Adjuvant Tamoxifen Therapy
Costantino JP, Kuller LH, Ives DG, et al (Univ of Pittsburgh, Pa)
J Natl Cancer Inst 89:776–782, 1997   15–9

Introduction.—The results of randomized clinical trials suggest that giving tamoxifen to women with breast cancer may not only improve survival but also reduce the risk of coronary heart disease. Data from the National Surgical Adjuvant Breast and Bowel Project (NSABP) were analyzed to determine mortality from coronary heart disease among tamoxifen-treated patients with early breast cancer.

Methods.—The analysis included 2,885 patients from the NSABP protocol B-14 trial of tamoxifen therapy. In the first phase of the trial, all patients were randomized to receive either tamoxifen or placebo for 5 years. Records were received to classify causes of heart disease–related death: deaths from definite fatal myocardial infarction, death from definite fatal coronary heart disease or possible myocardial infarction, and death from possible fatal coronary heart disease. The findings were compared by treatment group according to the average annual hazard rates and the corresponding relative hazard of death.

Results.—Patients receiving tamoxifen had a lower average annual rate of death from coronary heart disease, but not significantly so. Eight patients receiving tamoxifen died of definite heart-related causes, for an average annual rate of 0.62 per 1,000 patients. Twelve patients in the placebo group died of definite heart-related causes, for an average annual rate of 0.94 per 1,000 patients. Relative hazard of death from definite fatal heart disease was thus 0.66. Another 11 deaths in the tamoxifen group and 10 deaths in the placebo group were regarded as possibly caused by fatal coronary heart disease. On combined analysis of the possible and definite cases, the average annual rate of heart disease–related deaths was 1.48 per 1,000 in the tamoxifen group and 1.73 per 1,000 in the placebo group. Relative hazard of death was 0.85.

Conclusions.—Analysis of randomized trial data supports the notion than tamoxifen therapy for early breast cancer may reduce the rate of death from coronary heart disease. Final conclusions will require longer follow-up of patients from the NSABP and trials of preventive tamoxifen therapy. One key question will be whether stopping tamoxifen after 5 years affects the subsequent risk for coronary artery disease.

▶ Here is another interesting study designed to answer 1 question that raises the possibility of improving health in another, unexpected dimension. We now have 3 trials, all suggesting that tamoxifen reduces cardiovascular mortality. The point estimates consistently show a protective effect, but the confidence intervals still cross 1.0 for the relative risk, so the finding is not statistically significant. The good news is that the answer will probably be forthcoming as the parent tamoxifen trials continue to follow up patients for breast cancer recurrence, and in the trials of breast cancer prevention now under way using tamoxifen. If the relative risk (in the range of 0.8) holds up with further study, tamoxifen could be an important addition to cardiovascular disease prevention.

A.O. Berg, M.D., M.P.H.

Menopause and Hormone Replacement Therapy

Effect of Postmenopausal Hormone Therapy on Body Weight and Waist and Hip Girths
Espeland MA, for the Postmenopausal Estrogen/Progestin Interventions Study Investigators (Wake Forest Univ, Winston-Salem, NC)
J Clin Endocrinol Metab 82:1549–1556, 1997   15–10

Objective.—Despite the common belief that hormone use causes weight gain, study results indicate that hormone therapy decreases the rate of age-related increases in women's postmenopausal body weight and girth. Results of the 3-year, randomized, placebo-controlled Postmenopausal Estrogen/Progestin Interventions (PEPI) study were presented.

Methods.—The women were randomly assigned to receive placebo (N = 174), 0.625 mg daily conjugated equine estrogen (CEE) (N = 175), CEE plus 2.5 mg daily medroxyprogesterone acetate (MPA) (N = 174), CEE plus 10 mg MPA daily on days 1–12 (N = 174), and CEE plus 200 mg daily micronized progesterone on days 1–12 (N = 178). Height, weight, and waist and hip girth were measured at baseline and every 6 months at follow-up. Girths were measured at 12 and 36 months. Body mass index

TABLE 2.—Mean Changes in Weight, Girth, and Girth Ratios Between Randomization and Last Measurement by Treatment Assignment

Measure	Placebo (n = 166)	Unopposed CEE (n = 170)	CEE + MPA$_{(cyclical)}$ (n = 169)	CEE + MPA$_{(continuous)}$ (n = 170)	CEE + MP$_{(cyclical)}$ (n = 172)
Weight (kg)	2.1 ± 0.4	0.7 ± 0.4	1.3 ± 0.4	0.9 ± 0.3	1.3 ± 0.3
Waist girth (cm)	2.8 ± 0.4	1.1 ± 0.4	1.6 ± 0.5	1.5 ± 0.4	1.7 ± 0.4
Hip girth (cm)	1.1 ± 0.5	0.3 ± 0.4	0.3 ± 0.4	0.4 ± 0.4	0.4 ± 0.4
Waist/hip ratio	0.018 ± 0.004	0.009 ± 0.004	0.012 ± 0.004	0.011 ± 0.004	0.013 ± 0.003

Values are the mean ± standard deviation.

Abbreviations: CEE, conjugated equine estrogen; *MPA*, medroxyprogesterone acetate; *MP*, micronized progesterone.

(Courtesy of Espeland MA, for the Postmenopausal Estrogen/Progestin Interventions Study Investigators: Effect of postmenopausal hormone therapy on body weight and waist and hip girths. *J Clin Endocrinol Metab* 82(5):1549–1556, copyright 1997, The Endocrine Society.)

and waist-to-hip girth were calculated. Group measurements were compared statistically.

Results.—The impact of hormone therapy on weight and girth changes were analyzed an average of 2.97 years after the beginning of therapy (Table 2). Women taking CEE with or without progestins gained less weight (average, 1 kg less) and added less to waist measurements (1.2 cm less) and hip measurements (0.3 cm less). When weight was controlled for, changes in girth were not significant. Multivariate analysis determined that hormone therapy, older age, and greater physical activity were independently associated with less weight gain. Smaller increases in waist girth were associated with increased physical activity and Hispanic ethnicity. Smaller increases in hip girth were associated with activity at work and increased alcohol consumption. The effects of hormone therapy were comparable across treatment groups except for baseline physical activity level at home and baseline smoking status.

Conclusion.—Women taking postmenopausal hormone therapy gain less weight and add less girth to waist and hips. Smoking negates these effects.

▶ I have been asked so many times about whether hormone replacement therapy makes women gain weight that I am happy to provide a definitive answer based on a randomized controlled trial. The answer is *no*. In fact, the women on active treatment gained less weight than the women on placebo. Perhaps providing women with these facts will increase compliance with hormone replacement therapy. Just as with the bone mass changes, women who smoked did not receive this benefit. This is the well-known, large PEPI trial, which is, overall, well designed and completed.

M.A. Bowman, M.D., M.P.A.

A Randomized, Double-blind, Placebo-controlled, Crossover Study on the Effect of Oral Oestradiol on Acute Menopausal Symptoms
Chung TKH, Yip SK, Lam P, et al (Prince of Wales Hosp, New Territories, Hong Kong; Chinese Univ of Hong Kong, New Territories)
Maturitas 25:115–123, 1996   15–11

Background.—Acute menopausal symptoms are more common in white women than in Asian women. Although estrogen replacement treatment has been shown to be effective in controlling white women's acute symptoms, its effect in Asian women is not well researched.

Methods.—Eighty-three Hong Kong Chinese women who had had a surgical menopause were enrolled in a randomized, double-blind, placebo-controlled, crossover study of the effects of oral estradiol on the incidence of acute menopausal symptoms. One group received oral estradiol, 2 mg daily, for the first 6 months and placebo for the second 6 months; group 2 received placebo first and the same estradiol treatment second.

Findings.—Estradiol concentrations were noted to be significantly increased in the active treatment period compared with the placebo period. However, the reporting of symptoms did not differ significantly between the treatment and placebo periods.

Conclusion.—The reasons for estrogen's apparent lack of effect on acute menopausal symptoms in Chinese women are not clear. It may be related to the generally low incidence of symptoms in this population or to this population's greater dietary intake of phytoestrogens. Further research is needed to better explain the findings.

▶ This is a cultural difference that I had failed to appreciate. Asian women have fewer hot flashes at menopause, and this study suggests that they may not get relief from what symptoms they do have with a common estrogen dose. The authors speculate that the Asian women's high intake of phytoestrogens through soy products may explain these findings; alternatively, the women need a higher dose! And this was a group of younger patients (average age, 44 years) with surgical menopause—a characteristic of women who usually get more symptoms.

M.A. Bowman, M.D., M.P.A.

Effects of Alcohol Ingestion on Estrogens in Postmenopausal Women
Ginsburg ES, Mello NK, Mendelson JH, et al (Brigham and Women's Hosp, Boston; McLean Hosp, Belmont, Mass)
JAMA 276:1747–1751, 1996   15–12

Introduction.—Estrogen replacement therapy (ERT) and moderate alcohol consumption both have been linked to an increase in the risk of breast cancer. This raises concern about a possible additive effect of the 2. There is little information about potential interactions between ERT and alcohol in postmenopausal women. Both factors may be associated with elevated plasma estradiol, which has been implicated in the development of breast cancer. The effects of moderate alcohol intake on circulating estradiol levels were assessed in postmenopausal women taking ERT.

Methods.—The randomized, double-blind, placebo-controlled trial included 2 groups of healthy postmenopausal women. One group was taking ERT, consisting of estradiol, 1 mg/day, and medroxyprogesterone acetate. The other group was not taking ERT. In random order on consecutive days, the women drank a 0.7-g/kg dose of alcohol and an isocaloric placebo. The effects of alcohol ingestion on plasma estradiol and estrone levels were analyzed. The ERT group was studied during the estrogen-only portion of their ERT, with estrogen administered each night at 9:00 PM.

Results.—In the ERT group, alcohol ingestion was associated with a 3-fold increase in circulating estradiol. The estradiol increase was from 297 to 973 pmol/L, and occurred within 50 minutes during the ascending limb of the blood alcohol curve. Estradiol remained significantly elevated for 5 hours after alcohol ingestion. The non-ERT group had no significant change in estradiol. The ERT group had a significant decline in estrone level after both alcohol and placebo. There was no difference between groups in blood alcohol level, which peaked at 21 mmol/L within 1 hour after the start of drinking. The increase in estradiol in the ERT group was significantly correlated with the changes in blood alcohol level on both the ascending and descending curve.

Conclusions.—In women taking ERT, acute alcohol ingestion may produce a substantial and lasting rise in circulating estradiol level. The increase may be 3 times higher than the target values for ERT. More study is needed to see how this effect influences the risk-benefit ratio of ERT.

▶ This may be an article that takes me a while to digest its clinical importance. I am a firm believer that ERT is an excellent choice for many postmenopausal women, improving many aspects of their health. However, this article clearly shows that alcohol increases plasma estradiol and estrone levels. Alcohol and estrogens both have been implicated in breast cancer. But the whole picture is not yet making sense to me. If alcohol raises estrogen levels generally, and estrogens increase bone mass, then why is alcohol ingestion not associated with higher bone mass? Perhaps it is just a "peak" effect, and the influence of the higher peak is different on bone and breast. In any event, I am not ready to change my clinical practice much but may be more wary of using ERT in women who drink substantially.

M.A. Bowman, M.D., M.P.A.

Hormone Replacement Therapy After Transcervical Resection of the Endometrium
Istre O, Holm-Nielsen P, Bourne T, et al (Central Hosp of Hedmark County, Hamar, Norway; Univ Hosp, Aarhus, Denmark)
Obstet Gynecol 88:767–770, 1996   15–13

Introduction.—Transcervical resection of the endometrium often is used in the treatment of menometrorrhagia. Because most of the women referred for the procedure are premenopausal, hormone replacement therapy (HRT) subsequently may be prescribed. The effect of HRT on residual endometrial tissue is a concern, however. A double-blind, randomized study was conducted to determine whether women can be treated safely with estrogens alone after transcervical resection of the endometrium.

Methods.—The 62 women who entered the trial had requested HRT for menopausal symptoms or prophylaxis against osteoporosis and cardiovascular disease. Twenty-one had menopausal symptoms at the time of transcervical resection of the endometrium and 38 were recruited at an average of 20 months after the procedure. In the latter group, a second resection was performed before study entry to remove any residual endometrium. Thirty-one women were randomly assigned to receive unopposed estrogen therapy and 31 to receive combined HRT. Three women, all from the unopposed estrogen group, were excluded from analysis. Clinical and US examinations were performed every 3 months for 1 year. Hysteroscopically standardized endometrial biopsies were obtained at the conclusion of follow-up.

Results.—Sweating and flushing both were markedly reduced in both the unopposed (17β-estradiol 2 mg) and combined (17β-estradiol 2 mg plus norethisterone 1 mg) treatment groups. The mean number of bleeding days, compared for the first and last days of the study period, differed significantly between the 2 groups. The unopposed estrogen group experienced an increase from 6.8 to 11.8 days, whereas bleeding days in the combined therapy group were reduced from 2.2 to 0.9. After 1 year, endometrial hyperplasia without atypia was found in 6 women and proliferative endometrium in 8 women in the estrogen-only group. Neither condition was detected in the combined therapy group. Endometrial thickness was significantly greater in the single-agent therapy group.

Conclusions.—Women who undergo transcervical resection of the endometrium may have residual endometrium that retains the ability to proliferate during postmenopausal HRT. Because the use of unopposed estrogen in such women may be associated with the same potential risk of endometrial cancer as in women with an intact uterus, progestagen should be included in HRT. Combined therapy also has other advantages, including decreased bleeding.

▶ Endometrial resection of the uterus is becoming more common, so the question of HRT will become more common. Does resection remove the need for the concurrent progesterone in HRT? At least for now, the answer is no; endometrial hyperplasia still develops, even in women who had amenorrhea after the endometrial resection. Thus, even with a history of endometrial resection, progesterone should be used if hyperplasia is to be avoided.

M.A. Bowman, M.D., M.P.A.

The Influence of Oestrogen Replacement on Faecal Incontinence in Postmenopausal Women

Donnelly V, O'Connell PR, O'Herlihy C (Univ College Dublin; Mater Misericordiae Hosp, Dublin)
Br J Obstet Gynaecol 104:311–315, 1997   15–14

Background.—Fecal incontinence, occurring mainly in women, usually becomes manifest after menopause. Cumulative obstetric injury is apparently compensated by the integrity of the pelvic floor connective tissues until trophic estrogen support declines with the cessation of reproductive ovarian function. The value of hormone replacement therapy (HRT) in postmenopausal women with fecal incontinence was investigated.

Methods.—Twenty postmenopausal women, aged a mean of 61 years, were studied. All had demonstrable fecal incontinence and had not previously received HRT. The subjects completed a bowel function questionnaire and underwent anorectal physiologic assessment before and after 6 months of standard estrogen HRT.

Findings.—All women had significant symptoms of anorectal dysfunction before treatment, whereas 25% were free of symptoms after treatment. Another 65% had improvements in flatus control, urgency, and fecal staining. Although bowel frequency and stool consistency were unchanged after HRT, social activity was much improved. Anal resting pressures and voluntary squeeze increments were increased significantly after treatment. However, there were no differences in anal canal vector symmetry index. Changes in threshold volume of rectal sensation and volume of defecatory urge were not significant, but maximum tolerated rectal volume was significantly changed after 6 months. Treatment had no effect on anal canal electrosensitivity and pudendal nerve terminal motor latency. Thirty-five percent of the women had an identifiable anal sphincter defect on anal endosonography. However, the outcome in this group was not significantly different from that among women with an intact anal sphincter.

Conclusion.—Estrogen replacement therapy may be beneficial in postmenopausal women with symptoms of impaired fecal continence. This hypothesis now needs to be tested in a prospective, randomized, controlled trial.

▶ This is good news for the estimated 4% of postmenopausal women with fecal incontinence. Ninety percent experienced at least some improvement, and one quarter were "cured." Anal manometry improved, as did social functioning. All around, great results! I suspect that women with lesser degrees of incontinence than those in this study would also experience improvement, although perhaps not as dramatically.

M.A. Bowman, M.D., M.P.A.

Hormone Replacement Therapy and Risk of Venous Thromboembolism: Population Based Case-Control Study
Gutthann SP, Rodríguez LA, Castellsague J, et al (Universidad Complutense, Madrid)
BMJ 314:796–800, 1997   15–15

Background.—The negative effect of contraceptive estrogens on the risk of venous thromboembolism is sometimes attributed to postmenopausal replacement estrogens as well, but there are little data to support this. Early epidemiologic studies did not show a higher risk of venous thromboembolism in women given hormone replacement therapy, but the results were limited by small study populations and inadequate control of confounding factors.

Methods.—Hormone replacement therapy and risk of venous thromboembolism were studied in a cohort of 347,253 women with no major risk factors for venous thromboembolism. The patients were between 50 and

79 years of age. There were 292 case patients with idiopathic venous thromboembolism, 97 with pulmonary embolism, and 195 with deep venous thrombosis. There were 10,000 control patients.

Results.—The adjusted odds ratio of venous thromboembolism for women who used hormone replacement therapy was 2.1 compared with nonusers of hormone replacement therapy. The higher risk was restricted to the first 12 months of estrogen therapy. The odds ratio was 4.6 during the first 6 months and 3.0 during the second 6 months. There were no major differences in risk between high and low doses of estrogen, unopposed and opposed treatment, or oral and transdermal treatment. In women who did not use hormone replacement therapy, the risk of venous thromboembolism was 1.3 per 10,000 women per year.

Discussion.—The risk of idiopathic venous thromboembolism is slightly higher in women who use hormone replacement therapy than in women who do not. This results in 1 or 2 additional cases of venous thromboembolism per 10,000 women per year. This higher risk is only in the first 12 months of such hormone replacement therapy. This is the largest study to date of the risk of venous thromboembolism associated with hormone replacement therapy.

▶ Generally, standard-dose hormone replacement therapy has been thought not to increase the risk of thromboembolism, although high-dose estrogen has a well-known association with thrombotic events. This is a very large study, but the study methodology (case-control) is not the ideal randomized controlled trial.

The results suggest a rate of thromboembolism about twice as high as for those taking estrogens, although the actual number of events was still quite low. Importantly, this risk seemed to appear only in the first year of use. There are other recent studies with similar findings. Thus, I think we should warn the patients of the risk and include it in our information of benefits and costs of estrogen replacement therapy. However, the numbers continue to suggest that the benefits of hormone replacement therapy on overall morbidity/mortality outweigh the risks for many patients.

M.A. Bowman, M.D., M.P.A.

Effects of Hormonal Replacement Therapy on the Postural Balance Among Postmenopausal Women

Hammar ML, Lindgren R, Berg GE, et al (Univ Hosp, Linköping, Sweden)
Obstet Gynecol 88:955–960, 1996   15–16

Introduction.—The bone loss that accelerates around the time of menopause is known to contribute to an increased risk of fractures, especially hip fractures. Loss of estrogen also may affect other risk factors for fractures resulting from falls, including impaired protective reflexes and balance. The effects of hormone replacement therapy on balance performance were studied in healthy postmenopausal women.

Methods.—The 19 study participants were recruited when they sought advice for vasomotor symptoms. The median age of the group was 54 and the median time since menopause was 3 years. Exclusion criteria were serious illness, a history of vertigo or dizziness, and use of drugs that could interfere with balance, coordination, or reactivity. The women were treated for 12 weeks with transdermal 17β-estradiol (50 µg/day), then had oral medroxyprogesterone acetate (5 mg/day) added for 2 weeks to induce withdrawal bleeding. They were asked to keep a diary of vasomotor symptoms during the 2 weeks before treatment and the 14-week period of hormone replacement therapy. Dynamic posturography assessment was conducted at baseline and at weeks 4, 12, and 14. The assessment comprised 2 main tests—a sensory organization test and a movement coordination test. Because dynamic posturography is designed for patients with balance problems and vertigo, some more challenging tests were added in order that therapy-related changes might be seen in a normal group.

Results.—An increase in serum estradiol and a decrease in follicle-stimulating hormone concentrations were observed with treatment, and hormone therapy significantly decreased the number of hot flushes and climacteric symptoms. Although all women had normal balance performance for age before treatment, 4 weeks of estrogen therapy led to a highly significant improvement in the most difficult sensory organization tests. This improvement was sustained throughout the treatment period, after which women were offered continued hormone replacement therapy.

Discussion.—Women with menopausal symptoms and normal stability demonstrated increased stability after 4 weeks of hormone replacement therapy. This improvement suggests that the central integration performed in the brain stem, cerebellum, or both may be affected by estrogen-progestagen. The addition of progestagen did not counteract the effects of estrogen.

▶ This article is yet 1 more on the positive side of the estrogen debate. Estrogen improves balance in postmenopausal women, which could lead to fewer falls. This is consistent with some other small studies. Of note, however, is that this occurred in women who had vasomotor symptoms. Another small study found that estrogen increased the cross-sectional area of the thoracic aorta; with the combination of progesterone and estrogen, there was no change in size.[1] This sounds like a good effect, but the clinical significance is unknown.

M.A. Bowman, M.D., M.P.A.

Reference

1. Giraud DG, Morton MJ, Wison RA, et al: Effects of estrogen and progestin on aortic size and compliance in postmenopausal women. *Am J Obstet Gynecol* 174:1708–1718, 1996.

Effect of Hormone Replacement Therapy on Bone Mineral Density in Postmenopausal Women With Mild Primary Hyperparathyroidism: A Randomized, Controlled Trial
Grey AB, Stapleton JP, Evans MC, et al (Univ of Auckland, New Zealand; Yale Univ, New Haven, Conn)
Ann Intern Med 125:360–368, 1996   15–17

Background.—Because primary hyperparathyroidism is asymptomatic in at least 50% of patients, most of whom are elderly women, a conservative management approach is often recommended. There is evidence, however, that the disorder is associated with osteopenia, and this finding is considered an indication for surgical intervention. A controlled trial was conducted to evaluate the effect of hormone replacement therapy for osteopenia in primary hyperparathyroidism.

Patients and Methods.—Forty-two postmenopausal women entered the double-blind trial and were randomly assigned to receive either continuous combined therapy with conjugated equine estrogens, 0.625 mg/day, and medroxyprogesterone acetate, 5 mg/day, or identical placebo tablets. Treatment was to continue for 2 years, but 9 women withdrew before the trial had ended. Bone mineral density was measured every 6 months, and findings recorded for the whole body, lumbar spine, proximal femur, and forearm. A food-frequency questionnaire was used to determine calcium intake. Fasting blood samples and urine samples were collected at baseline, at 6 months, and at 2 years to assess biochemical indices of bone turnover and calcium metabolism.

Results.—The hormone replacement therapy group demonstrated decreases in markers of both bone turnover and bone resorption during the treatment period. The mean serum total alkaline phosphatase, a marker of osteoblast function, was 22% lower than baseline level at 2 years. Two-year mean decreases were 38% for urine hydroxyproline excretion, 60% for N-telopeptide excretion, and 33% for urinary calcium excretion. Although urinary markers of bone resorption did not change between baseline and 6 months in the placebo group, this group did have decreases in excretion of N-telopeptide and calcium at between 6 months and 2 years (both of these markers decreased to a greater extent in the hormone replacement group). Bone mineral densities decreased in the placebo group and increased in the hormone replacement group. At the end of the study, between-group differences were significant at all sites except for the Ward triangle (Fig 2). Levels of serum ionized calcium and of intact parathyroid hormone were unchanged in those receiving hormone replacement therapy.

Conclusion.—Hormone replacement therapy suppressed bone turnover, reduced calcium excretion, and increased bone mineral density at most skeletal sites in postmenopausal women with mild primary hyperparathy-

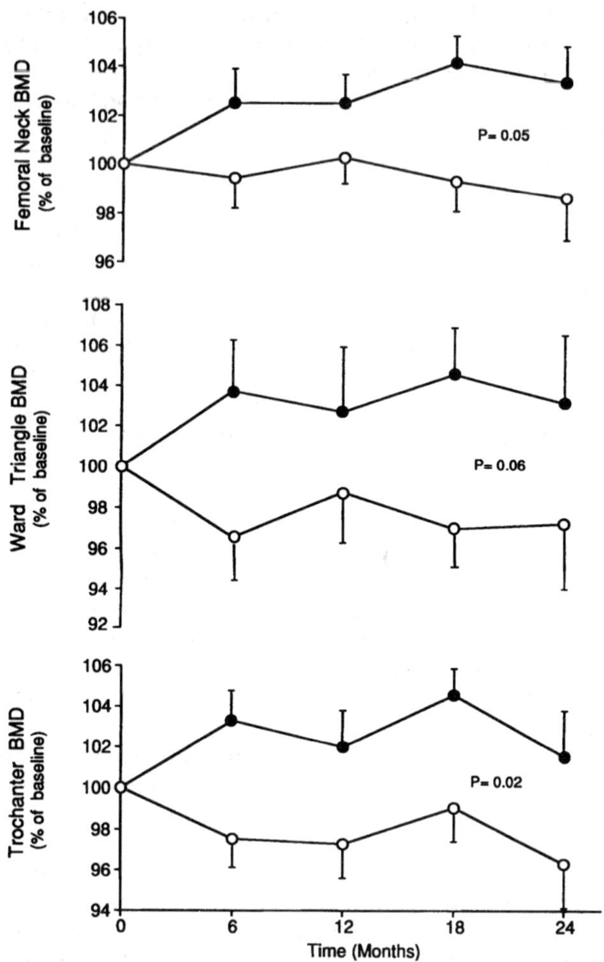

FIGURE 2.—Mean (±standard error) bone mineral density (*BMD*) of the proximal femur in postmenopausal women with primary hyperparathyroidism who received hormone replacement therapy (*black circles*) or placebo (*white circles*) for 2 years. The results are expressed as a percentage of the baseline values. Changes in bone mineral density of the femoral neck and trochanter were significantly more positive in patients receiving hormone replacement therapy than in patients receiving placebo. Changes in the bone mineral density of the Ward triangle tended to be more positive in the hormone replacement therapy group. (Courtesy of Grey AB, Stapleton JP, Evans MC, et al: Effect of hormone replacement therapy on bone mineral density in postmenopausal women with mild primary hyperparathyroidism: A randomized, controlled trial. *Ann Intern Med* 125:360–368, 1996.)

roidism. The treatment was well tolerated and may be protective against cardiovascular disease as well as fractures.

▶ Mild primary hyperparathyroidism is common, and whether or when to perform surgery remains unclear. This well-done study shows that hormone replacement therapy (continuous combined estrogen and progesterone) can improve the bone mass of women with this particular metabolic abnormality, and surgery should not be required solely on the basis of the presence of osteopenia. The amount of increase in bone mass looked to be similar to that in women without hyperparathyroidism, although that was not studied. The authors suggest a randomized, controlled trial comparing the effects of surgery vs. hormone replacement therapy, which would be a good idea.

M.A. Bowman, M.D., M.P.A.

Long-term Compliance of Continuous Combined Estrogen and Progestogen Replacement in Postmenopausal Women

Dören M, Schneider HPG (Westfälische Wilhelms-Universität Münster, Germany)
Maturitas 25:99–105, 1996   15–18

Background.—For many women, the uterine bleeding associated with hormonal replacement therapy is unacceptable. Data on compliance and bleeding patterns in 1 group of women taking oral replacement therapy were reviewed.

Methods and Findings.—The subjects were 70 women receiving daily estradiol, 2 mg; estriol, 1 mg; and norethisterone acetate, 1 mg, given in a continuous combined manner to avoid withdrawal bleeding. Compliance was 97% at 1 year, 76% at 5 years, and 58% at 9 years. Spotting was the most common reason for abandoning treatment. Women with and without bleeding did not differ significantly in reproductive history, body weight, pretreatment estradiol, or follicle-stimulating hormone concentrations. The probability of maintaining amenorrhea with hormone replacement therapy did not increase with the length of postmenopausal interval or weight. One woman was found to have highly differentiated in situ adenocarcinoma of the endometrium on endometrial histologic examination. Women with bleeding had significantly higher induced serum estradiol levels and lower pretreatment sex hormone–binding globulin levels than did women without bleeding.

Conclusion.—The compliance rates documented in this study appear to provide an alternative as to when to counsel patients receiving long-term hormone replacement therapy. However, the absence of parameters for patient selection and the problem of irregular bleeding at the start of treatment do not permit continuous combined hormone replacement therapy to be considered as first-line therapy for long-term hormone replacement treatment.

▶ Once again, the long-term compliance with combined hormone replacement therapy was mediocre. Of note, the authors were unable to determine any factors that seemed associated with the spotting, but the spotting was clearly the main factor in stopping the medication. The paper also reports the first adenocarcinoma of the endometrium reported in the literature in a woman receiving combined therapy; this woman had recurrent spotting. The ideal regimen has obviously not been found, and the appropriate surveillance for spotting is unknown.

M.A. Bowman, M.D., M.P.A.

Dysfunctional Bleeding

Endometrial Biopsy in DUB

Ash SJ, Farrell SA, Flowerdew G (Dalhousie Univ, Halifax, NS, Canada)
J Reprod Med 41:892–896, 1996   15–19

Background.—The incidence of abnormal endometrial histologic findings in women with dysfunctional uterine bleeding (DUB) has not been established. This incidence was determined and the predictive value of risk factors for endometrial cancer in women with DUB was assessed.

Methods and Findings.—Three hundred ten women with DUB undergoing endometrial biopsy were included in the retrospective review. Endometrial biopsy results were abnormal in 6.7%. Independently significant risk factors for abnormal endometrial histology included menstrual cycle irregularity, age of 40 years or more, and hypertension. Premenopausal women with DUB and regular cycles had a less than 1% probability of abnormal endometrial histologic findings. Menstrual cycle irregularity increased the probability of abnormal endometrial histology to 14.3% of patients. (Table 3).

Conclusion.—Regardless of age, patients initially seen with DUB and a history of menstrual cycle irregularity should undergo endometrial biopsy. The current clinical emphasis on age in decision making regarding endometrial biospy in women with DUB is not justified.

▶ In practice, I had come to about the same conclusion as the authors, although I was not nearly as systematic in my observations. It seemed that if I just followed the rule that age over 40 years plus DUB required an endometrial biopsy, I was performing a lot of biopsies with negative results

TABLE 3.—Rate of Abnormal Endometrial Histology in Women With Dysfunctional Uterine Bleeding

| | | | % Patients with abnormal biopsy | | | |
| | | | Observed | | | |
Irregular menses	Hypertension*	Age ≥40 yr	No.	%	Predicted (%)†	95% CI
0	0	0	(0/93)	0.0	0.2	(0.0, 1.5)
0	0	1	(0/111)	0.0	0.9	(0.2, 4.1)
0	1	0	(0/3)	0.0	1.1	(0.2, 7.5)
0	1	1	(2/18)	11.1	4.3	(0.8, 20.1)
1	0	0	(4/27)	14.8	14.3	(5.8, 31.1)
1	0	1	(13/30)	43.3	39.8	(24.6, 57.3)
1	1	0	(1/2)	50.0	45.1	(12.3, 82.8)
1	1	1	(1/3)	33.3	76.6	(38.0, 94.6)

*0 indicates risk factor is absent; 1 indicates risk factor is present.
†Predicted by logistic regression model.
(Courtesy of Ash SJ, Farrell SA, Flowerdew G: Endometrial biopsy in DUB. *J Reprod Med* 41:892–896, 1996.)

and feeling as though I had put the women through an unneeded procedure. The next question regarding this study is whether it was rigorous enough and had enough patients to make it sufficiently generalizable so that these findings could be implemented in practice. To this, I would answer a qualified "yes." The patients were from a general gynecology practice, but I gather that it was a teaching practice and may have been at the medical school; if anything, this could make the likelihood of pathology higher.

Menopausal women were appropriately excluded. The authors did not consider family history, which I would have considered important. There were very low numbers of patients in some of the statistical cells; for example, there was only 1 abnormal histologic result in a patient with irregular menses, hypertension, and age over 40 years. However, this affirms the authors' point that there were few abnormal biopsy results.

Another important point concerning the authors' results is that they used the term 'irregular menses' for menometrorrhagia, metrorrhagia, oligomenorrhea, and amenorrhea (i.e., either abnormal bleeding amounts or menstrual length) and only when the irregularity had been the predominant pattern in the previous year. A woman with spotting and regular menses would not be considered to have irregular menses, but a woman with spotting and prolonged bleeding and a regular cycle length would be so considered. The bottom line: women over 40 years with DUB who are otherwise low risk do not need endometrial biopsies; the overwhelming risk factor was menstrual irregularity (irregular cycle length or bleeding amounts), with other risk factors probably including hypertension, diabetes, and obesity—to which I would add a family history of endometrial cancer. Perhaps we should simply change our definition of DUB to the authors' definition of menstrual irregularity, instead of including simple spotting or 1 to 2 abnormal periods as DUB, and then continue our old, frequently used adage for determining when to do biopsies.

M.A. Bowman, M.D., M.P.A.

Add-back Therapy for Long-term Use in Dysfunctional Uterine Bleeding and Uterine Fibroids
Thomas EJ (Princess Anne Hosp, Southampton, England)
Br J Obstet Gynaecol 103:18–21, 1996   15–20

Background.—Dysfunctional uterine bleeding (DUB) and uterine fibroids are common problems that are effectively treated by gonadotrophin-releasing hormone (GnRH) agonists. However, because these agents have adverse effects on bone mass, they have been used for short courses only. One way to minimize the hypoestrogenic effects of GnRH agonists without countering the therapeutic benefits of the agonists may be to give add-back hormone replacement therapy. Previous studies of GnRH agonists plus add-back hormone replacement therapy for the treatment of DUB and uterine fibroids are reviewed.

Findings.—One study evaluated the effects of add-back therapy with cyclic estradiol–norgestrol combined with goserelin acetate for 21 women with subjective DUB. Add-back therapy significantly reduced the duration of menstruation, the number of days of heavy bleeding, and the objectively measured blood loss. Symptoms also improved significantly. Another study used combined estrogen–progestogen therapy for 21 months after 3 months of GnRH agonist treatment in 51 women with symptomatic uterine fibroids. The treatment did not promote fibroid regrowth; in contrast, women assigned to treatment with progestogen only had a gradual increase in uterine volume.

Discussion.—In women with DUB or uterine fibroids, add-back combined hormone replacement therapy appears effective in maintaining the therapeutic benefits of GnRH agonists. This treatment approach does not reduce bone mineral density but does decrease hypoestrogenic vasomotor and other menopausal side effects. Giving HRT add-back therapy allows more extended treatment with GnRH agonists and thus may be especially helpful for patients who are not candidates for surgery or who wish to avoid hysterectomy.

▶ GnRH agonists work well to decrease the size of fibroids in the uterus. However, because they so negatively affect bone mass and so frequently cause disabling hot flashes, they can only be used for a few months. Currently, they are often used to shrink symptomatic fibroids to increase the likelihood of a vaginal rather than an abdominal hysterectomy. This study suggests that early GnRH-agonist treatment (given for 3 months) followed by combined hormone replacement therapy for 21 months did not encourage regrowth of the fibroids. Perhaps intermittent GnRH can be given, with hormone replacement therapy used to prevent bone loss. The add-back hormone replacement therapy to GnRH is known to prevent bone loss, but I think a study incorporating all aspects (fibroids and bone mass) for longer periods are needed.

M.A. Bowman, M.D., M.P.A.

Spontaneous Abortion

Tree-based, Two-stage Risk Factor Analysis for Spontaneous Abortion
Zhang H, Bracken MB (Yale Univ, New Haven, Conn)
Am J Epidemiol 144:989–996, 1996   15–21

Background.—The risk factors for spontaneous abortion are difficult to investigate epidemiologically. The epidemiology is distinct in cases of abortion resulting from errors in fetal development caused by genetic or chromosomal anomaly, developmental anomaly in a chromosomally normal fetus, and anatomical problems of the uterus or placenta. Research also is difficult because of the failure to detect the majority of spontaneous abortions and the many confounding risk factors that must be evaluated.

Methods.—Data from more than 2,800 women who had a singleton live-birth or spontaneous abortion were analyzed. Interviews were conducted during 5 to 16 weeks of pregnancy. The possible risk factors were as follows: employment; standing, walking, or sitting more than 2 hours at work; exposure to vibration at work; commuting to work; reaching over the shoulders at work; carrying loads greater than 9 kg at work; drinking alcohol or coffee during the first month of pregnancy; and gynecologic problems before pregnancy. The possible confounding factors were as follows: age, marital status, education, race, mother's height, tobacco use, tobacco use before pregnancy, use of or passive exposure to marijuana, chronic conditions, cocaine use, use of birth control, number of pregnancies, infertility, induced abortion, stillbirth, spontaneous abortion, and ectopic pregnancy.

Results.—Carrying loads of more than 9 kg at least once a day increased the risk of spontaneous abortion by 70%. The risk of spontaneous abortion also was increased by drinking 3 or more cups of coffee per day in the first month of pregnancy. The risk of spontaneous abortion was slightly increased by reaching over the shoulders at least once per day.

Discussion.—This strategy, which combines tree-based analyses with the method of Mantel-Haenszel and logistic regression, can efficiently analyze new risk factors for spontaneous abortion, which already has many possible confounding factors. This method may be helpful for a wide range of epidemiologic studies.

▶ Spontaneous abortion of a desired pregnancy is distressing to the patient and frustrating to the physician. When the problem recurs, there is often a search for answers and a desire for advice for having a successful pregnancy. Large epidemiologic studies such as this may provide helpful information but should not be considered conclusive. From this study, one would advise a woman to avoid carrying weight over 20 lbs (implications at home and at work) and to avoid drinking 3 or more cups of coffee a day. Reassurance can be given about the long list of other activities that were not shown to be risk factors for spontaneous abortion.

J.E. Scherger, M.D., M.P.H.

A Medical Approach to Management of Spontaneous Abortion Using Misoprostol
Chung T, Leung P, Cheung LP, et al (Chinese Univ of Hong Kong; Prince of Wales Hosp, Sha Tin, Hong Kong)
Acta Obstet Gynecol Scand 76:248–251, 1997   15–22

Background.—A number of studies have reported the use of misoprostol in the management of spontaneous abortion. It was hypothesized that, by extending misoprostol treatment to a maximum of 48 hours, the number of evacuations of retained products of conception (ERPCs) could be further reduced without unacceptable morbidity.

Methods.—Three hundred fifty-four women hospitalized because of spontaneous abortion were enrolled in the prospective, observational study. Two hundred twenty-five with retained products of conception were given misoprostol for up to 48 hours. One hundred one women were excluded from this treatment because transvaginal scan (TVS) showed an empty uterus, and another 28 were excluded because they were not suitable candidates for conservative therapy. One hundred thirty-seven women undergoing routine ERPC after TVS evidence of retained products of conception comprised a comparison group.

Findings.—In the misoprostol group, uterine evacuation occurred within 24 hours in 107 women and at 48 hours in 148. Three uterine curettages were performed up to 14 days after hospital discharge because of persistent bleeding ($n = 1$) and pelvic infection ($n = 2$). In 1 woman, ectopic pregnancy was diagnosed at follow-up. The overall complication rates in the misoprostol and control groups were 1.7% and 6.6%, respectively.

Conclusions.—A 48-hour regimen of misoprostol for the management of spontaneous abortion in women with TVS-documented retained products of conception markedly reduces the need for surgery. Subsequent morbidity associated with this treatment is low.

▶ Basically, 2 of 3 women avoided surgical evacuation of their uterus after spontaneous abortion by having an ultrasound and receiving misoprostol for 2 days if the uterus was not empty. Fewer than half who avoided surgery had no retained products of conception at the time of ultrasound; most of the remainder had an empty uterus within 48 hours. Of those who had products of conception after 24 hours, 42% emptied their uterus in the next 24 hours. There was no control group of women who were observed and did not receive misoprostol. The misoprostol patients were more likely to require analgesia than the postoperative patients. A cost comparison was not done. As 1 recent study[1] of expectant management found an 80% evacuation rate at 3 days with no intervention, it is unclear how much the misoprostol is adding to nature. Another recent study[2] found that those who spontaneously evacuated had lower progesterone and human chorionic gonadotropin values. More direct comparisons of misoprostol with observation only should be undertaken.

M.A. Bowman, M.D., M.P.A.

References

1. Nielsen S, Hahlin M: Expectant management of first-trimester spontaneous abortion. *Lancet* 345:84–86, 1995.
2. Nielsen S, Hahlin M, Oden A: Using a logistic model to identify women with first-trimester spontaneous abortion suitable for expectant management. *Br J Obstet Gynaecol* 103:1230–1235, 1996.

Fertility After a Randomised Trial of Spontaneous Abortion Managed by Surgical Evacuation or Expectant Treatment

Blohm F, Hahlin M, Nielsen S, et al (Sahlgrenska Univ, Göteborg, Sweden)
Lancet 349:995, 1997
15–23

Background.—A previous study reported that expectant management and primary surgical evacuation of the uterus for miscarriages of less than 13 weeks' gestation yield the same short-term outcomes. After 2 years, an attempt was made to contact the participants of this study who had indicated a desire for future pregnancy to assess fertility.

Methods.—A questionnaire was sent to 127 of the previous study's participants, eliciting data on fertility in the 24 months after their spontaneous abortions. The response rate was 89%.

Findings.—The cumulative conception rates and pregnancy outcomes were comparable in the surgical and expectant management groups (figure). Three of the women originally managed expectantly had had pelvic inflammatory disease; the 2 available for follow-up had given birth. Pelvic inflammatory disease had also been diagnosed in 5 women in the

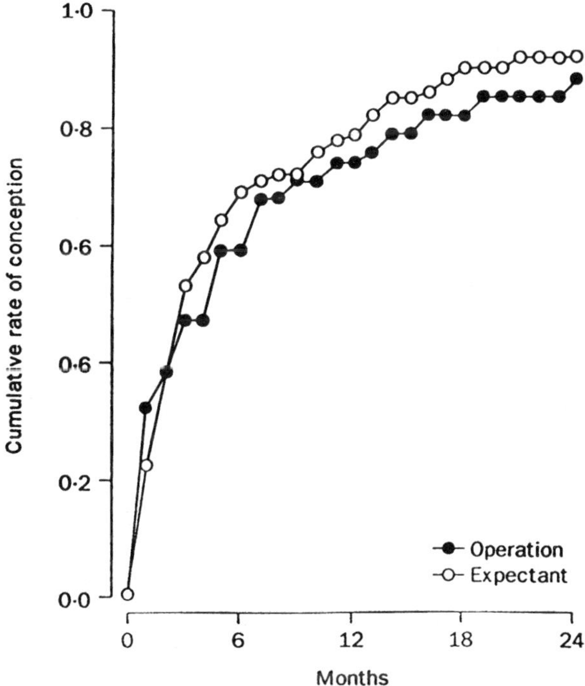

FIGURE.—Comparison of cumulative conception rates. During the 24 months after spontaneous abortion managed by surgical evacuation (N = 34) or expectant treatment (N = 72). There is no significant difference between conception rates. (Courtesy of Blohm F, Hahlin M, Nielsen S, et al: Fertility after a randomised trial of spontaneous abortion managed by surgical evacuation or expectant treatment. *Lancet* 349:995, copyright 1997 by The Lancet Ltd.)

original surgical group, 3 of whom were available for follow-up and 2 of whom had given birth. The cumulative conception rate in women trying to get pregnant who were managed expectantly but later needed surgical evacuation was 93%; in women managed expectantly only, it was 91%, and in those undergoing primary evacuation, it was 88%.

Conclusion.—Expectant management of spontaneous abortion does not affect fertility in the 24 months after the abortion. Cumulative conception rates and pregnancy outcomes in women managed expectantly were similar to those in women treated surgically.

▶ This is the shortest study (1 page) that I have selected in all my years with the YEAR BOOK. However, the question the authors attempt to answer is important. As expectant management of spontaneous abortions is coming back into vogue, the question of the effect on fertility is, once again, highlighted. The number of patients in the study was high enough (113) to be reassuring, and the fertility rate was excellent.

M.A. Bowman, M.D., M.P.A.

Androgen Excess

Prostate-specific Antigen in Female Serum, a Potential New Marker of Androgen Excess
Melegos DN, Yu H, Ashok M, et al (Univ of Toronto; Univ of Southern California, Los Angeles)
J Clin Endocrinol Metab 82:777–780, 1997   15–24

Introduction.—Prostate-specific antigen (PSA) was believed to be absent from female tissues until it was recently detected in female breast tissue. The production of PSA by steroid hormone receptor-positive breast cancer cells is regulated by steroid hormones via action of steroid hormone receptors. Because there is a relationship between PSA production and androgen regulation, PSA may be a marker of androgen action in women. A highly sensitive PSA assay was used to measure serum PSA levels in normal women and women with hirsutism to determine whether serum PSA is associated with hyperandrogenic states in women.

Methods.—Serum PSA levels were compared between 22 women with hirsutism and a Ferriman-Gallwey score higher than 8 and 50 women without hirsutism. The distribution of PSA, age, and 3α-androstanediol glucuronide (3α-AG) was calculated for both groups. Serum testosterone levels were measured in 14 patients.

Results.—Compared with controls, women with hirsutism had higher PSA levels. There was a positive correlation between levels of PSA and 3α-AG. There was a negative correlation between PSA and 3α-AG values and patient age. In patients in whom serum testosterone was measured, there was a positive correlation between serum testosterone and 3α-AG and PSA and a negative correlation between PSA and α-AG and age. The 3α-AG was a slightly better marker of androgen excess than PSA.

Conclusion.—Serum PSA levels were significantly higher in women with hirsutism. There was a significant positive correlation between PSA levels and 3α-AG and a negative correlation with age. Serum PSA may be considered a biochemical marker of androgen action in females.

▶ Finasteride has been used successfully for hirsutism in women; this study helps us to understand why. Prostate-specific antigen has been thought to be produced only by men, but with a newer, more sensitive test, it has now been found in women, and it is higher in hirsute women. High PSA could suggest which women would respond to finasteride. Whether PSA will become a common test in hirsute women awaits further studies.

M.A. Bowman, M.D., M.P.A.

Outcome of Long-term Treatment With the 5α-reductase Inhibitor Finasteride in Idiopathic Hirsutism: Clinical and Hormonal Effects During a 1-year Course of Therapy and 1-year Follow-up
Castello R, Negri C, Tosi F, et al (Univ of Verona, Italy)
Fertil Steril 66:734–740, 1996   15–25

Background.—The competitive 5α-reductase inhibitor finasteride converts testosterone to its active metabolite dihydrotestosterone, and is widely used for the treatment of benign prostatic hyperplasia. Increased 5α-reductase activity is involved in several common skin disorders, including idiopathic hirsutism and baldness. The long-term outcomes of finasteride treatment in women with idiopathic hirsutism were evaluated.

Methods.—Fourteen women, with a mean age of 23, received 12 months of treatment with finasteride, 5 mg once daily. At baseline, all had a modified Ferriman-Gallwey hirsutism score of 9 or greater. The women were followed up through treatment, and 9 for 1 year after treatment. Outcome measures included the Ferriman-Gallwey score, serum sex hormone levels, and serum and urinary markers of 5α-reductase activity.

Results. At the end of treatment, the mean Ferriman-Gallwey score had dropped from 11.8 to 4. Serum markers of 5α-reductase activity had declined, whereas urinary steroid metabolite ratios had consistently increased. All these hormonal changes reverted to normal after the end of treatment. There were no serious adverse effects. Although hirsutism scores increased in the year after finasteride therapy, they remained lower than baseline (Fig 1).

Conclusions.—Finasteride is an effective and well-tolerated therapy for idiopathic hirsutism in women. For most patients, this treatment produces sustained reduction in hair growth. 5α-Reductase inhibition appears to be the most rational treatment approach for hirsute women with normal serum androgen levels. They must receive careful contraception during therapy.

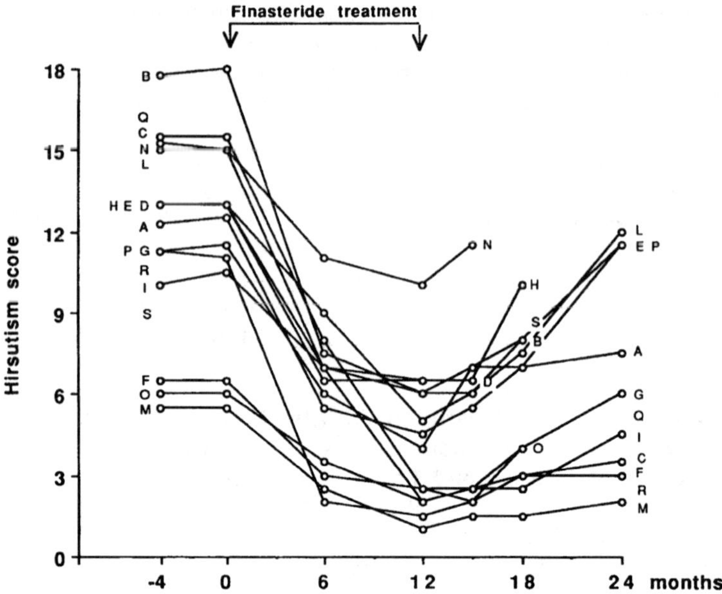

FIGURE 1.—Changes in individual Ferriman-Gallwey scores of the 14 women under study, indicated by the letters *A* to *P*. Evaluations were performed twice at baseline (−4 and 0 months), after 6 and 12 months of treatment, and after 3, 6, and 12 months of follow-up. (Courtesy of Castello R, Negri C, Tosi F, et al: Outcome of long-term treatment with the 5α-reductase inhibitor finasteride in idiopathic hirsutism: Clinical and hormonal effects during a 1-year course of therapy and 1-year follow-up. *Fertil Steril* 66:734–740, 1996. Reproduced with permission of the publisher, the American Society for Reproductive Medicine [formerly The American Fertility Society].)

▶ I continue to be fascinated by the increasing possibilities for improving idiopathic hirsutism, a frequent cosmetic concern for mostly middle-aged women. Finasteride has been shown to provide good improvement in hirsutism with few side effects in a few small studies, and is probably better than spironolactone for this. This study is also small, but it provided longer follow-up than previous studies. The finding that some of the hirsutism effect persisted for 1 year after 1 year of therapy is encouraging, because one fear concerns the long-term effects of the use of finasteride in women. Much of the improvement in hirsutism on finasteride occurred in the first 6 months, which may mean that shorter, intermittent treatment could be used. I have not used this treatment and am unlikely to do so except in a severe and otherwise unresponsive case, and then I would inform the patient that it was experimental. From what I have seen and heard, the new laser treatment for hirsutism is also encouraging.

M.A. Bowman, M.D., M.P.A.

Miscellaneous

Normal Findings in Vulvar Examination and Vulvoscopy

van Beurden M, van der Vange N, de Craen AJM, et al (Academic Med Centre, Amsterdam, Netherlands Cancer Inst, Amsterdam)
Br J Obstet Gynaecol 104:320–324, 1997   15–26

Background.—The vulvoscope, introduced to aid in the assessment of vulvar complaints, has been used in the management of vulvar intraepithelial neoplasia (VIN) to remove all visible lesions. Whether vulvoscopy has the same predictive value as colposcopy is unknown. To obtain a reference value for vulvar examination and vulvoscopy in the diagnostic workup of women with vulvar complaints, vulvar findings by vulvoscopy and naked-eye examination in healthy, asymptomatic women were documented.

Methods and Findings.—Forty volunteers with no vulvar complaints, aged 21 to 56 years, were included. Naked-eye vulvar assessment revealed vestibular papillomatosis in 33% of the women and vestibular erythema in 43%. In 53% of women with vestibular erythema, the touch test was positive. Vulvoscopy was performed after the application of 5% acetic acid. An acetowhite vestibule was noted in all women. Thirty percent had acteowhite lesions outside the vestibule, and 15% were positive for human papillomavirus (HPV) DNA. The finding of HPV DNA was uncorrelated with vestibular erythema and vestibular papillomatosis. The occurrence of acetowhite lesions outside the vestibule was weakly correlated with HPV DNA. In this group, younger women were significantly more likely to have vestibular papillomatosis, and smokers more often had a genital HPV infection.

Conclusion.—In these healthy women, vestibular papillomatosis was normal and could disappear with age. Vestibular erythema with a positive touch test was also common. Thus, it is questionable whether every acetowhite lesion in women with VIN III contains dysplastic epithelium.

▶ Knowing what is normal is key to knowing what is abnormal. Although we all see many normals every day in the practice of family medicine, it is often still difficult to know whether a finding is normal or represents pathology that requires treatment. Thus, this article adds to our knowledge of the normal vulva, particularly with acetic acid and vulvoscopy. I have long believed erythema, sebaceous glands, and some papillomatosis seems normal, which the authors confirm. In addition, the touch test, often used for the diagnosis of vestibulitis (chronic vestibular pain of unknown cause), produced abnormal results in over half of those with erythema. The authors also found that all women had an acetowhite vestibule after the application of acetic acid— although the vestibule looked anatomically consistent and symmetric; however, some acetowhite lesions were not HPV, suggesting the need for biopsy confirmation.

M.A. Bowman, M.D., M.P.A.

An Updated Basal Body Temperature Method

Frank E, White R (Emory Univ, Atlanta)
Contraception 54:319–321, 1996

15–27

Introduction.—Many women monitor their basal body temperatures (BBT) in an effort to conceive or avoid conception. However, many factors besides hormones can affect BBT, including the time of day, sleep, ambient temperatures, and voluntary and involuntary activities. These activities were adjusted for by measuring BBT in a control participant who has exogenous influence similar to a woman's but no hormonal changes: the woman's husband.

Methods.—A married, cohabiting couple each took their temperature using the same BBT thermometer. Temperatures were measured each day on first awakening for 2 months.

Results.—The husband's and wife's temperatures showed substantial covariability. When an unexplained change in the wife's temperature occurred, a similar change was seen in the husband's temperature. An enlarged gap between the temperatures occurred in the postovulatory period, consistent with the results of home and laboratory tests (Figs 1–5).

Conclusions.—Use of a noncycling control who is exposed to the same exogenous influences (i.e., the woman's husband) could represent a new approach to BBT monitoring. This method is inexpensive, simple, and painless and may improve the accuracy of BBT monitoring. Larger studies are warranted.

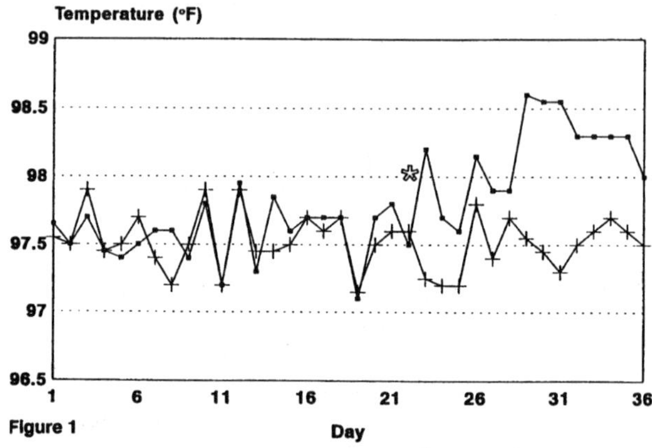

FIGURES 1–5.—Basal body temperatures during 5 cycles in consecutive months of a 34-year-old woman and a 36-year-old male control exposed to similar environmental influences. *Abbreviations: EF,* Erica Frank; *LH,* luteinizing hormone; *RFW,* Randell White. (Courtesy of Frank E, White R: An updated basal body temperature method. *Contraception* 54:310–321. Copyright 1996, Elsevier Science, Inc.)

(Continued)

FIGURE 1-5 (cont.)

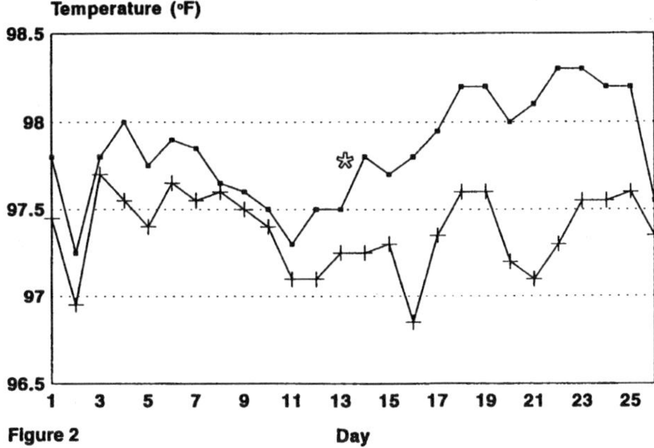

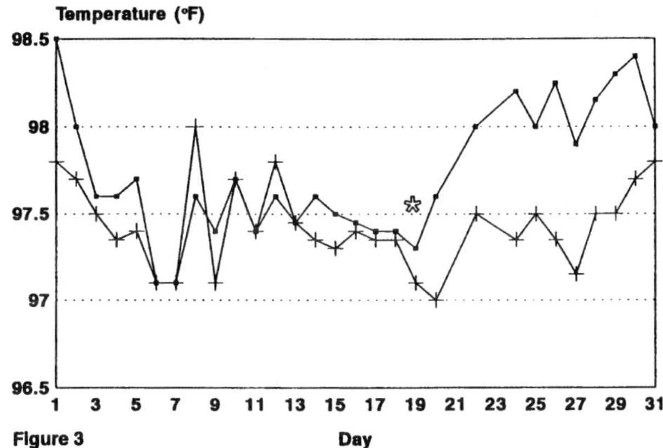

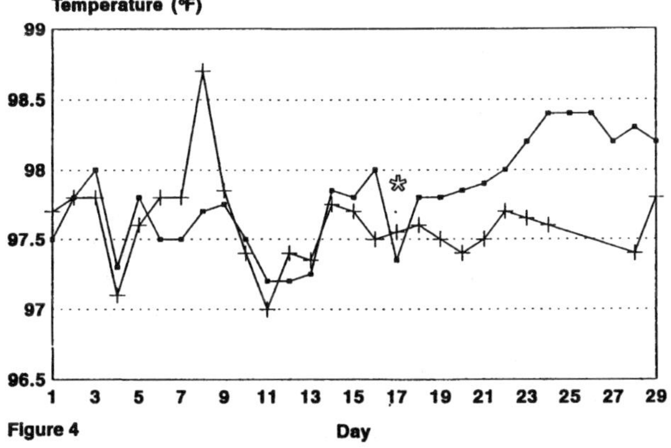

(Continued)

FIGURE 1-5 (cont.)

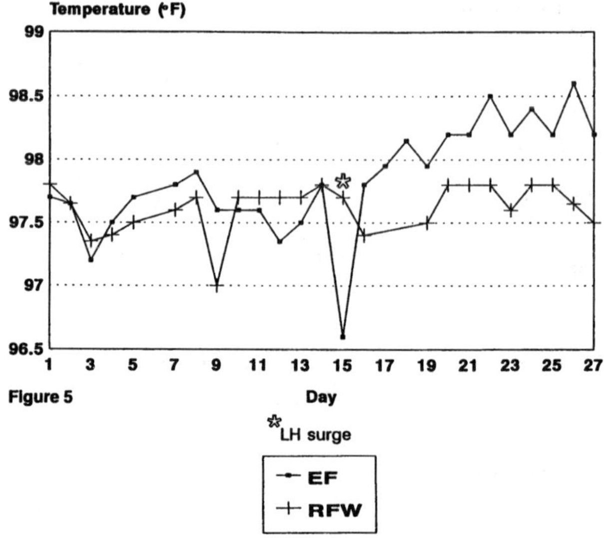

▶ Here is a new way to get the potential father-to-be involved! This is a case report, but an interesting one to family medicine. It is common to use BBTs to ascertain the presence or absence of ovulation. However, this physician couple clearly shows that the woman's BBT varies with that of her husband's and that ovulation is even clearer when the two BBTs are compared.

M.A. Bowman, M.D., M.P.A.

Vaginal Douching and the Risk of Ectopic Pregnancy Among Black Women

Kendrick JS, Atrash HK, Strauss LT, et al (Emory Univ, Atlanta, Ga)
Am J Obstet Gynecol 176:991–997, 1997

15–28

Background.—For unknown reasons, the number of ectopic pregnancies has increased markedly in recent years, especially among black women and women of other minority groups. Douching is a potential but little-studied risk factor for ectopic pregnancy. Vaginal douching was studied as a risk factor for ectopic pregnancy in black women.

Methods.—The case-control study included 197 black women seen at a public hospital with surgically confirmed ectopic pregnancy. Two control groups of black women were studied, 882 who delivered live or stillborn infants and 237 who were seeking pregnancy termination. As part of a larger interview, each woman was asked about douching.

Results.—Women with ectopic pregnancy were more likely to have a history of ever having douched, with an adjusted odds ratio of 3.8. Ectopic pregnancy risk rose along with the number of years of douching at least once a month (Fig 1). All douching practices, even douching for routine

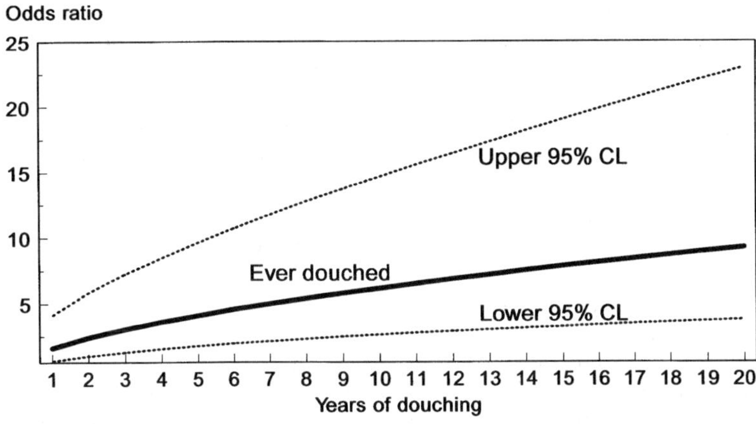

FIGURE 1.—Risk of ectopic pregnancy by years of douching at least once per month. *CL,* Confidence limit; *Asterisk,* Odds ratio for ever douching compared with never douching, adjusted for marital status, parity, smoking, and infertility. (Courtesy of Kendrick JS, Atrash HK, Strauss LT, et al: Vaginal douching and the risk of ectopic pregnancy among black women. *Am J Obstet Gynecol* 176:991–997, 1997.)

cleanliness, increased the risk of ectopic pregnancy. It is estimated that two thirds of black women douche, and the findings suggest that as many as 65% of ectopic pregnancies among these women are related to douching.

Conclusions.—Douching appears to be a modifiable risk factor for ectopic pregnancy among black women. The reasons that women douche may involve complex psychosocial issues involving product marketing and women's perceptions of their bodies and sexuality. Douching has been linked to other gynecologic conditions as well; no form of douching appears to be safe.

▶ Black women have more ectopic pregnancies and are more likely to douche. This study attempted to see whether there was a link between these facts. From the study results and the estimate that two thirds of black women douche, the authors claim that 65% of ectopic pregnancies in black women may be associated with douching. We could add a question about douching to our routine questionnaires, and we should consider warning black women about the association with ectopic pregnancies. Although I suspect that the same association may be true for white women, they were not included in this study.

M.A. Bowman, M.D., M.P.A.

Oral Contraception and the Recognition of Endometritis
Ness RB, Keder LM, Soper DE, et al (Univ of Pittsburgh, Pa; Magee Women's Hosp, Richmond, Va; Med College of Virginia, Richmond; et al)
Am J Obstet Gynecol 176:580–585, 1997
15–29

Objective.—The use of oral contraceptives is associated with a lower incidence of pelvic inflammatory disease (PID) and a higher incidence of chlamydial cervicitis. To explain this apparent contradiction, an investigation was made of women with histologic findings of endometritis but without clinical findings of PID, comparing them with women with clinically recognized PID and endometritis.

Methods.—In the multicenter, case-control study, biopsy specimens were obtained from 100 women without clinical signs of PID and from 219 women with recognized PID. In the unrecognized PID group, 43 women had endometritis, and in the PID group, 111 had endometritis. Oral contraceptive use and other risk factors were determined and analyzed statistically.

Results.—Compared with women with recognized endometritis, women with unrecognized endometritis were significantly less likely to report a history of PID or of sexually transmitted diseases or to have a positive cervical culture for *Neisseria gonorrhoeae.* Twelve of 43 women with unrecognized endometritis and 10 of 111 women with recognized endometritis used oral contraceptives. When these results were adjusted for potentially confounding factors, oral contraceptive use among women with unrecognized endometritis was 4.3 times that of women with recognized endometritis.

Conclusion.—Oral contraceptive use appears to have a mediating effect on endometritis, possibly by reducing the inflammatory reaction associated with infection of the upper genital tract. The relationship between oral contraceptive use and sexually transmitted disease needs further investigation.

▶ These women had positive cultures for *Neisseria gonorrhoeae* or *Chlamydia trachomatis* or a male partner culture positive for the same organisms. All the women had endometrial biopsies to identify endometritis. The women taking oral contraceptives had a greater rate of unmatched physical evidence and histologic evidence of PID. Why would women taking oral contraceptives have less signs of tenderness with endometritis? The authors theorize that oral contraceptives reduce the inflammatory response or that fewer organisms get into the upper track and, thus, the endometritis is less severe. The long-term outcome regarding infertility is unknown. Similarly, the implications for endometritis caused by organisms other than *Neisseria* or *Chlamydia* are unknown. However, this should heighten our awareness of potential missed PID in women taking oral contraceptives.

M.A. Bowman, M.D., M.P.A.

16 Obstetrics

Introduction

This chapter contains a small but significant number of randomized clinical trials, somewhat unusual in obstetrics. The opening section covers risks of work, exercise, obesity, and stress on pregnancy outcome. Clinical trials of sweeping membranes and use of misoprostol in labor induction follow. Two randomized trials of selective amniotomy and labor position, and an American Academy of Family Physicians clinical policy (based on randomized trials) of trial of labor in women with prior cesarean section comprise the section on the second stage. Articles documenting the hazards of episiotomy are reviewed in the next section, followed by a couple of studies in the postpartum period on eating habits and depression.

The organization and delivery of obstetric services is covered in 3 articles with good things to say about nurse-midwives. Two studies on risk of post-term birth and the birth outcomes of in vitro fertilization in a large cohort appear in the final short section.

Randomized controlled trials: Abstracts 16–6, 16–8, 16–9, and 16–10.

Alfred O. Berg, M.D., M.P.H.

Prenatal Care

Reproductive Hazards of the American Lifestyle: Work During Pregnancy
Gabbe SG, Turner LP (Univ of Washington, Seattle; Ohio State Univ, Columbus)
Am J Obstet Gynecol 176:826–832, 1997   16–1

Introduction.—Nearly all women who have worked before pregnancy now continue their employment into the third trimester. A review of the literature relating to the impact of working on perinatal outcome was designed to address concerns about possible adverse effects, particularly for American women who work during pregnancy.

Methods.—Data examined for the study included U.S. Department of Labor reports, the 1988 National Maternal and Infant Health Survey, a questionnarie study of nurses in the Association of Women's Health, Obstetrical, and Neonatal Nurses, and journal articles. Topics considered were characteristics of the working woman in the United States, adverse outcomes related to working during pregnancy, workplace exposures, the significance of stress, and the role of the obstetrician-gynecologist in improving pregnancy outcomes for working women.

Results.—Approximately 70% of women who work are employed in technical, sales, and administrative occupations (44.4%) or in managerial and professional areas (26.2%). In contrast to nonworking women, pregnant women who are employed are more likely to be educated, have a higher income, start prenatal care earlier, and gain more weight during pregnancy. Working women are also less likely to have a low–birth-weight infant and significantly less likely to have a preterm birth. One study found a relationship between preterm birth and indices of occupational fatigue (based upon components of activity, including posture, work on an industrial machine, physical exertion, mental stress, and working environment). In general, an increase in preterm and low–birth-weight infants is observed in women with stressful or physically demanding jobs and those exposed to hazardous substances. Women with less strenuous occupations or who can modify their work activity during pregnancy have fewer adverse outcomes.

Conclusion.—Most working pregnant women have good perinatal outcomes, but various factors can increase the risk for preterm birth and delivery of a low–birth-weight infant. Physicians should ask specific questions about employment, particularly concerning prolonged periods of standing, strenuous work, and exposure to hazardous substances. Modification of job requirements or a leave from work may be needed to assure a good outcome.

▶ Today, most pregnant women are working outside the home. Overall, work during pregnancy is not associated with an increased risk of adverse perinatal outcomes. However, a woman whose occupation requires prolonged periods of standing and long working hours may be at increased risk for preterm birth and the delivery of a low–birth-weight infant. Mental stress at work also increases risk. The family physician should provide support and guidance to working pregnant women. Physician-ordered frequent breaks, including elevation of the legs, may help the mother balance her working environment with her pregnancy.

J.E. Scherger, M.D., M.P.H.

Physical Activity and Pregnancy Outcome: Review and Recommendations
Sternfeld B (Kaiser Permanente Med Care Program, Oakland, Calif)
Sports Med 23:33–47, 1997   16–2

Background.—Historically, recommendations for physical activity during pregnancy have been based on social standards rather than on scientific evidence. The American College of Obstetrics and Gynecologists issued recommendations for exercise during pregnancy in 1985 and revised these recommendations in 1994 to acknowledge the growing body of evidence indicating that exercise does not harm fetal growth and development during a normal pregnancy. The evidence regarding exercise during pregnancy was reviewed and practical guidelines for safe exercise were presented.

Physiologic Factors.—The dual stresses of pregnancy and exercise can create conflicting physiologic demands that can adversely affect pregnancy outcome. The redistribution of uterine blood flow and possible fetal hypoxia, hyperthermia and risk of teratogenic effects, decreased carbohydrate availability for the fetus, and increased uterine contractility with a potential increase in risk for preterm labor have all been recognized as potential threats to fetal growth and development. However, for each of these physiologic problems, there appear to be compensatory mechanisms that protect the fetus.

Studies of Physical Activity and Pregnancy Outcome.—A large body of evidence has accumulated in the last 20 years on the effects of exercise on outcome of pregnancy. Case studies of pregnant athletes, laboratory studies of physical fitness, exercise intervention studies, and epidemiologic studies of recreational and occupational activity have analyzed the effects of activity during pregnancy on birth weight and gestational age. Results generally indicate that physical activity is safe for healthy, well-nourished women during a normal pregnancy. Exceptions include a higher risk of premature birth associated with prolonged standing and decreased birth weight associated with undernutrition and limited weight gain.

Recommendations.—An exercise program for pregnant women has the same elements as other exercise programs. It should be individualized and should take into account the health status, interests, and needs of the individual. The exercise design should cover aerobic conditioning, muscular strength, endurance, flexibility, warm up, and cool down.

Discussion.—Most studies have found little or no association between exercise and birth weight or gestational age. Exercise is safe for healthy women during a normal pregnancy. The public health message is probably that women may exercise during pregnancy and not that they should exercise.

▶ This well-balanced article describes the risks and benefits of exercise, both documented and potential, during pregnancy. The literature review is extensive, and the discussion is detailed and specific. This article might be copied and given to patients wanting extensive information. The "bottom line" is quite reassuring, i.e., for healthy, well-nourished women, exercise during pregnancy is safe and subject to few restrictions.

J.E. Scherger, M.D., M.P.H.

Lowering the Threshold for the Diagnosis of Gestational Diabetes

Rust OA, Bofill JA, Andrew ME, et al (Univ of Mississippi, Jackson; Carolinas Med Ctr, Charlotte, NC)
Am J Obstet Gynecol 175:961–965, 1996   16–3

Introduction.—A carbohydrate intolerance of varying severity with onset or diagnosis during pregnancy is known as gestational diabetes mellitus. With a reported incidence of 3% of all gestations, it is the most common metabolic disorder of pregnancy. There has been some debate over the recommendations for the diagnostic criteria of gestational diabetes mellitus on the basis of whole blood glucose determinations. Whether lowering the diagnostic threshold for gestational diabetes mellitus on 3-hour 100-g oral glucose tolerance testing would select a population at risk for adverse perinatal outcome was determined.

Methods.—A standardized 3-hour oral glucose tolerance test was given to 434 women with an abnormal 50-g glucose screen result of 140 mg/d or greater. The results were stratified according to the lower diagnostic threshold and maternal weight. The primary perinatal outcome variables analyzed were birth weight and rate of macrosomia. Retrospectively, the patients were divided into 4 groups. One group had gestational diabetes mellitus diagnosed by 2 abnormal values by the standard National Diabetes Data Group/American College of Obstetricians and Gynecologists (ACOG) criteria; the second group would have had gestational diabetes mellitus diagnosed only if the Sacks criteria were used; the third group had only 1 abnormal value by any criteria, and the fourth group had all normal glucose values by all criteria.

Results.—Patients who would have been newly diagnosed with gestational diabetes mellitus according to the Sacks criteria, were older and heavier. Statistical significance was not achieved with any other variable comparisons. When the same patients were stratified according to prepregnancy weight, overweight patients were older, had had cesarean section more often, gained less weight during the third trimester, and had higher cumulative maternal morbidity. Macrosomia was not predicted, nor was birth weight influenced by the degree of hyperglycemia, according to regression analysis. Macrosomia was associated with prepregnant maternal body mass index.

Conclusion.—Maternal prepregnant body mass index influences fetal macrosomia. Overdiagnosis of gestational diabetes mellitus would be the result of lowering the glucose tolerance test threshold, and this would not improve perinatal outcome. Until a more sensitive criteria set can be determined with respect to perinatal outcome, the National Diabetes Data Group/ACOG criteria should be maintained as the diagnostic threshold for gestational diabetes mellitus.

▶ I welcome this article as a counterbalance to the trend of lowering the threshold for the diagnosis of gestational diabetes, which results in many more diagnoses. Data such as these should keep us from having many normal women burdened by this diagnosis, reserving the extensive testing and intervention for those patients who truly have the problem.

J.E. Scherger, M.D., M.P.H.

The Preterm Prediction Study: Maternal Stress Is Associated With Spontaneous Preterm Birth at Less Than Thirty-five Weeks' Gestation

Copper RL, and the National Institute of Child Health and Human Development Maternal-Fetal Medicine Units Network (Natl Inst of Child Health, Bethesda, Md)

Am J Obstet Gynecol 175:1286–1292, 1997   16–4

Introduction.—Increased rates of prematurity and low birth weight (LBW) are linked with such psychosocial factors as stress, depression, and low self-esteem. These factors are also associated with poor health behaviors during pregnancy, such as smoking and substance abuse. This study examined the hypothesis that women with stress during pregnancy have higher rates of spontaneous preterm delivery, LBW, and intrauterine growth restriction (IUGR). It was also hypothesized that women with poor psychosocial status have increased rates of substance use, and that such behavior is more prevalent among women who deliver preterm or LBW babies.

Methods.—Participants were part of a larger prospective study of numerous predictors of spontaneous prematurity. Those eligible were identified at or before 24 weeks' gestation during an uncomplicated (as confirmed by US at 15 to 24 weeks) singleton pregnancy. Psychosocial assessments were administered to the women at a mean gestational age of 26.1 weeks; the lowest quartile scores were used to define poor psychosocial status. Women with high and low scores were compared for percentage of spontaneous preterm birth, LBW, and IUGR.

Results.—The study population was 63% black and 35% white; mean maternal age was 22.6 years. Tobacco use was reported by 30%, alcohol use by 12%, and illicit drug use by 5%. Most of the women were unmarried (72%) and had government insurance (94%). One hundred women (3.9%) had a spontaneous preterm birth at <35 weeks of gestation; the rate of preterm birth at <37 weeks was 15.5%. Rates of LBW and IUGR were 11.1% and 5.1%, respectively. The only psychosocial characteristic significantly associated with spontaneous preterm birth, IUGR, or LBW was high stress. Characteristics linked with poor psychosocial status (anxiety, low self-esteem, lack of mastery, and depression) were more likely to be present in women with these pregnancy outcomes, but the association was not statistically significant.

Conclusion.—Even after adjustment for maternal demographic and behavioral characteristics, stress was found to be associated with spontaneous preterm birth, IUGR, and LBW. Black race also proved a strong risk factor for these outcomes. Interventions targeted toward relieving emotional stress, enhancing self-esteem, and changing adverse health behaviors could improve pregnancy outcomes.

▶ Preterm birth is the number one cause of infant morbidity and mortality, and it carries extraordinary health care costs. Consequently, it is the number one public health target in perinatal care. Social factors may play a greater role than medical factors in its origin. As with so many other important public health problems of today, such as asthma, heart disease, and cancer, lifestyle and social factors must be addressed to achieve success.

J.E. Scherger, M.D., M.P.H.

Association Between Pre-pregnancy Obesity and the Risk of Cesarean Delivery

Crane SS, Wojtowycz MA, Dye TD, et al (State Univ of New York, Syracuse)
Obstet Gynecol 89:213–216, 1997　　　　　　　　　　　　　　　16–5

Background.—Currently, more than 32 million women in the United States are overweight, and 40% of young adult women are obese. Overweight and obesity carry a risk of diabetes, hypertension, dyslipidemia, cardiovascular disease, stroke, menstrual irregularities, and some types of cancer. Prepregnancy obesity is associated with gestational diabetes, macrosomia, shoulder dystocia, multiple gestation, and operative risks. Prepregnancy obesity may also be associated with a higher risk of cesarean delivery.

Methods.—The subjects were 19,699 women who had a live birth after 20 weeks' gestation. The mode of delivery in women who were obese before pregnancy was compared with that of women who were not obese before pregnancy. A separate analysis was made of women with singleton pregnancies and no prior cesarean deliveries.

Results.—Obesity was defined as a body mass index greater than 29. In a subset of 16,391 women who had a singleton pregnancy and no prior cesarean deliveries, 16.6% were obese before pregnancy, and 21.5% of these had cesarean delivery, compared with 13.5% of women who were not obese before pregnancy. In this subset, the overall rate of cesarean delivery was 14.8%. In the entire sample, 18.2% of women were obese before pregnancy, and 33.8% of these had cesarean delivery, compared with 20.2% of women who were not obese before pregnancy. For the entire sample, the overall rate of cesarean delivery was 22.7%. Increased age, increased parity, pregnancy-induced hypertension, diabetes mellitus, birth weight greater than 4,000 g, multiple gestation, and prior cesarean delivery were confounding variables.

Discussion.—These findings indicate that women who are obese before pregnancy have a higher risk of having a cesarean delivery. Before pregnancy, obese women should receive counseling on proper diet and activity to help them lose weight. A decrease in obesity before pregnancy may lower the rate of cesarean delivery.

▶ Preconception care is still not commonly practiced for women of child-bearing age. Obesity is a legitimate chronic disease, and with newer treatments leading to more successful management, the prepregnancy treatment of obesity is now more feasible than ever. This study underscores the importance of treating obesity before pregnancy to reduce the risk of pregnancy complications, including the need for cesarean section.

J.E. Scherger, M.D., M.P.H.

Labor Induction

The Effectiveness of Sweeping Membranes at Term: A Randomized Trial
Crane J, Bennett K, Young D, et al (Mem Univ of Newfoundland, St John's, Canada)
Obstet Gynecol 89:586–590, 1997   16–6

Introduction.—Sweeping or stripping membranes has long been used to initiate labor, but the benefits of this procedure have not been confirmed in a well-designed trial. A randomized study of 150 patients at low risk at 38 to 40 weeks of gestation examined the rate of spontaneous labor within 7 days of sweeping membranes.

Methods.—The healthy women recruited for the trial had no pregnancy complications or contraindications to vaginal delivery. Duration of gestation was based on firm dates of last menstrual period or early US findings. The women were randomly assigned to sweeping or control groups and stratified within these groups according to the status of the cervix (open vs closed) at pelvic examination. For those assigned to sweeping, as much membrane as possible was separated from the lower uterine segment by sweeping the examiner's index finger twice in a circumferential manner. In addition to the rate of spontaneous labor, reported outcomes included mode of delivery, analgesia use, maternal infection, and neonatal morbidity.

Results.—Seventy-six women were randomly assigned to the sweeping group (61 with cervix open and 15 with cervix closed) and 74 to the control group (60 with cervix open and 14 with cervix closed). The 2 groups were similar in baseline variables, including maternal age and Bishop score. Sweeping and control groups did not differ significantly in the proportion of women who entered spontaneous labor within 7 days of study entry (33% vs 38%, respectively). Outcomes were similar when only women with open cervices were included in the analysis (23 of 61 in the sweeping group and 22 of 60 in the control group) and after stratification on the basis of parity. Sweeping did not appear to increase spontaneous rupture of the membranes before the onset of labor or the rates of forceps or vacuum and cesarean deliveries. There were no serious maternal complications in either group, but significantly more women in the sweeping group received epidural analgesia. Multivariate analysis revealed that a Bishop score <7 predicted spontaneous labor within 1 week; gestational age at enrollment predicted spontaneous labor before 41 weeks and the overall rate of spontaneous labor.

Conclusion.—In contrast to previous studies, in which sweeping and control groups may have differed at baseline, this randomized trial found that sweeping membranes once at 38 to 40 weeks of gestation was of little value in initiating labor within 7 days.

▶ Sweeping or stripping the membranes has had renewed popularity because of the increased desire to avoid delayed delivery. These authors criticize previous studies showing effectiveness of this procedure[1, 2] and offer a randomized, controlled trial. My criticism of this study is that patients were selected between 38 and 40 weeks of gestation, often with a cervix that was not ripe. Experience shows that the success of sweeping membranes is directly related to the ripeness of the cervix, as the success of shaking an apple tree to harvest apples depends on the ripeness of the fruit. The study documents that sweeping membranes early in term (38 to 40 weeks) has little value and should be reserved for the period after 40 weeks, in an attempt to avoid going beyond 42 weeks.

J.E. Scherger, M.D., M.P.H.

References

1. Wiriyasirivaj B, Vutyavanich T, Ruangsri RA: A randomized controlled trial of membrane stripping at term to promote labor. *Obstet Gynecol* 87:767–770, 1996.
2. Berghella V, Rogers RA, Lescale K: Stripping of membranes as a safe method to reduce prolonged pregnancies. *Obstet Gynecol* 87:927–931, 1996.

Fetal Fibronectin: A New Tool for the Prediction of Successful Induction of Labor

Garite TJ, Casal D, Garcia-Alonso A, et al (Univ of California, Irvine; Hosp de Gineco-Obstetrica "Luis Castelazo-Ayala, Mexico City)
Am J Obstet Gynecol 175:1516–1521, 1996   16–7

Background.—There have been recent reports regarding an isoform of human fibronectin, called fetal fibronectin, that seeps from the choriodecidual interface through the cervix into the vagina 1 to 2 weeks before labor. An assay for cervicovaginal fetal fibronectin has been developed to identify patients with signs of premature labor who may be in true labor. This test may also be useful for predicting the success of labor induction.

Methods.—The study took place at a large hospital in Mexico City, Mexico, chosen for its large number of obstetric patients and its common practice of inducing labor. A vaginal swab from 160 women at 36 weeks' gestation was tested for fetal fibronectin at the time of initiation of prostaglandin for cervical ripening or initiation of oxytocin.

Results.—Test results for fetal fibronectin were positive in 108 patients and negative in 52. The rate of cesarean section was lower in patients with positive test results. These patients also had shorter intervals to delivery, including the interval from first dose of prostaglandin to delivery and first stage of labor. These findings were also seen in nulliparous women with a

Bishop score of 5 or less, in patients with positive test results having a statistically shorter interval to delivery and similar differences in cesarean section rate. In this subgroup of patients, more than 50% of women with negative test results had not delivered after 24 hours and were given a second dose of prostaglandin. Only 2 of 53 women with positive test results had not delivered after 24 hours and were given a second dose of prostaglandin. The predictive value of a positive test of fetal fibronectin was independent of the Bishop score.

Discussion.—Detection of fetal fibronectin in patients at 36 weeks' gestation before induction of labor may allow identification of patients who have a shorter interval to delivery, have shorter labor, and are less likely to need cesarean section. This test may also be used in patients with low Bishop scores.

▶ Fibronectin has emerged as an exciting new compound which, when present, is very predictive of ready onset of labor and feasibility of induction. This study presents an amazing finding. Even with intact membranes, women ripe for labor have a fetal compound present in the vagina. I have spoken with Dr. Garite, and exactly how this fetal compound gets into the vagina is open to speculation. It will be interesting to see whether this simple chemical measurement will replace the Bishop score, which has been used for decades yet is not well remembered by occasional providers of obstetric care.

J.E. Scherger, M.D., M.P.H.

A Comparison of Differing Dosing Regimens of Vaginally Administered Misoprostol for Preinduction Cervical Ripening and Labor Induction

Wing DA, Paul RH (Univ of Southern California, Los Angeles)
Am J Obstet Gynecol 175:158–164, 1996   16–8

Introduction.—The ideal labor induction is still unknown. Labor induction with an unfavorable cervix can be prolonged and tedious. Misoprostol is a synthetic prostaglandin E_1 analogue that has been used for preinduction cervical ripening and induction of labor in patients with Bishop scores of 4 or less. It is as effective as dinoprostone, the only drug approved by the Food and Drug Administration. The efficacy and safety of 2 differing dosing regimens of vaginally administered misoprostol were studied to minimize contractile problems.

Methods.—A total of 522 women with indications for induction of labor and unfavorable cervices were randomly assigned to one of 2 dosing regimens of vaginally administered misoprostol. The regimens were either 3-hourly applications in the posterior vaginal fornix to a maximum of 8 doses of 25 microgram tablets or 6-hourly applications to maximum of 4 doses. Regardless of the number of misoprostol doses administered, the maximal period of cervical ripening was 24 hours. Medication was not given after spontaneous rupture of membranes or at the beginning of active labor.

Results.—In the 3-hour dosing group, the average interval from start of induction to vaginal delivery was shorter (903.3 ± 482.1 minutes) when compared with the 6-hour dosing group (1,410 ± 869.1 minutes). In the 6-hour group, oxytocin augmentation of labor occurred more commonly (51.4%) than in the 3-hour group (41.8%). There were no significant differences between routes of delivery. Cesarean section was performed on 108 patients (20.8%). In the 3-hour group, there was a slightly higher prevalence of tachysystole (6 or more uterine contractions in a 10-minute window for 2 consecutive 10-minute periods) than in the 6-hour group; the difference was not statistically significant. There were no significant differences in the frequency of uterine hyperstimulation or hypertonus. There were no significant differences between the groups in the frequency of abnormal fetal heart rate tracings, meconium passage, 1- or 5-minute Apgar scores of more than 7, admissions to the neonatal ICU, or neonatal resuscitations.

Conclusion.—For cervical ripening and induction of labor, vaginally administered misoprostol is an effective agent. Women who were given the 3-hour dosing had shorter intervals to delivery, required oxytocin augmentation less frequently, and had fewer failed inductions than patients in the 6-hour group. More studies are needed to further characterize the safety of misoprostol, an inexpensive and simple-to-administer drug.

▶ It is difficult to keep up with the changing methods for cervical ripening and induction of labor. Prostaglandin gel now comes in different forms and differing applications. New in this area is the curious use of a medication that was designed to protect the stomach in patients taking nonsteroidal anti-inflammatory agents. Misoprostol has been shown to stimulate uterine contractions at any time during pregnancy. It appears to be comparable to prostaglandin gel in its safety and efficacy for cervical ripening and induction of labor. Oral regimens of this drug are also being studied for the same purpose.

J.E. Scherger, M.D., M.P.H.

Labor and Delivery

Randomised Trial Comparing a Policy of Early With Selective Amniotomy in Uncomplicated Labour at Term
Johnson N, Lilford R, Guthrie K, et al (St James's Univ, Leeds, England; Leeds Univ, England)
Br J Obstet Gynaecol 104:340–346, 1997   16–9

Introduction.—Some practitioners and hospitals follow a policy of leaving the membranes of women in labor at term intact for as long as possible; others rupture the membranes before full dilation. A randomized, controlled clinical trial was designed to compare these 2 management policies.

Methods.—Enrollment in the trial took place between January 1988 and August 1991. Eligible women were admitted to the labor ward after the 36th completed week of pregnancy. All were in normal, uncomplicated, spontaneous labor and had intact membranes. The primary null hypothesis was that artificial rupture of membranes would not affect duration of labor. Other outcome measures examined were Apgar score, fetal and maternal morbidity, mode of delivery, epidural rates, and the number of vaginal examinations in the first stage of labor after amniotomy. Membranes were ruptured in women randomly assigned to the no amniotomy group only if a specific reason was present (selective amniotomy).

Results.—Maternity statistics were available for 1,540 women, 875 randomly assigned to routine amniotomy and 665 to selective amniotomy. The mean interval from admission to study entry was 40 minutes in both groups. The 2 groups were also similar in mean age, median time of painful contractions before admission, and median cervical dilation (4 cm) at time of random assignments. For parous women, a policy of routine rupture of the membranes on admission when in labor shortened the duration of labor by only 4 minutes. Among nulliparous women, however, routine amniotomy shortened the interval between random assignment and delivery by 50 minutes. Results of the analysis were not affected after exclusion of women who were probably not in established labor at the time of random assignment. The cesarean rate was slightly higher in the routine amniotomy group (3.1%) than in the selective amniotomy group (1.8%), and more vaginal examinations were performed after membrane rupture in the routine group. No differences were noted in oxytocin use, fetal condition at birth, retained placenta rates, blood loss, pain, or analgesia requirements.

Conclusion.—Routine amniotomy in women in normal labor at term may shorten the duration of the first labor, but not subsequent ones. There may be some harm associated with the practice, because the risk of cesarean section appears to be increased.

▶ The timing of amniotomy to facilitate labor is highly variable, with uncertain risks and benefits. Some providers consider it the first thing to do when a decision to proceed to labor is made, others reserve it until after the establishment of active labor. Empirical experience suggests that early amniotomy facilitates labor and may result in less need for oxitocin. This randomized, controlled trial from Great Britain sheds light on the issue. No benefit of early amniotomy was seen for women who had had previous children. The benefit for primiparous women was 1 hour of shorter labor, which must be balanced against an increased risk of cesarean section and infection. The wisest course is the safest one, and amniotomy should be reserved until active labor has been established.

J.E. Scherger, M.D., M.P.H.

Randomised Trial Comparing the Upright and Supine Positions for the Second Stage of Labour

de Jong PR, Johanson RB, Baxen P, et al (Univ of Cape Town, South Africa; Keele Univ, Stoke on Trent, Staffordshire)

Br J Obstet Gynaecol 104:567–571, 1997

16–10

Background.—Both the upright (squatting) and the supine (dorsal or recumbent) positions for delivery have their advantages and disadvantages. Both methods were examined in terms of specific maternal and neonatal measurements.

Methods.—Five hundred seventeen low-risk pregnant women were randomized into 2 groups: 257 were assigned to the upright position for delivery and 260 to the supine position. Predelivery variables (e.g., maternal age, gestation) did not differ between the groups. The afternoon after delivery, a midwife ignorant of the mode of delivery interviewed the mother for her subjective comments about the delivery.

Findings.—All women assigned to deliver in the supine position indeed delivered in this position, whereas 97% of the women in the upright position group maintained this position during the second stage of labor and 89% delivered in this position. The 2 groups did not differ significantly in the duration of labor, the amount of blood loss, or the number of women with perineal trauma that required suturing; however, the patients in the upright position group did have significantly fewer episiotomies. Furthermore, fetal and neonatal outcomes (including abnormal fetal heart rate and Apgar scores at 1 minute) did not differ between the 2 groups. However, fewer women in the upright position group reported pain during delivery.

Conclusions.—Use of the upright birthing position does not adversely affect the outcome of labor, and it is associated with fewer episodes of discomfort and pain in the second stage of labor. However, not all women in the upright position group delivered in the position in which they started. Pregnant women should continue to be counseled about the benefits of the upright posture.

▶ Studies comparing positions for the second stage of labor and delivery have been conflicting, but all suggest that there is no single preferred labor and birth position. Upright positions have advantages as described in this study from South Africa. The art of labor management includes helping the woman find the most comfortable and most effective position for delivering her baby. This is often different from the position preferred by the nurse to get external monitor tracings, or by the physician wanting maximum comfort delivering the baby. Nurses and physicians should be flexible and defer their comfort to the best option for the mother.

J.E. Scherger, M.D., M.P.H.

Vacuum-assisted Vaginal Delivery
Paluska SA (Univ of Michigan, Ann Arbor)
Am Fam Physician 55:2197–2203, 1997   16–11

Introduction.—Although physicians in the United States are often unwilling to use the vacuum extractor to assist vaginal deliveries, this method has replaced forceps as the instrument of choice in many other countries. The modern vacuum instrument has undergone a number of refinements to reduce the risk of injury to the mother and fetus. Various issues related to use of the vacuum extractor include indications and contraindications, technique, and potential complications.

Vacuum Extractor Versus Forceps.—Vacuum extraction has both advantages and disadvantages in comparison with forceps (Table 1). Most studies report no difference in effectiveness or in neonatal outcomes, but significantly more women require greater anesthesia for forceps delivery. Forceps are associated with a higher risk of maternal birth canal trauma and fetal facial injury, whereas neonatal jaundice not requiring phototherapy and neonatal retinal hemorrhages have occurred more frequently with vacuum extraction. Soft cups make the extractors easier to use and reduce the risk of fetal scalp trauma.

Indications and Contraindications.—Prerequisites for vacuum extraction are similar to those for forceps-assisted delivery (Table 2). Maternal factors include preexisting disease, exhaustion, and a prolonged second stage of labor; fetal jeopardy is another common reason for hastening delivery. Certain situations require that vacuum-assisted delivery be discontinued and forceps-assisted delivery or cesarean section considered (Table 3).

TABLE 1.—Comparison of Vacuum Extractor and Forceps

Advantages of vacuum extractor over forceps
Easier application
Less force applied to fetal head
Less anesthesia required
Less maternal soft tissue injury
Fewer fetal injuries
Less parental concern
Fetal head remains free to rotate

**Disadvantages of vacuum extractor compared
  with forceps**
Traction applied during contractions only
Possibly longer delivery than forceps
Small increase in cephalohematomas
Higher prevalence of neonatal jaundice
Lack of operator familiarity and experience
Difficulty in maintaining effective vacuum
Only used for term/near-term vertex infants

Information from Robinson JC: Forceps and vacuum extraction. *Curr Opin Obstet Gynecol* 6:414–416, 1994.
(Courtesy of Paluska SA: Vacuum-assisted vaginal delivery. *Am Fam Physician* 55:2197–2203, 1997. Reprint from the May 1997 issue of *American Family Physician*, published by the American Academy of Family Physicians.)

TABLE 2.—Requirements for Vacuum-assisted Delivery

Operational
Cesarean delivery staff available
Informed consent obtained
Experienced operator

Maternal
Clinical pelvimetry assessed
Maternal anesthesia provided
Bladder and rectum emptied
Amniotic membranes ruptured
Uterine cervix fully dilated

Fetal
Term or near-term fetus
Head deeply engaged
Skull has reached the pelvic floor
Scalp is visible at the introitus without separating
  the labia
Sagittal suture is in the anteroposterior diameter
  or right or left occiput anterior or posterior
  position
Postion and station of head known to be at or on
  the perineum and rotation does not exceed 45
  degrees
Vertex presentation

Information from Cunningham FG, MacDonald PC, Gant NF, et al. In Cunningham FG, Williams JW (eds): *Williams Obstetrics*, ed 19. Norwalk, Conn, Appleton & Large, 1993, pp 555–576. Information from Lucas MJ: The role of vacuum extraction in modern obstetrics. *Clin Obstet Gynecol* 37:794–805, 1994.

(Courtesy of Paluska SA: Vacuum-assisted vaginal delivery. *Am Fam Physician* 55:2197–2203, 1997. Reprint from the May 1997 issue of *American Family Physician*, published by the American Academy of Family Physicians.)

Technique.—The mother is positioned securely in the stirrups, with an empty bladder and adequate anesthesia. The integrity of the vacuum extractor is checked by generating negative pressure with the cup pressed against a flattened palm. Folding of the cup in the operator's hand facilitates its insertion and contact with the fetal head. The cup is placed as close as possible to the fetal occiput along the sagittal suture to promote flexion of the head. Finger sweeps are repeated to ensure that no vaginal tissue is included between the scalp and the cup. Traction attempts should be inter-

---

TABLE 3.—Indications for Discontinuing Vacuum-assisted Delivery

Three detachments of vacuum cup from the fetal
  head
Prolonged trial in excess of 30 minutes without
  success
Maximal vacuum force applied for more than 10
  minutes
Fetal scalp trauma after cup detachment

(Courtesy of Paluska SA: Vacuum-assisted vaginal delivery. *Am Fam Physician* 55:2197–2203, 1997. Reprint from the May 1997 issue of *American Family Physician*, published by the American Academy of Family Physicians.)

mittent and should coincide with contractions and maternal pushing. Negative pressure is reduced between contractions and rapidly
increased to maximum pressure (400 to 600 mm Hg) with each
subsequent contraction. Total time of maximum pressure should
not exceed 10 minutes. Once the head crowns, the extractor is
pulled upward at a 45-degree angle to the floor. Once the head
crosses the perineum, negative pressure is released, and the extractor cup gently is disengaged.

Complications.—Fetal injuries are more common than maternal injuries
during vacuum extraction. Retinal hemorrhage occurs most often in infants who are small for gestational age. Cephalohematomas, reported in as
many as 15% of vacuum-assisted deliveries, are usually self-limiting. Sub-
aponeurotic bleeding is a rare and potentially fatal complication. An
experienced operator and sound technique are essential to the success of
vacuum extraction.

▶ Vacuum-assisted deliveries have largely replaced the use of forceps and
can easily be done by providers of low-risk obstetric care, such as family
physicians and certified nurse-midwives. The technique is often taught right
in the delivery area, usually in a "see one, do one, teach one" mode. The
technique is generally simple and safe; however, there is an art to achieving
success, and the risk of fetal scalp injury is very real. This article describes
the appropriate use and method of this technique in detail. My only disagreement with the presentation concerns the requirements described in
Table 2. Maternal anesthesia is not necessary, and the vacuum may be
applied to the fetal skull before it has fully reached the pelvic floor. Sometimes this technique is helpful in assisting the fetal head with the position
change necessary for a successful delivery.

J.E. Scherger, M.D., M.P.H.

Trial of Labor or Repeated Cesarean Section: The Woman's Choice
Roberts RG, Bell HS, Wall EM, et al (Univ of Wisconsin, Madison; Univ of
Washington, Seattle; Oregon Health Sciences Univ, Portland; et al)
Arch Fam Med 6:120–125, 1997   16–12

Background.—Many studies have been published on vaginal birth after
cesarean section. However, no one has attempted to demonstrate which
approach is preferred after accounting for all outcomes previously reported, women's preferences, and the costs of each approach.
Methods.—Through MEDLINE searches and references from retrieved
articles, 759 citations were found. Among these, 202 articles with primary
outcomes data contrasting trial of labor (TOL) and elective repeat cesarean section (ERCS) were identified. Data were extracted by at least 2
investigators using a structured form.

Findings.—Trial of labor increased the risk for uterine rupture, and ERCS increased the risk for infection and bleeding. Among infant outcomes, only 5-minute Apgar scores of less than 7 differed. These were more likely to occur in infants whose mothers underwent TOL. Two thirds of the women desired TOL, and one third preferred ERCS. The cost of ERCS was 1.7–2.4 times greater.

Conclusions.—Clinicians should counsel women about the risks, benefits, and costs of TOL and ERCS. Although guidelines should recommend TOL, a woman's preference for ERCS should be respected.

▶ This article is the synthesis of the extensive clinical policy developed by a task force of the American Academy of Family Physicians. This review of vaginal birth after cesarean section is quite extensive, and goes a long way to support TOL instead of ERCS. However, the power of this article is in the argument that women should have a right to choose ERCS for personal reasons, without economics or medically controlled policies getting in the way. Demanding TOL may be just as inappropriate as demanding ERCS.

J.E. Scherger, M.D., M.P.H.

Episiotomy

Is There a Benefit to Episiotomy at Operative Vaginal Delivery? Observations Over Ten Years in a Stable Population

Ecker JL, Tan WM, Bansal RK, et al (Univ of California, San Francisco)
Am J Obstet Gynecol 176:411–414, 1997   16–13

Background.—Episiotomy is often done at operative vaginal delivery, although some have suggested that its use is associated with greater perineal morbidity. For spontaneous vaginal deliveries, time series analysis suggested that a decrease in the episiotomy rate was associated with a decrease in the rate of third- and fourth-degree perineal lacerations. The relationship between episiotomy rate and vaginal and perineal morbidity during operative (vacuum or forceps) vaginal delivery was examined.

Methods.—Between 1984 and 1994, 2,041 operative deliveries (976 vacuum and 1,065 forceps) met the inclusion criteria and were included in the study. Inclusion criteria included the delivery of a singleton term infant via cephalic presentation. Standard definitions of perineal lacerations were applied; third-degree lacerations involved partial tears of the anal sphincter. An intact perineum was defined as the absence of an episiotomy or lacerations of any degree.

Findings.—During the 10 years of the study, the episiotomy rate for operative vaginal deliveries declined significantly (from 93.4% to 35.7%). The overall vaginal laceration rate increased significantly (from 16.1% to 40.0%), yet the number of women with intact perinea (neither episiotomy nor lacerations) also increased significantly (2.2% to 2.7%). The rate of third-degree lacerations did not change significantly, although there were significantly fewer fourth-degree lacerations. These statistical relationships remained when data were stratified according to parity and type of instrument used.

Conclusions.—During the 10 years of the study, with the significant decrease in episiotomy rate came an increase in the rate of vaginal lacerations, yet also an increase in the rate of women with intact perinea. Such lacerations, although they require repair and cause postpartum blood loss and pain, are generally associated with minimal morbidity. The use of episiotomy at operative vaginal delivery must be balanced between the increase in vaginal lacerations and the decrease in fourth-degree lacerations.

▶ Until recently, episiotomy has been routinely done during vaginal delivery. For operative vaginal delivery (vacuum and forceps), the usual instructions are to perform an episiotomy. I have even seen this recommendation expressed as a "generous episiotomy." It has been assumed that, with operative vaginal delivery, the more room available the better. This study casts serious doubt on the use of episiotomy for vacuum or forceps delivery. It is noteworthy that during the period studied during this retrospective analysis, the use of episiotomy decreased for operative deliveries from 93.4% to 35.7%. In my own experience, I avoid the use of episiotomy for vacuum deliveries and rarely do forceps deliveries. Whereas the results of this study are inconclusive, family physicians should realize that episiotomy is not necessary for operative delivery, and that there will be many fewer fourth-degree lacerations from avoiding the procedure.

J.E. Scherger, M.D., M.P.H.

Association Between Median Episiotomy and Severe Perineal Lacerations in Primiparous Women

Labrecque M, Baillargeon L, Dallaire M, et al (Laval Univ, Québec; Centre de Santé Publique de Québec)
Can Med Assoc J 156:797–802, 1997   16–14

Objective.—Episiotomies are widely used to prevent severe perineal tears in primiparous women. For many years, studies have questioned whether having a median episiotomy actually increases the frequency of perineal lacerations. However, the relationship between an episiotomy and severe perineal lacerations is still unclear. The effects of a median episiotomy on the risk of severe perineal tears were analyzed in primiparous women, and adjustment was made for factors previously identified as potential confounders.

Methods.—The retrospective cohort study included 6,522 primiparas who delivered a single live baby in cephalic presentation during an 8½-year period. Information on a broad range of factors related to the labor and delivery were entered into a computerized database. Factors related to the attending physician were considered as well. The frequency of severe perineal lacerations was determined for women who did and did not undergo median episiotomies.

Results.—Sixty-seven percent of the women underwent median episiotomies, and 15% had third- or fourth-degree perineal lacerations. The rate of lacerations was 21% in women undergoing episiotomies vs. 4.5% in those not undergoing episiotomies, which yielded a relative risk of 4.58. After stratified analysis for type of delivery and birth weight, the risk of lacerations was still higher in women undergoing episiotomies, (relative risk, 3.3). The relationship held after logistic regression for type of delivery, birth weight, epidural analgesia, shoulder dystocia, baby's head circumference, physician experience, and year of delivery (odds ratio, 3.58).

Conclusions.—Performing median episiotomies during delivery in primiparous women greatly increases the frequency of third- and fourth-degree lacerations. It is important to prevent these injuries to the greatest extent possible, as they are associated with a risk of short- and long-term sequelae. Not performing median episiotomies would probably reduce the rate of severe perineal tears, although it would not eliminate them completely.

▶ I include this as another study that demonstrates that episiotomies are associated with severe lacerations after delivery. Physicians learning to avoid performing episiotomies will often begin with multiparous women and will remain reluctant to avoid the procedure in primiparous women. This study focuses on women having their first children, and the avoidance of an episiotomy is especially important in this population. They are generally younger, and the trauma often spontaneously occurs with subsequent births.

J.E. Scherger, M.D., M.P.H.

How Can Second-stage Management Prevent Perineal Trauma? Critical Review

Flynn P, Franiek J, Janssen P, et al (BC's Women's and Children's Hosps, Vancouver, BC, Canada)

Can Fam Physician 43:73–84, 1997

16–15

Background.—The best methods for clinicians to assist childbirth have not been determined. Much of the morbidity after a normal birth results from perineal trauma. Dyspareunia and urinary incontinence, 2 long-term consequences of perineal trauma, were examined. The literature was reviewed for reports of perineal management.

Methods.—Randomized, controlled trials and cohort studies of perineal trauma pattern, sexual dysfunction or satisfaction, urinary incontinence, and pelvic floor function were identified. Factors that can affect perineal integrity and that may be modifiable by pregnant women and physicians were studied.

Results.—Of 80 papers identified, 16 were analyzed in detail. Five factors that can affect perineal integrity were identified: episiotomy, third-trimester perineal massage, mother's position during second stage labor, method of pushing, and epidural anesthesia. Routine episiotomy does not improve perineal outcome. Studies of third-trimester perineal massage were inadequate. Studies of mother's position in birth chairs and recumbent vs. upright positions were also inadequate, and no recommendations were made. Studies of methods of pushing were limited and uncontrolled, and, again, no recommendations were made. Epidural anesthesia can also affect perineal integrity, but this topic is beyond the scope of this paper.

Discussion.—An analysis of the literature revealed that much of the way second stage labor is managed by physicians and midwives is based on opinion, not scientific evidence. Routine use of episiotomy has no place in childbirth and should be reduced. Women should be encouraged to use the position of their choice and push less urgently, unless there is concern for the fetus. Long holding of the breath while pushing can interfere with placental function. Most alternatives to traditional positions and pushing methods do no harm. Further studies of these factors that can affect perineal integrity are needed.

▶ This is an excellent review and, I hope, will add another nail to the coffin of routine episiotomy. Most of what we learned in hospitals 10 to 20 years ago about the second stage of labor needs to be forgotten. Women should push spontaneously, rather than with prolonged breath holding. They should assume whatever position is most comfortable. Most importantly, the infant should be delivered over an intact perineum, resulting in frequent superficial skin trauma but much less perineal trauma.

J.E. Scherger, M.D., M.P.H.

Postpartum Issues

Eating Habits and Attitudes in the Postpartum Period

Stein A, Fairburn CG (Leopold Muller Univ, London; Univ of Oxford, England)
Psychosom Med 58:321–325, 1996   16–16

Purpose.—Although major changes in body shape and weight occur in the 6 months after pregnancy, there has been little or no research into the changes in women's eating habits and attitudes during this time. Mothers may find it difficult to lose the weight they gained during pregnancy. If the mother's eating patterns become disrupted, it may cause problems with the baby's feeding. Changes in women's eating habits and attitudes during the 6 months after pregnancy were studied, with a focus on signs of eating disorders.

Methods.—The study included a general population sample of 97 primigravidas, participants in a previous study of eating habits during pregnancy. The women were followed up for 6 months after delivery to assess changes in their eating habits and weight after childbirth. Particular attention was paid to the behaviors and attitudes associated with clinical

TABLE 1.—Changes in the Psychopathologic Features of Eating Disorders During Pregnancy and the Postnatal 6 Months

	Before conception* mean (SD)	Late pregnancy† mean (SD)	3 Months postnatal mean (SD)	6 Months postnatal mean (SD)	Effect of time‖ P
Concern about shape	0.91 (0.75)	1.14 (0.89)	1.34 (1.07)	1.08 (0.86)	4.80††
Concern about weight	0.96 (0.94)	0.80 (0.60)	1.34 (1.24)	1.63 (1.19)	15.27‡‡
Concern about eating	0.13 (0.50)	0.04 (0.29)	0.15 (0.32)	0.09 (0.23)	3.68**
Dietary restraint	0.94 (1.42)	0.90 (1.36)	1.08 (1.10)	0.90 (1.00)	2.25¶
Global EDE‡	0.60 (0.61)	0.58 (0.46)	0.79 (0.67)	0.77 (0.56)	5.67††
Weight (kg)	58.1§ (7.69)	70.9 (8.54)	62.0 (8.48)	59.9 (8.82)	70.00‡‡

*Immediately before pregnancy.
†At 32 weeks of pregnancy.
‡Average score of Eating Disorder Subscales.
§Maternal report.
‖Significance level of effect of time: ¶ = $P < 0.1$; ** = $P < 0.5$; †† = $P < 0.01$; ‡‡ = $P < 0.001$.
(Courtesy of Stein A, Fairburn CG: Eating habits and attitudes in the postpartum period. *Psychosom Med* 58(4):321–325, 1996.)

eating disorders. Assessments included an eating disorder examination and the Symptom Check List.

Results.—During the first 3 months postpartum, the women showed a significant rise in eating disorder symptoms, including concern about shape, concern about weight, and concern about eating. Overall symptoms leveled off during the next 6 months. However, concern about weight continued to increase up to 6 months postpartum, whereas concern about shape fell off (Table 1). Many of the women found their residual weight gain after pregnancy to be particularly distressing. By 6 months postpartum, there were 4 cases of "eating disorder not otherwise specified" that appeared to be related to concern over weight. The research subjects indicated that they would have liked to receive advice about changes in eating, weight, and shape after pregnancy.

Conclusions.—Symptoms of eating disorders appear to increase during the 6 months after delivery. The increase in psychopathologic behaviors appears to be related mainly to weight gain, not to the postpartum period per se. Education or advice regarding postpartum changes in eating, weight, and shape may help to reduce the risk of eating disorders after pregnancy.

▶ One of the distressing problems that may occur after childbirth is the excess residual weight that the mother gains. The joy of childbirth may be dampened by the realization that the mother has not returned to the weight and shape present before pregnancy. This study documents the psychopathologic eating behaviors that often occur in the first 3 months postpartum. Weight concerns in the postpartum period should be addressed as part of prenatal education and should receive particular attention in the management of the early postpartum period.

J.E. Scherger, M.D., M.P.H.

Screening for Postpartum Depression: An Antepartum Questionnaire

Posner NA, Unterman RR, Williams KN, et al (Albany Med College, NY; Maimonides Med Ctr, Brooklyn, NY; Union College, Schenectady, NY)
J Reprod Med 42:207–215, 1997   16–17

Background.—Postpartum depression is a common occurrence that is often underdiagnosed and undertreated. Antepartum identification of women at greatest risk of depression after birth may enable earlier treatment and ultimately reduce the morbidity associated with postpartum depression. These authors developed a questionnaire to be completed before birth that can assess the degree of depression after birth.

Methods.—Two phases with 2 different samples of women were used to refine the questionnaire. In phase I, 125 women were interviewed during the second trimester and given a 61-item questionnaire to assess depression risk factors. These women were also evaluated by the Beck Depression Inventory 3 days, 4–6 weeks, and approximately 12 weeks after birth. Stepwise linear regression identified the 24 test items most predictive of

Directions
For questions 1–23 check the one answer that most closely applies to you.

1. Marital information:
   0 ( ) married and living with husband
   4 ( ) other (for example—single, separated, divorced)

2. I was separated from my mother when I was a child or teenager:
   4 ( ) yes
   0 ( ) no

3. When I was growing up, my relationship with my mother was:
   1 ( ) very close
   2 ( ) close
   3 ( ) fairly close
   4 ( ) sometimes distant
   5 ( ) distant

4. I believe that when I was growing up, my mother:
   1 ( ) was very happy about being a mother
   2 ( ) was satisfied with being a mother
   3 ( ) accepted her role as a mother
   4 ( ) was disappointed and frustrated in her role as a mother
   5 ( ) was very unhappy in her role as a mother

5. When I was growing up, if I needed help or advice, I knew that I could count on my father:
   1 ( ) almost always
   2 ( ) usually
   3 ( ) sometimes
   4 ( ) hardly ever
   5 ( ) never

6. When I was growing up, I felt that I was a worthwhile and important member of my family:
   1 ( ) almost always
   2 ( ) often
   3 ( ) sometimes
   4 ( ) hardly ever
   5 ( ) never

7. When I am NOT pregnant, I feel that my general emotional state is:
   1 ( ) excellent
   2 ( ) good
   3 ( ) fair
   4 ( ) poor
   5 ( ) very poor

8. When I am NOT pregnant, I generally feel sad:
   5 ( ) almost always
   4 ( ) often
   3 ( ) sometimes
   2 ( ) hardly ever
   1 ( ) never

9. At the present time I feel good about myself as a person:
   1 ( ) almost all of the time
   2 ( ) most of the time
   3 ( ) some of the time
   4 ( ) hardly ever
   5 ( ) none of the time

10. Before pregnancy, when I menstruated, most of the time:
    1 ( ) I felt comfortable enough to go about my normal routine
    2 ( ) I may have had to take a few hours off for one day
    3 ( ) I may have had to take a day off
    4 ( ) I may have had to take two or more days off
    5 ( ) I may have had to take off for my entire period

11. After the birth of one or more of my children, I:
    5 ( ) was very depressed and had to have medical attention
    4 ( ) was very depressed but did not have medical attention
    3 ( ) was moderately depressed for more than a week
    2 ( ) had a few days of the blues
    1 ( ) was not depressed
    4 ( ) this is my first child

12. So far in this pregnancy, I have had nausea or vomiting:
    2 ( ) almost all the time
    1 ( ) often
    0 ( ) sometimes
    1 ( ) hardly ever
    2 ( ) not at all

13. During this pregnancy I felt nervous and anxious:
    5 ( ) almost all of the time
    4 ( ) often
    3 ( ) sometimes
    2 ( ) hardly ever
    1 ( ) not at all

(Continued)

FIGURE 1 (cont.)

14. During this pregnancy I have generally felt sad:
    5 ( ) almost all of the time
    4 ( ) often
    3 ( ) sometimes
    2 ( ) hardly ever
    1 ( ) not at all

15. At the present time I am satisfied with the amount of education that I have had:
    1 ( ) almost always
    2 ( ) usually
    3 ( ) sometimes
    4 ( ) hardly ever
    5 ( ) never

16. I feel that I can manage on my present income:
    1 ( ) almost always
    2 ( ) usually
    3 ( ) sometimes
    4 ( ) hardly ever
    5 ( ) never

17. At the present time, my relationship with my mother is:
    1 ( ) very close
    2 ( ) close
    3 ( ) fairly close
    4 ( ) sometimes distant
    5 ( ) distant
    3 ( ) My mother is not living

18. My mother criticizes me:
    2 ( ) almost all the time
    1 ( ) too often
    0 ( ) sometimes
    1 ( ) hardly ever
    2 ( ) never
    3 ( ) My mother is not living

19. At the present time, when I really need help, I know that I can count on my father:
    1 ( ) almost always
    2 ( ) usually
    3 ( ) sometimes
    4 ( ) hardly ever
    5 ( ) never
    6 ( ) My father is not living

20. At the present time, my relationship with my father is:
    1 ( ) very close
    2 ( ) close
    3 ( ) fairly close
    4 ( ) sometimes distant
    5 ( ) distant
    6 ( ) My father is not living

21. At the present time my relationship with my husband or boyfriend is usually:
    1 ( ) excellent
    2 ( ) good
    3 ( ) fair
    4 ( ) poor
    5 ( ) very poor

22. If I need help or advice, I know that I can count on my husband or boyfriend:
    1 ( ) almost always
    2 ( ) usually
    3 ( ) sometimes
    4 ( ) hardly ever
    5 ( ) never

23. At the present time I feel good about my life:
    1 ( ) almost all the time
    2 ( ) most of the time
    3 ( ) some of the time
    4 ( ) hardly ever
    5 ( ) none of the time

24. At the present time, if I need help or advice, I can count on the following people: (Check all that apply)
    −1 ( ) my mother
    −1 ( ) my father
    −1 ( ) my husband or boyfriend
    −1 ( ) a sister, brother, or relative
    −1 ( ) another person
     0 ( ) no one

FIGURE 1.—Antepartum questionaire. Directions for scoring: 1. Add algebraically the numerical value of the responses checked for all 24 questions. 2. A score of 46 or more suggests clinical potential for the development of postpartum depressive symptoms. (Courtesy of Posner NA, Unterman RR, Williams KN, et al: Screening for postpartum depression: an antepartum questionnaire. *J Reprod Med* 42:207–215, 1997.)

postpartum depression, and these items constituted the final antepartum questionnaire. This questionnaire was administered to a different group of 125 women (phase II), who also were evaluated by the Beck Depression Inventory according to the same schedule as in phase I. Scores were determined by adding the numerical value for each of the 24 items (Fig 1).

Findings.—Women with antepartum questionnaire scores $\geq$ 46 were considered at risk of postpartum depression. In phase II, the antepartum questionnaire retrospectively identified 12 of the 15 women who had depressive symptoms based on the total Beck Depression Inventory scale (sensitivity 80%). Furthermore, 64 of 84 women classified as asymptomatic on the total Beck Depression Inventory were also classified as asymptomatic by the 24-item antepartum questionnaire (specificity 82%). Among all women in both phases, based on the Beck Depression Inventory, the incidence of depression increased from 10% shortly after delivery, to 17% at 4 to 6 weeks, and then declined to 15% at approximately 12 weeks. The severity of the depression increased with time.

Conclusions.—The 24-item antepartum questionnaire was useful in screening women prospectively for postpartum depression. A pregnant woman with an antepartum questionnaire score of 46 or more should be evaluated before delivery and followed up closely for signs of depression.

▶ The 24 questions presented here will provide a wealth of information for the physician caring for a pregnant mother before and after birth. The validation of this questionnaire as a screen for postpartum depression is good. There are more good questionnaires available in family practice than one could ever possibly use. However, women visit their physicians 8–12 times during pregnancy, which includes a lot of time in the waiting room. Such a questionnaire can easily be administered by the office staff and interpreted by a nurse, social worker, or physician, who as a team may address the issues that will be identified.

J.E. Scherger, M.D., M.P.H.

Organization of Obstetric Services

Interspecialty Differences in the Obstetric Care of Low-risk Women
Rosenblatt RA, Dobie SA, Hart LG, et al (Univ of Washington, Seattle; Univ of Rochester, NY; Washington-Georgetown Univ, DC)
Am J Public Health 87:344–351, 1997   16–18

Background.—Despite the importance of obstetric care, which accounts for >10% of hospital discharges in the United States, there is considerable controversy regarding the optimal management of pregnancy. Enormous differences exist, for example, in the way healthy women with low-risk pregnancies are treated by obstetricians, general and family physicians, and certified nurse-midwives. Such interspecialty differences were examined with stratified random sample of obstetric providers.

Methods.—Study participants were drawn from all urban obstetric providers in the state of Washington who routinely provided obstetric care in hospital settings during 1988. Patient data were based on women who delivered between February 10, 1989, and April 26, 1990. All prenatal and intrapartum care was assigned to the provider with whom the patient initiated care. Of the 1,680 obstetric providers identified, 461 were obstetricians, 1,134 were family physicians, and 85 were certified nurse-midwives. Analyses are based on data from 54 obstetricians, 54 family physicians, and 43 certified nurse-midwives.

Results.—Obstetricians tended to be older than members of the other provider groups. All certified nurse-midwives were women, whereas 80% of physicians were men. The typical patient at low-risk was white, married, multiparous, privately insured, and in her mid 20s. Birth outcomes were similar across the provider groups, as were birth weights and mean 5-minute Apgar scores. Patients of obstetricians were much more likely to undergo amniocentesis (6.8%) than were patients of either family physicians (1.4%) or midwives (2.2%). The 3 provider groups were similar in their use of US. Major differences existed, however, in intrapartum management. Certified nurse-midwives were significantly less likely to induce labor, use continuous electronic monitoring and epidural anesthesia, or perform episiotomies. Cesarean rates were 15.1% for family physicians, 13.6% for obstetricians, and 8.8% for nurse-midwives. Costs of obstetric care were 12.2% higher for obstetricians than for nurse-midwives.

Conclusion.—Obstetricians and family physicians showed similar practice patterns in their management of low-risk pregnancies. Certified nurse-midwives' patients at low risk received fewer obstetric interventions, had lower cesarean section rates, and incurred lower costs than did similar patients in the care of obstetricians and family physicians.

▶ This study reports on the value that certified nurse-midwives bring to obstetric care. The midwifery approach to childbirth includes treating labor and delivery as a normal process and providing personal attention to the woman throughout labor. This attitude and behavior result in use of fewer obstetric technologies. Family physicians would do well to adopt a midwifery approach toward labor and delivery management for women at low risk.

J.E. Scherger, M.D., M.P.H.

Comparisons of Outcomes of Maternity Care by Obstetricians and Certified Nurse-Midwives

Oakley D, Murray ME, Murtland T, et al (Univ of Michigan, Ann Arbor)
Obstet Gynecol 88:823–829, 1996   16–19

Introduction.—Nurse-midwife care is recognized as a reasonable option for pregnant women at low risk, although physicians deliver more than 94% of the 4 million births each year in the United States. An earlier study found that neonates born to women in the physician group weighed 94 g more on average than those born in the midwife group, and that the proportion of women with third- and fourth-degree perineal lacerations was significantly higher in the physician group. When statistical controls took alternative explanations into account, a comparison was made to determine whether infant and maternal outcomes differ according to obstetrician or certified nurse-midwife care.

Methods.—A comparison of pregnancy outcomes was made for 710 women cared for by private obstetricians and 471 cared for by certified nurse-midwives. The study compared infant and maternal mortality, 30 clinical indicators, satisfaction with care, and monetary charges. Random assignment was precluded because consumer choice of provider was honored.

Results.—For 7 clinically important outcomes, significant differences between the obstetrician and nurse-midwife groups were found. There were 7% infant abrasions in the obstetrician group and 4% in the midwife group (Table 1); 15% of infants remained with the mother for the entire

TABLE 1.—Infant Outcomes by Provider

Outcome	Obstetrician (*n* = 710)	Nurse-midwife (*n* = 471)	*P*
Gestational age (wk)	39.42 ± 1.70	39.45 ± 1.57	NS
Hematocrit (%)	56.78 ± 7.45	57.45 ± 7.13	NS
Length (cm)	51.60 ± 2.65	51.80 ± 2.65	NS
Head circumference (cm)	34.82 ± 1.69	35.04 ± 1.66	NS
1-minute Apgar score <7	109 (15.4%)	66 (14.0%)	NS
5-minute Apgar score <7	16 (2.3%)	11 (2.3%)	NS
Infant bruised	153 (21.5%)	86 (18.3%)	NS
Respiratory difficulty	88 (12.4%)	60 (12.8%)	NS
Abrasions	49 (6.9%)	17 (3.6%)	.04
Slow, lethargic	35 (5.0%)	27 (5.8%)	NS
Anything abnormal	22 (3.1%)	27 (5.8%)	.02
Eye problem	20 (2.8%)	18 (3.8%)	NS
Fontanelle problem	7 (1.0%)	4 (0.9%)	NS
Clavicle problem	3 (0.4%)	2 (0.4%)	NS
Birth weight (g)			
<2500	20 (2.8%)	14 (3.0%)	
2500–4000	598 (84.2%)	367 (77.9%)	
>4000	93 (13.1%)	88 (18.7%)	
Breast-fed at delivery	584 (82.2%)	432 (91.7%)	<.001
Stayed with mother	101 (14.2%)	124 (26.3%)	<.001
To neonatal intensive care unit	33 (4.6%)	30 (6.4%)	
To moderate care nursery	37 (5.3%)	31 (6.6%)	
To observation or newborn nursery	519 (73.1%)	275 (58.4%)	

Note: There are a few cases of missing data on 1 or 2 characteristics. Outcomes shown were counted only when specifically noted in the charts. Data are presented as mean ± standard deviation or N (%). Infant bruised = bruising described on any assessment of infant, includes cephalohematomas; respiratory difficulties = grunting, nasal; abrasions = abrasions on initial assessment; slow, lethargic = initial assessment of activity level, compared with alert, active, responsive, vigorous, or no data; anything abnormal = abnormalities noted in chart at delivery or before discharge; eye problem = hemorrhagia or other eye problem; fontanelle problem = closed or building; clavicle problem = evidence of fracture; stayed with mother = no transfer to the alternatives shown (moderate care included triage to an intensive care observation nursery) and, if transferred to more than 1 location, assignment was made in coding to the highest level of care received.

Abbreviation: NS, not significant.

(Reprinted with permisson from American College of Obstetricians and Gynecologists, courtesy of Oakley D, Murray ME, Murtland T, et al: Comparisons of outcomes of maternity care by obstetricians and certified nurse-midwives. *Obstet Gynecol* 88:823–829, 1996.)

hospital stay in the doctors group and 27% did so in the midwife group; there were 23% third- or fourth-degree perineal lacerations in the doctor group compared with 7% in the midwife group; there were 0.7 complications in the doctor group compared with 0.4 in the midwife group (Table 2); satisfaction with care was lower in the doctor group (4.23 ± 0.65) than in the midwife group (4.23 ± 0.62) on a 5-point scale; hospital charges were $5,427 for the doctor group compared to $4,296 for the midwife group; and the average professional fee for the doctor group was $3,425 compared with $3,237 for the midwife group. Significantly more infants in the midwife group were breast fed immediately after delivery.

TABLE 2.—Maternal Complications by Provider

Complication	Obstetrician ($n = 710$)	Nurse-midwife ($n = 471$)	P
Postpartum hemorrhage	179 (25.2%)	67 (14.2%)	<.001
Major perineal laceration (vaginal deliveries only)	134 (23.3%)	27 (6.6%)	<.001
Infection	42 (5.9%)	17 (3.6%)	NS
Medical complication	32 (4.5%)	20 (4.2%)	NS
Delayed bleeding	28 (3.9%)	22 (4.7%)	NS
Readmission within 6 wk	24 (3.4%)	9 (1.9%)	NS
Anesthesia complications	10 (1.4%)	2 (0.4%)	NS
Spinal headache	2 (0.3%)	2 (0.4%)	NS
Severe problem	6 (0.8%)	4 (0.8%)	NS
Postpartum anemia	4 (0.6%)	4 (0.8%)	NS
Respiratory complications	4 (0.6%)	1 (0.2%)	NS
Neurological complications	2 (0.3%)	0	NS
Phlebitis	2 (0.3%)	1 (0.2%)	NS
Average no. of complications	0.67 ± 0.88	0.37 ± 0.75	<.001

Note: Postpartum hemorrhage = blood loss >500 mL if vaginal delivery or >1,000 mL if cesarean; major perineal laceration = third or fourth degree; infection = 100°F temperature for at least 4 hours plus antibiotics prescribed; delayed bleeding = definite chart record so labeled; readmission within 6 weeks = readmission data in chart; anesthesia complications = hypotension, seizure, aspiration, or other definite chart record so labeled; spinal headache = definite chart record so labeled or blood patch; severe problem = disseminated intravascular coagulation, seizure, uterine inversion, embolus, cardiac arrest, shock, hypertensive crisis, uterine rupture, respiratory arrest, and the like; postpartum anemia = first postpartum hematocrit <22%; respiratory or neurologic complications or phlebitis = definite chart record so labeled; average number of complications = a count of those listed in the table (shown as the mean ± standard deviation).

Abbreviation: NS, not significant.

(Reprinted with permisson from American College of Obstetricians and Gynecologists, courtesy of Oakley D, Murray ME, Murtland T, et al: Comparisons of outcomes of maternity care by obstetricians and certified nurse-midwives. *Obstet Gynecol* 88:823–829, 1996.)

Conclusion.—There were differences in outcomes between obstetrician and midwife care, although most outcomes were equally good.

▶ I admire an obstetrics-gynecology journal for publishing these data which strongly support intrapartum care delivered by certified nurse-midwives. Many family physicians practice a "midwifery model" of obstetric care. We can also celebrate these data and use them to reinforce a low-intervention style of obstetric care.

J.E. Scherger, M.D., M.P.H.

Access to Maternity Care in Rural Washington: Its Effect on Neonatal Outcomes and Resource Use

Nesbitt TS, Larson EH, Rosenblatt RA, et al (Univ of California-Davis, Sacramento; Univ of Seattle, Washington)
Am J Public Health 87:85–90, 1997

16–20

Background.—The number of providers of obstetric health care services in rural areas in the United States decreased by 20% between 1984 and 1989. The proportion of rural family physicians providing obstetric health care was 43% in 1988 and 37% in 1992. Decreased access to local obstetric and neonatal services in rural areas raises the question of how health care resources should be made available locally to rural populations. The effect of limited access to local obstetric care on neonatal outcome and use of health care resources was studied.

Methods.—Data from birth certificates were linked to data from hospital records of women and their newborns. Data from 29,809 births to residents of rural areas were analyzed. Information from residents of rural areas where more than two thirds of women traveled to larger communities for health care was compared with information from residents of rural areas where less than one third traveled to larger communities to obtain health care.

Results.—For patients who were privately insured and those who received Medicaid, there was an association between poor local access to health care in rural areas and a significantly higher risk of having a nonnormal neonate. Poor local access to health care was associated with longer hospital stay and increased cost only for privately insured patients.

Discussion.—The risk of having a nonnormal newborn is higher in women in rural areas with poor local access to obstetric health care. Women who travel to a larger community for health care are more likely to have longer hospital stays and higher charges for neonatal care compared with nonrural patients. Local providers of obstetric services in rural areas serve as an entry point into the regionalized system of perinatal health care. Without access to such services, the outcome of high-risk infants is lowered.

▶ This article is essentially a rewrite of an important study originally published in 1990.[1] As the number of family physicians providing obstetric care remains low, the public health consequences in rural areas are worth repeating. Many believe that there is little need for family physicians to provide obstetric care in this era of an ample supply of obstetricians/gynecologists and a growing supply of certified nurse-midwives. However, in rural America, family physicians have been the mainstay of obstetric care. Lacking a continuation of this situation, increasing numbers of women do not have access to local care, and birth outcomes are adversely affected.

J.E. Scherger, M.D., M.P.H.

Reference

1. Nesbitt TS, Connell FA, Hart LG, et al: Access to obstetric care in rural areas: Effect on birth outcomes. *Am J Public Health* 80:814–818, 1990.

Miscellaneous

Post-term Birth: Risk Factors and Outcomes in a 10-year Cohort of Norwegian Births

Campbell MK, Østbye T, Irgens LM (Univ of Western Ontario, London, Canada; Univ of Bergen, Norway)
Obstet Gynecol 89:543–548, 1997

16–21

Background.—Post-term birth is defined as birth after 42 weeks of gestation. A study was performed to identify risk factors associated with post-term birth and with adverse outcomes.

Study Design.—The data was derived from the Medical Birth Registry of Norway for the period 1978 to 1987. Gestational age was based on the mother's last menstrual period. There were 379,445 term births and 65,796 post-term births.

Findings.—After controlling for covariates, there was a slightly increased risk of perinatal mortality in post-term births compared with term births. Among post-term births, the risk factors for perinatal mortality were small size for gestational age (SGA) and older maternal age, whereas large size for gestational age (LGA) was protective. These were also risk factors for perinatal mortality in term births. Fetal distress was associated with SGA and post-term birth. Labor dysfunction and obstetric trauma were associated with LGA and post-term birth. Shoulder dystocia and maternal hemorrhage were associated with LGA.

Conclusions.—The increased maternal complications associated with post-term births in a large birth registry were generally associated with increased fetal size. The increased fetal complications associated with post-term birth were in infants who were small for gestational age. Once other factors were taken into account, the evidence for an adverse impact of post-term birth on perinatal mortality was weak.

▶ Scandinavian studies of incredibly large sample size often shed light on questions in obstetric care. Much fuss and intervention are currently devoted to avoiding allowing pregnancies to go beyond 42 weeks. However, many normal pregnancies extend beyond this arbitrary cut-off point. In this study of over 400,000 births, the risk of pregnancy beyond 42 weeks is small in women who do not have other risk factors. Patient choice based on informed consent should be honored to allow the option of spontaneous labor and delivery after 42 weeks in otherwise low-risk women.

J.E. Scherger, M.D., M.P.H.

Evolution of Pregnancies and Initial Follow-up of Newborns Delivered After Intracytoplasmic Sperm Injection

Palermo GD, Colombero LT, Schattman GL, et al (New York Hosp/Cornell Med Ctr)

JAMA 276:1893–1897, 1996

16–22

Background.—Intracytoplasmic sperm injection (ICSI) in human in vitro fertilization (IVF) is a major advance in assisted reproductive technology. Although evidence of its safety has been reassuring, there is still concern about the possible risk of genetic abnormalities with this treatment. The in vivo development of embryos conceived after ICSI was studied, along with obstetric outcomes, the occurrence of chromosomal abnormalities, and the rate of congenital malformations in neonates conceived in this manner.

Methods.—Seven hundred fifty-one couples were studied retrospectively. In all couples, the cause of repeated failed IVF attempts was presumed to be the male partner, or semen parameters were found to be unacceptable for conventional IVF treatment. Pregnancies resulting from 987 ICSI cycles were analyzed.

Findings.—Overall, the clinical pregnancy rate was 44.3%. The delivery rate per ICSI cycle was 38.7%. Cytogenetic data available for 8 of 11 miscarriages showed autosomal trisomy. Another 7 pregnancies were terminated after the prenatal diagnosis of chromosomal abnormality. One hundred ninety-two infants were born vaginally, and 190 by cesarean delivery. Of the 578 neonates born after ICSI, 2.6% had congenital abnormalities, a lower rate than in children born after standard IVF. Also, there were no differences in the frequency of miscarriages or in the rate of congenital malformations between ICSI and IVF babies.

Conclusions.—The evolution of pregnancy and the occurrence of congenital malformations after ICSI treatment are comparable to those associated with other assisted reproductive technology procedures. Careful monitoring of the technique and continued, meticulous obstetric and pediatric follow up will help alleviate safety concerns.

▶ When male infertility exists, standard IVF is done with donor sperm. This deprives the father of having a biological child. Intracytoplasmic sperm injection provides the opportunity for a father with a low sperm count or dysfunctional sperm to still have biological offspring with risks similar to spontaneous pregnancy.

J.E. Scherger, M.D., M.P.H.

17 Geriatrics

Introduction

The importance of falls is recognized in the opening section, with a handy screening test for assigning risk, a discussion of environmental hazards, and a randomized trial of an intervention. The 3 articles that follow on Alzheimer's disease address prognosis and a randomized trial of a family intervention that delayed nursing home placement. Studies on the beneficial effects of exercise on sleep, the use of nonsteroidal anti-inflammatory drugs to prevent cognitive decline, use of benzodiazepines, and a very useful article on inappropriate prescribing practices round out the chapter.

Randomized controlled trials: Abstracts 17–4, 17–5, 17–8, and 17–10.

Alfred O. Berg, M.D., M.P.H.

Falls

"Stops Walking When Talking" as a Predictor of Falls in Elderly People
Lundin-Olsson L, Nyberg L, Gustafson Y (Umeå Univ, Sweden)
Lancet 349:617, 1997   17–1

Introduction.—Some frail elderly individuals stop walking when talking because they cannot do both at once. The usefulness of "stops walking when talking" as a predictor of falls was studied in elderly residents in a group home who could walk with or without assistance.

Methods.—Fifty-eight residents (72% women), with an average age of 80.1 years, who could follow instructions were observed by a physiotherapist who noted whether they stopped walking when talking, their ability to walk safely, and the number of falls during the following 6 months.

Results.—Ten of 12 individuals who stopped walking when talking fell during the observation period, and 21 of 58 fell at least once. Significantly more of those who stopped walking when talking fell (Figure). The positive and negative predictive values were 83% and 76%, respectively. The specificity was 95% but the sensitivity was only 48%. Those who stopped walking when talking had a significantly less safe gait and were slower and more dependent in the activities of daily living.

Conclusion.—Elderly individuals who stop walking when talking are at increased risk for falling.

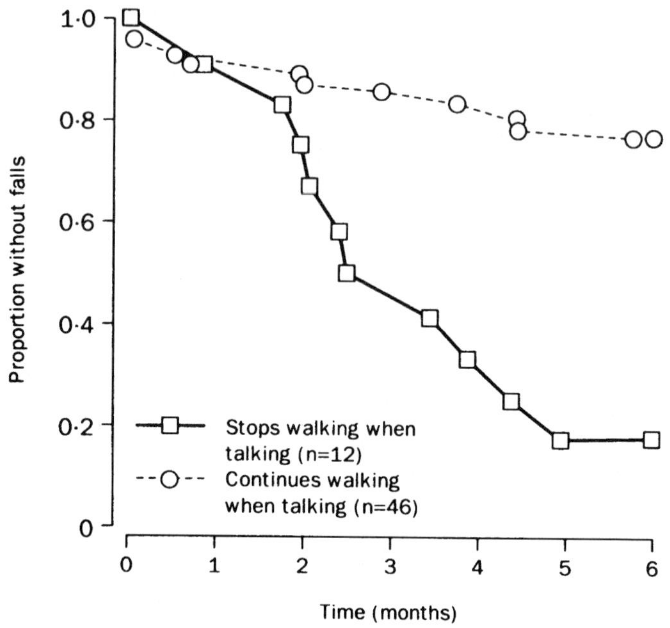

FIGURE.—Kaplan-Meier curves for falls during 6 months. (Courtesy of Lundin-Olsson L, Nyberg L, Gustafson Y: "Stops walking when talking" as a predictor of falls in elderly people. *Lancet* 349:617, 1997. Copyright by The Lancet Ltd. 1997.)

▶ I imagine that this is the way useful and simple items of the history or physical examination are discovered: a thoughtful physician sees significance for something that has always been there but had never struck anyone else as remarkable. The figure is included because the results are so striking. This finding might be useful in both the history (ask the patient or family members) and the physical examination (direct observation). In any case, a "positive" result might prompt a more careful assessment of fall risk, including environmental modification for prevention.

A.O. Berg, M.D., M.P.H.

One-leg Balance Is an Important Predictor of Injurious Falls in Older Persons

Vellas BJ, Wayne SJ, Romero L, et al (Univ of New Mexico, Albuquerque; CHU Toulouse-Purpan, France; GRECC, Sepulveda, Calif)
J Am Geriatr Soc 45:735–738, 1997   17–2

Introduction.—A simple, accurate, reproducible indicator of fall risk in elderly adults is needed. One-leg balance was prospectively analyzed for its ability to predict falls in healthy older adults living in the community.

Methods.—A total of 316 volunteers older than 60 years with no known serious medical conditions underwent the following: an interview, physical examination, the Iowa Self Assessment Inventory, and assessment of gait and balance performance. Volunteers were asked to stand unassisted on one leg for 5 seconds. Falls and injurious falls were recorded over a period of 36 months.

Results.—The mean age of the 316 volunteers was 72.7 years. At baseline, 84.5% of volunteers were able to perform one-leg balance. Over a 3-year follow-up period, 71% of volunteers experienced falls. Of these, 22% were injurious falls. Age greater than 73 years at baseline was the only significant independent predictor of all falls. Impaired one-leg balance was the only significant independent predictor of injurious falls.

Conclusion.—One-leg balance was a significant predictor of injurious falls, but not of all falls. This test is easy to administer and could become part of a routine geriatric assessment.

Clinical Significance.—These findings should be viewed with the understanding that there are many diverse factors involved in falling. It may be that there is no single factor accurate enough to become a sole predictor of fall risk or fall injury risk.

▶ The ability to predict older patients who are at high risk for a fall could be valuable to patients and their families. These authors evaluated a simple office-based diagnostic test. They asked their older patients to stand for 5 seconds on one leg. Of the 316 senior citizens evaluated by this one-leg balance test, 84% were judged to have "passed" the test. Of those who were unable to maintain their balance for 5 seconds, the risk for an injurious fall was more than double the risk for patients who were able to pass the test.

I think the real value in this test is its simplicity and its ability to be used when safety issues in the home are being evaluated. Individuals who are unable to maintain their balance might warrant intervention by the family or caregivers toward a more supervised living situation or at least toward a reduction of fall risks in the home environment. This test is certainly easy to administer. It seems worthwhile for select patients.

R.C. Davidson, M.D., M.P.H.

Environmental Hazards and Hip Fractures
Parker MJ, Twemlow TR, Pryor GA (Peterborough District Hosp, England; Univ of Aberdeen, Scotland)
Age Ageing 25:322–325, 1996   17–3

Introduction.—A fractured femoral neck in the elderly is a very common and expensive problem. Although previous studies have examined the environmental hazards or seasonal factors involved in falls, none have looked at both factors during a specified time. The types of environmental hazards associated with falls leading to hip fractures were examined during a 3-year period.

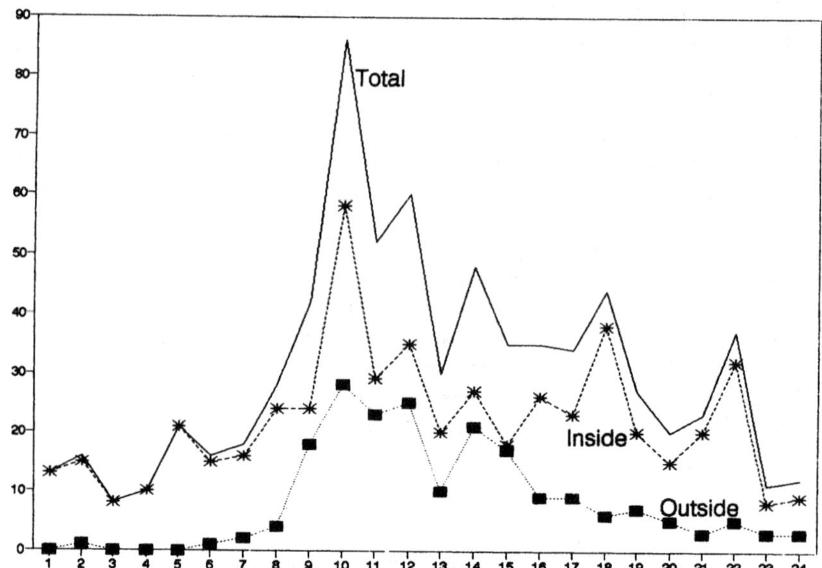

FIGURE 1.—Number of falls for each hour of the day. (Courtesy of Parker MJ, Twemlow TR, Pryor GA: Environmental hazards and hip fractures. *Age Ageing* 25:322–325, 1996. By permission of Oxford University Press.)

Methods.—The study included all patients admitted to 1 district hospital with hip fractures. The patients were asked about the circumstances when the falls occurred, what they were doing before the falls, where the falls occurred, and any environmental hazards involved.

Findings.—There were a total of 787 patients with hip fractures. Thirty-two had pathologic fractures related to tumors or Paget's disease, and 26 had spontaneous hip pain without a fall. The patients' average age was 79 years, and three fourths were women. Seventy-one percent were living at home. The most common time for falls was between 9:00 AM and noon (Fig 1). More than half of the patients who could describe the fall in detail could identify an environmental hazard. A total of 51 different hazards were reported, including getting out of a car, walking on stones or gravel, tripping over a stool or chair, and dancing. Blackouts and epileptic attacks were also mentioned. About one fourth of patients who normally used a walking aid were not using it when they fell.

Conclusions.—Many different environmental hazards can contribute to falls by the elderly. These factors are highly diverse, which suggests that measures to remove environmental hazards are unlikely to reduce the rate of hip fractures significantly. For unknown reasons, the greatest number of falls occurs in the morning hours.

▶ Although the methodology used in this study does not allow strong conclusions, there are 2 very interesting findings.

This is a retrospective study of 787 consecutive patients with hip fractures. There is no comparison group, and the study population is not representative except for this particular practice setting. However, the issue is important enough for primary care physicians that I included this article.

The authors found that almost half of these falls would not have been preventable by any environmental change. I'm not sure whether the glass is half empty or half full. An interesting finding is the frequency distribution by hour of the day. This came as a bit of a surprise to me. Of course, the nighttime sleeping hours would show a much smaller incidence, but the peak in the morning hours was a bit surprising. The message I take from this article is to remind myself to ask about environmental hazards when I interview my elderly patients. I'm not sure what to do about the peak in the morning hours as I don't know what it's caused by.

R.C. Davidson, M.D., M.P.H.

A Randomized Trial of a Consultation Service to Reduce Falls in Nursing Homes

Ray WA, Taylor JA, Meador KG, et al (Vanderbilt Univ, Nashville, Tenn; Belmont Univ, Nashville, Tenn; Duke Univ, Durham, NC)
JAMA 278:557–562, 1997   17–4

Background.—Falls and the resulting injuries are an important public health issue in nursing homes. Though interventions to reduce the risk of falls have been shown to work in the community setting, there is no proven intervention to reduce falls among nursing home residents. An intervention to prevent falls and fall-related injuries among nursing home residents at high risk was studied in a randomized, controlled trial.

Methods.—The study included 482 residents of 14 middle Tennessee nursing homes. The homes were randomly assigned in pairs to the study intervention or a control group. All residents studied were at high risk for falls and had a potential safety problem amenable to correction by the study intervention. Nursing homes assigned to the intervention underwent a structured, comprehensive assessment leading to specific safety recommendations. The recommendations were geared toward correcting suboptimal practices related to environmental and personal safety, wheelchairs, psychotropic drugs, and transfer and ambulation. Nursing home staff members were encouraged to act on the recommended interventions and to improve the overall safety of their nursing home. The 2 groups of homes were compared for the mean proportion of recurrent fallers and the incidence of injurious falls for 1 year after the intervention.

Results.—Nursing homes assigned to the study intervention had a 19% mean proportion of recurrent fallers, compared with 54% in the control facilities. The mean rate of injurious falls was about 14/100 person-years in the intervention facilities vs. 20/100 person-years in the control facilities. The difference was not significant, however. The intervention appeared to be most beneficial to residents for whom the study interventions were carried out and those who had at least 3 falls in the preceding year.

Conclusions.—This randomized, controlled trial suggests that nursing home intervention can reduce the mean proportion of recurrent fallers by 44% and the rate of injurious falls by 31%. In the nursing home setting, falls and resultant injuries are not necessarily inevitable. Rather, structured safety programs can significantly reduce these adverse outcomes.

▶ Yes, we can reduce various unfortunate events, or increase appropriate events, if we spend enough time, resources, and highlight the goal. We can increase the provision of preventive services, and we can prevent falls. But just what does it take? And how long can we sustain it? Do we manage to get everyone flu shots this year, prevent falls the next year, and have our patients with diabetes see ophthalmologists the next? Despite the intervention in this study, about half of the patients fell again. This intervention thus may have been better than others that had no reported improvement in the number of falls, but there remains great potential for improvement. The authors do not report the cost, nor did they provide any measure of sustainability beyond 1 year. Perhaps they are on the right track, but other interventions would obviously be needed to reduce falls to a level that would feel safe.

M.A. Bowman, M.D., M.P.A.

Alzheimer's Disease

A Family Intervention to Delay Nursing Home Placement of Patients With Alzheimer Disease: A Randomized Controlled Trial
Mittelman MS, Ferris SH, Shulman E, et al (New York Univ, New York; Columbia Univ, New York; New York State Psychiatric Inst, New York)
JAMA 276:1725–1731, 1996   17–5

Objective.—Although deterioration occurs in every patient with Alzheimer's disease (AD), the rate of progression varies. Most families prefer to keep the patient out of the nursing home if possible, but this requires considerable assistance for the caregiver. Previous studies have suggested that psychosocial interventions may be able to prevent or delay nursing home placement of patients with AD. A comprehensive support and counseling program for the families of patients with AD was studied for long-term effectiveness in postponing or preventing nursing home placement.

Methods.—The randomized, controlled trial included 206 spouse-caregivers of patients with AD. All patients were living at home at the start of the study. The families came from a broad range of socioeconomic backgrounds. The caregivers were randomly separated into treatment and control groups. The treatment group received 6 counseling sessions, 2 individual and 4 family. Counseling was task-oriented, with a focus on promoting communication, teaching problem-solving techniques, and improving support for the caregiver. All patients in the treatment group were required to join a regular support group. In addition, counselors were continuously available to help in crises and as the patient's symptoms changed. The control group received the normal services offered to the families of patients with AD. The 2 groups were compared for the time until the family member with AD was admitted to a nursing home.

Results.—On Kaplan-Meier survival analysis, the median adjusted time to nursing home placement was 1,203 days for the treatment group vs. 874 days for the control group. By intention-to-treat analysis in a Cox proportional hazard model, the adjusted relative risk (RR) of nursing home placement was 0.65 for the treatment group. Thus, caregivers in the treatment group were two-thirds as likely to place their family member in a nursing home as were those in the control group, after adjustment for caregiver sex, patient age, and patient income. The treatment program had the largest effect on placement rate for patients with mild to moderate dementia, RR 0.18 to 0.38, respectively.

Conclusions.—With comprehensive support and counseling, caregivers may be able to keep family members with AD out of the nursing home longer. Such programs are most likely to be effective for patients in the mild to moderate stages of dementia, when nursing home admission is least appropriate. The cost-effectiveness of the study intervention is being analyzed. Convincing the family members to take advantage of available counseling, education, and support will be a challenge for the future.

▶ I like this study because the intervention was sensible and modest, and not too hard to implement in a medical organization of any size. Further, the main finding was clinically and statistically significant: patients in the intervention group were able to stay at home almost a year longer than those in the control group. Good news in dealing with AD that can be implemented in an average practice is uncommon, but I think this qualifies. If I had many patients with AD in my practice, I would obtain more details about how this intervention actually worked.

A.O. Berg, M.D., M.P.H.

Predicting Time to Nursing Home Care and Death in Individuals With Alzheimer Disease

Stern Y, Tang M-X, Albert MS, et al (Columbia Univ, New York; Johns Hopkins Univ, Baltimore, Md; Harvard Med School, Boston)
JAMA 277:806–812, 1997   17–6

Background.—Patients with Alzheimer's disease (AD) and their families commonly want to know how long it will be until the patient needs nursing home admission or dies. These questions cannot be answered on the basis of empirical data. This study sought to use clinical features to predict such important outcomes in individual patients with AD.

Methods.—The study included 236 patients who met the National Institute of Neurological and Communicative Disorders and Stroke–Alzheimer's Disease and Related Disorders Association criteria for probable AD. The patients were 140 women and 96 men (mean age 73 years;

mean duration of AD was about 4 years). All had mild dementia at baseline, with no neuroleptic medications for at least 1 month. Patients with substance abuse, schizophrenia, schizoaffective disorder, previous electroconvulsive therapy, or evidence of stroke were excluded. The predictors evaluated included duration of illness, age at onset, extrapyramidal signs, and cognition. Starting in the sixth year of the study, apolipoprotein E genotype testing was offered as well. Outcomes evaluated were nursing home placement or its equivalent and death.

Results.—Although 28% of patients had abnormal medical findings at baseline, none were considered to be contributing to dementia. Sixty-nine percent of patients reached the point of needing nursing home care during the maximum follow-up of 7 years. Forty-two percent of patients died. Mortality was lower for women, patients with longer duration of higher Mini-Mental State Examination scores, and higher for patients with extrapyramidal signs. Prediction algorithms based on Cox proportional hazard models were used to generate survival curves for time to study outcomes. When predictor variables from a validation cohort of 105 patients were entered into the algorithms, predicted survival fell within the 95% confidence bands of survival curves.

Conclusions.—Prediction algorithms for time to nursing home admission or death for patients with AD are described. These algorithms represent an initial step toward providing prognoses for individual patients with AD. The described approach could be useful in the design and interpretation of clinical trials by providing an expected time course to be compared with the patient's actual course.

▶ The sophistication of these sadly necessary predictive indexes continues to improve. These 2 are quite simple to use and very successful in predicting the need for nursing home care and death. Family physicians caring for patients with AD should keep the indexes handy for use when questions about prognosis become pressing for patient or family.

A.O. Berg, M.D., M.P.H.

Predictors of Mortality in Patients Diagnosed With Probable Alzheimer's Disease
Bowen JD, Malter AD, Sheppard L, et al (Univ of Washington, Seattle)
Neurology 47:433–439, 1996   17–7

Introduction.—It has been difficult to predict mortality in patients with diagnosed Alzheimer's disease (AD). In many studies, either early or advanced cases are over-represented or patients with comorbid conditions have been eliminated from analysis. A large cohort of patients with recently diagnosed probable AD was followed up for a median of 3.3 years to identify baseline characteristics predictive of shorter survival.

Methods.—The longitudinal study included 327 patients who were enrolled within a geographically defined portion of a large HMO. Efforts are made to record all new cases of dementia in the Alzheimer's Disease Patient Registry (ADPR). Those who allow their names to be released to the ADPR and give informed consent undergo a standardized diagnostic evaluation. Cases categorized as probable AD were enrolled in the study. Data gathered included demographic variables, measures of dementia severity, and comorbid conditions. Proportional hazards regression techniques were used in the survival analysis.

Results.—The 327 patients had an average age of 79 and a mean Mini-Mental State Examination (MMSE) score of 20 at entry. Of the 93 patients who died during follow-up, 51 died within the first 2 years after diagnosis. The ratio of observed to expected deaths (given the geographic area, age, and gender distribution) was 2.1. Variables associated with shortened survival in univariate analysis were age, male gender, MMSE score, Blessed dementia rating scale (DRS) score, rate of symptom progression, wandering or agitation, and sensory impairment affecting hearing and reading. In the multivariate model, functional limitation as measured by the Blessed DRS had the strongest association with shortened survival. Mortality risk was higher for younger patients with high Blessed DRS scores than for the oldest patients with high Blessed DRS scores.

Discussion.—Patients with newly diagnosed probable AD had increased short-term mortality compared with general population groups of comparable age, gender distribution, and area of residency. Variables associated with increased mortality were measures of dementia severity and of general debility.

▶ Articles such as this one on predictors of mortality for AD are of interest because prognosis sometimes is the only thing we can offer patients (and their families) whose disease process is not much affected by our attempts at management. The cohort was large and the patient characteristics were similar to those we might see in a family practice setting. The fact that general debility and sensory impairment were strongly associated with decreased survival in the multivariate analysis should not obscure the clinically important univariate effects of age and male sex.

A.O. Berg, M.D., M.P.H.

Miscellaneous

Moderate-intensity Exercise and Self-rated Quality of Sleep in Older Adults: A Randomized Controlled Trial
King AC, Oman RF, Brassington GS, et al (Stanford Univ, Calif; Univ of Oklahoma, Oklahoma City; Emory Univ, Atlanta, Ga)
JAMA 277:32–37, 1997   17–8

Background.—Sleep problems are very common in middle age and thereafter. It generally is assumed that exercise helps to improve sleep quality; however, this rarely has been tested in controlled studies. A randomized, controlled trial of the effects of moderate exercise on sleep quality was reported.

Methods.—The study included 43 adults, aged 50 to 76 years, with moderate sleep complaints. Two thirds of the patients were women; all were sedentary and free of cardiovascular disease. They were assigned to 16 weeks of community-based, moderate-intensity exercise or a waiting-list control. The exercise group performed 4, 30- to 40-minute sessions of brisk walking per week, at 60% to 75% of their measured heart rate reserve. Changes in self-reported sleep quality were assessed on the Pittsburgh Sleep Quality Index.

Results.—At the end of the study, the exercise group had a significant improvement in global sleep score. Sleep onset latency improved by a mean of 11.5 minutes, whereas sleep duration improved by a mean of 42 minutes. The exercise adherence rate averaged 94%. As exercise time increased, time spent napping during the day decreased, along with sleep latency.

Conclusions.—Moderate exercise can improve self-reported sleep quality in older adults with moderate sleep complaints. It will be important to identify those subgroups of elderly people with sleep disruptions who stand to benefit from physical activity. In this study, it took more than 8 weeks of endurance exercise to produce a difference in sleep quality.

▶ We have known for quite awhile that individuals who exercise also sleep better, but the studies have been retrospective and descriptive, raising the question of whether exercise actually helps with sleep, or whether exercise and good sleep just go together in healthy individuals. This is the first randomized trial in a typical patient population with modest sleep problems, and it shows that exercise makes a difference. The intervention also is practical—basically vigorous walking 4 times a week. This is a useful study that can be implemented readily in practice.

A.O. Berg, M.D., M.P.H.

Protective Effect of Chronic NSAID Use on Cognitive Decline in Older Persons

Rozzini R, Ferrucci L, Losonczy K, et al (P Richiedei Hosp, Gussago, Italy; Natl Research Inst, Florence, Italy; Natl Inst on Aging, Bethesda, Md)
J Am Geriatr Soc 44:1025–1029, 1996   17–9

Purpose.—Studies in patients with rheumatoid arthritis and in others suggest that long-term use of nonsteroidal anti-inflammatory drugs (NSAIDs) may lower the risk of cognitive decline in the elderly. Use of NSAIDs may even affect cognitive decline in patients with Alzheimer's disease. However, many questions remain about the generalizability of this effect. Data from the Established Populations for Epidemiologic Studies of the Elderly (EPESE) were used to assess the protective effect of long-term NSAID use against cognitive decline in older adults.

Methods.—The prospective study included a population-based sample of 7,671 elderly individuals from 3 EPESE communities. All research

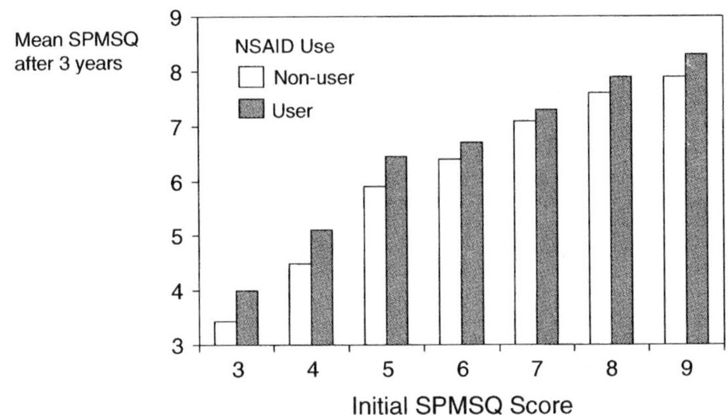

FIGURE 1.—Mean SPMSQ score at the end of the 3-year observation period according to SPMSQ score at beginning of period for long-term users and nonusers of nonsteroidal anti-inflammatory drugs (NSAIDs). *Abbreviation: SPMSQ,* Short Portable Mental Status Questionnaire. (Courtesy of Rozzini R, Ferrucci L, Losonczy K, et al: Protective effect of chronic NSAID use on cognitive decline in older persons. *J Am Geriatr Soc* 44(9):1025–1029, 1996.)

subjects were interviewed in person at their sixth annual follow-up. Twenty-one percent were using NSAIDs at the time of the interview and had used them for the 3 years before—they were considered long-term users. The rest were considered NSAID nonusers. Nonsteroidal anti-inflammatory drug status was compared with the longitudinal change in score on 1 nine-item version of the Short Portable Mental Status Questionnaire (SPMSQ).

Results.—At each score level measured at baseline, the SPMSQ score after 3 years of observation was higher in the long-term NSAID users. At the end of this time, and after adjustment for initial SPMSQ score and potential confounding factors, cognitive function was significantly better for the long-term NSAID users (Fig 1). Other factors independently associated with a lower SPMSQ score were older age, female sex, education, and history of cerebrovascular disease. Multivariate analysis suggested that long-term NSAID use conferred a protective benefit equivalent to an age difference of 3.5 years. During observation, long-term NSAID users were less likely to deteriorate below a given cutoff point than the nonusers. The adjusted relative risk of cognitive decline for long-term NSAID users was 0.82 for a decline in SPMSQ score below 8 and 0.80 for a decline below a score of 6.

Conclusions.—Long-term NSAID use may protect against cognitive decline in the elderly. Given the observational nature of this study, no causal relationship can be proved. A randomized, controlled trial is needed to tell definitively whether taking NSAIDs reduces the risk of cognitive decline.

▶ Dementia in older age has become more common as the population lives longer. The fact that most dementias in older age have no effective treatment makes this loss of cognitive function even more frightening. This interesting study joins several others in documenting the positive effect of the use of NSAIDs as a protection against cognitive decline in older individuals.

This was a well-designed study of 7,600 research subjects in the New England area of the United States. It was a prospective 3-year observational study. Although the results are not earth-shaking, there was a demonstrable reduction in loss of cognitive function with the use of NSAIDs. This effect occurred regardless of how bad the dementia was at the onset of the study. Unfortunately, this study did not document any of the potential side effects of the use of NSAIDs. The authors hypothesize 2 mechanisms for why NSAIDs might protect against cognitive decline. The first of these is an inflammatory origin of many dementias. The other argument involves the platelet anti-aggregation properties of aspirin and other NSAIDs.

Because there is often little more we can do with these patients in terms of their cognitive loss, I think the patient and their family should at least be informed of the possible positive effect of the use of NSAIDs, and, if there are no contraindications to their use, a trial should be begun.

R.C. Davidson, M.D., M.P.H.

Outpatient Geriatric Evaluation and Management: Results of a Randomized Trial

Toseland RW, O'Donnell JC, Engelhardt JB, et al (State Univ of New York, Albany; Albany Med College, NY)
Med Care 34:624–640, 1996

17–10

Introduction.—There is growing evidence that geriatric evaluation and management (GEM) is an effective approach to providing health care to frail elderly inpatients. It is not known whether GEM is similarly effective for outpatient care. The effectiveness and efficiency of GEM and usual primary care (UPC) were compared in frail elderly outpatients.

Methods.—One hundred sixty frail elderly patients were randomly assigned to receive either GEM or UPC. The patients were evaluated at baseline and 8 months for health and functional status, psychosocial well-being, quality of health and social care, use of inpatient and outpatient services, and cost of care.

Results.—Compared to UPC, patients receiving GEM had significantly reduced mortality, more patient satisfaction, and improved quality of health and social care. Geriatric evaluation and management was not more effective than UPC in decreasing health care use or cost.

Conclusions.—The greatest impact of outpatient GEM was observed in the quality of health and social care received by frail elderly patients. These findings have important implications for policy makers and health care providers. The GEM approach is more likely than UPC to provide an efficient and effective means of improving the care and well-being of the frail elderly. Now the long-time effects on patient health and the quality, use, and cost of outpatient GEM should be determined.

▶ For those who favor intensive geriatric services, one can find support in this article. For those who believe they are expensive and ineffective, one also can find support. Personally, I believe that many patients could use much more support in multiple ways than our medical system can provide; this is not limited to geriatric patients. Social factors affect health and medical utilization, yet we struggle with the medical system's role in social support. Where the line is drawn is basically a matter of what we wish to finance (or ration) and to whom.

M.A. Bowman, M.D., M.P.A.

Benzodiazepine Use and the Risk of Motor Vehicle Crash in the Elderly

Hemmelgarn B, Suissa S, Huang A, et al (McGill Univ, Montreal; Royal Victoria Hosp, Montreal)

JAMA 278:27–31, 1997   17–11

Objective.—Benzodiazepines are the drugs of choice for elderly individuals with anxiety and insomnia. Although these drugs are known to impair the ability to drive, the few epidemiologic studies conducted have yielded inconsistent results. The risk of motor vehicle crashes among elderly drivers after the initiation of treatment with long half life (> 24 hours) and short half life (≤ 24 hours) benzodiazepines, the time after initiation for this risk to become increased, and the duration of increased risk with prolonged use are reported.

Methods.—Driving records of all individuals in Quebec between the ages of 67 and 84 on June 1, 1990 were examined for motor vehicle accidents and injuries. The cohort of 224,734 individuals was followed for 3 years as a nested case-control study. Benzodiazepine exposure was ascertained via prescription records. The crash rate for benzodiazepine users was estimated from the odds ratio calculated with both conditional and unconditional logistic regression.

Results.—Insurance records were available for 5,579 of the 6,064 individuals involved as a driver in a motor vehicle crash with injuries. When these data were compared with data from a random sample of 10 control individuals per case selected from a subcohort of 13,256 individuals, the prevalence of exposure to benzodiazepines at least once in the year prior to the start of the study was 38.5% for the drivers and 36.2% for the controls. Current use of long half-life benzodiazepines was significantly associated with increased risk of an injurious crash (rate ratio 1.28), and the adjusted rate ratio (1.45) for the first week after beginning treatment was significantly increased. After 8 days, the rate ratios were no longer significant. There was no increased risk of injurious crash with short half-life benzodiazepines.

Conclusion.—Although this was not a randomized study, findings suggest that the use of long half-life benzodiazepines in the elderly significantly increase the risk of an injurious crash, particularly during the first week of use.

▶ With 225,000 in the database, this is a huge study that bears close scrutiny. The increased risk of motor vehicle accidents in those exposed to long-acting benzodiazepines is both statistically and clinically significant—clinically significant because the elderly are already at higher risk so that a relatively modest increase in relative risk causes a disproportionately large increase in absolute risk. Indications for the long half-life agents are few, if any, yet benzodiazepines are prescribed twice as often for the elderly as for any other age group. In this article, nearly 1 in 5 subjects was on a benzodiazepine on any given day, even though all package inserts counsel against use while driving a motor vehicle. This article provides more justification for cautious prescribing, using short-acting agents, if at all possible, and for the shortest possible term. In the long run, there will always be a tension between individual independence and mobility and concern for public safety in using these agents.

A.O. Berg, M.D., M.P.H.

Survival of Medicare Patients After Enrollment in Hospice Programs

Christakis NA, Escarce JJ (Univ of Chicago; Univ of Pennsylvania, Philadelphia)
N Engl J Med 335:172–178, 1996   17–12

Objective.—Hospice care, by palliating the patient's physical and mental suffering, can enhance the quality of the end of life. About 220,000 Medicare beneficiaries are enrolled in hospice programs each year. To be eligible, these patients must be certified as "terminally ill," with a life expectancy of less than 6 months. This 6-month cutoff point may be difficult for physicians to apply, however. The life expectancy of Medicare patients after hospice enrollment was studied.

Methods.—The study used 1990 Medicare claims data on 6,451 patients admitted to hospice programs in 5 large states. The patients' characteristics were analyzed, along with their survival after hospice enrollment. All were followed up for at least 27 months.

Findings.—The patients' mean age was 76 years, and 92% were white. Eighty percent had some type of cancer, the most common diagnoses being lung cancer (21%), colorectal cancer (10.5%), and prostate cancer (7%). The patients survived for a median of only 36 days after enrollment, including 16% who died within a week. About 15% of patients survived for longer than 6 months (Fig 1). Even after adjustment for age and comorbidity, survival was strongly affected by diagnosis. Crude survival was longest for patients with chronic lung disease, dementia, or breast cancer and shortest for those with renal failure, leukemia, or lymphoma. Patients in for-profit, larger, outpatient, or newer hospices had longer survival than those in other types of hospices.

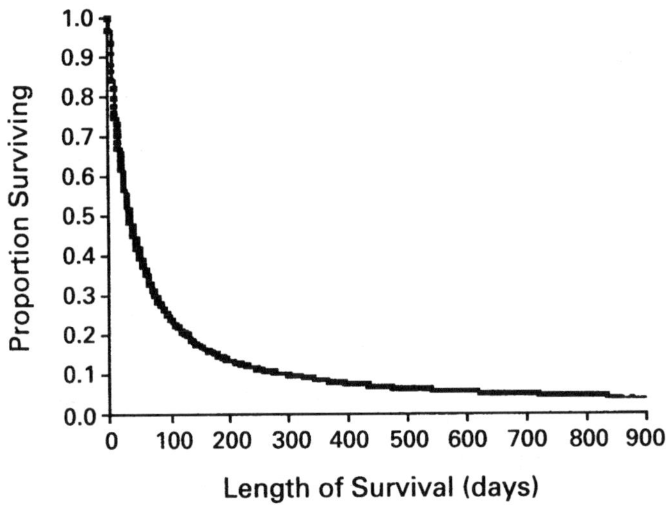

FIGURE 1.—Kaplan-Meier survival curve for 6,451 Medicare beneficiaries enrolled in hospice programs in 1990. Survival was measured from the day of enrollment in the hospice program to the day of death. (Courtesy of Christakis NA, Escarce JJ: Survival of Medicare patients after enrollment in hospice programs. *N Engl J Med* 335:172–178, 1996. Reprinted by permission of *The New England Journal of Medicine*, copyright 1996, Massachusetts Medical Society. All rights reserved.)

Conclusions.—Most Medicare patients in hospice programs are not enrolled until late in the course of their illness. The timing of enrollment is significantly affected by patient and hospice characteristics. Enrolling patients in hospices earlier on might be able to reduce health care spending while improving quality of care at the end of life.

▶ I chose this article because it provides useful basic data and supplies a counter-argument to those who fear long stays and high costs in implementing the Medicare benefit. The figure summarizes the survival data best. I am most impressed by the median survival of 36 days. The authors do a nice job of discussing whether we should treat this as too long or too short. I am on the "too short" end. It seems to me that the short length of stay for such a large proportion of patients means that the benefit is provided too late. I suspect (with the authors) that the requirement that patients not be admitted to a hospice unless their expected survival is less than 6 months dissuades patients and physicians from using the program sooner. For those with the shortest stays—less than a week—it seems unlikely that staff were able to get to know the patient and family well enough to provide much benefit. The fact that other countries do not have the 6-month rule, but have average lengths of residence well under 6 months, suggests that we could safely discard the rule. The authors point to other evidence that earlier admission provides more humane care and is cost-effecive besides.

A.O. Berg, M.D., M.P.H.

Defining Inappropriate Practices in Prescribing for Elderly People: A National Consensus Panel

McLeod PJ, Huang AR, Tamblyn RM, et al (McGill Univ, Montreal)
Can Med Assoc J 156:385–391, 1997   17–13

Background.—The elderly suffer from more illness and disability, are prescribed more medication, and have a greater likelihood of adverse effects from presciption medication than younger patients. Inappropriate prescription is a preventable cause of morbidity and mortality. A study of intervention to reduce inappropriate prescribing has been initiated. The first step in this project was the development of a list of inappropriate practices in prescribing for the elderly patient.

Study Design.—Inappropriate practices in the prescription of drugs for the elderly patient were divided into 3 categories: prescription of drugs contraindicated because of an unacceptable risk-benefit ratio, prescription of drugs that can cause adverse drug-drug interactions, and prescription of drugs that can cause drug-disease interactions. Only those practices that caused a substantial and clinically significant increase in the risk of serious adverse effect, had alternative effective therapies available, and were common enough that practice change could decrease morbidity were included in the list. An arbitrarily chosen expert panel of 32 specialists in clinical pharmacology, geriatrics, family medicine, and pharmacy were asked to examine the initial list and make suggestions to create the final list. The final list was returned to the experts so they could rate the clinical importance of the adverse effects caused by practices on the list.

Results.—The expert panel developed a list of 71 inappropriate practices in prescribing for the elderly patient (Table 4). For each inappropriate practice, alternative therapies were recommended. There was good agreement among the specialists on alternative therapies and on the significance of adverse reactions.

Conclusions.—A panel of specialists used a consensus method to derive a valid, relevant list of inappropriate practices in prescribing for the elderly, as well as a list of alternative therapies. This list will be used in a double-blind, controlled trial of an intervention to improve prescription practices for the elderly patient.

▶ The elderly are a vulnerable group when it comes to drug prescribing. They tend to be receiving more significant drugs with potential for adverse reactions and for serious drug-drug interactions. I am not usually a fan of consensus statements, but the 4 extended tables in this publication listing inappropriate prescriptions for the elderly patient are a quite reasonable summary of things to watch out for. The items in these tables follow the principle of "first do no harm." I spot checked the scientific evidence supporting the consensus statements and was pleased to find them well documented in the medical literature. I have included here the fourth table for miscellaneous drugs, but I would recommend tracking down this article

TABLE 4.—Inappropriate Practices in Prescribing Miscellaneous Drugs for Elderly Patients

Practice	Mean clinical significance rating	Risk to patient	Alternative therapy	% of panel members who agreed with alternative
Prescription of cimetidine to treat peptic ulcer for patients already receiving warfarin	3.47	May inhibit warfarin metabolism and increase the risk of bleeding	Other histamine (H_2)-receptor antagonist	84
Prescription of anticholinergic or antispasmodic drugs to treat irritable bowel syndrome for patients with dementia	3.41	May worsen cognitive and behavioural function	Nondrug and diet therapy, calcium-channel blocker to treat diarrhea	69
Prescription of dipyridamole to prevent stroke	3.30	Ineffective	ASA Ticlopidine	94 69
Long-term prescription of orally administered steroids to treat COPD for patients with a history of NIDDM	3.25	May worsen NIDDM	Inhaled steroids and bronchodilators with monitoring of blood glucose levels	97
Prescription of anticholinergic drugs to prevent extrapyramidal effects of antipsychotic drugs	3.16	May cause agitation, dilirium and impaired cognition	Decreased dosage of antipsychotic drugs or reassessment of need for these drugs	97
Long-term prescription of diphenoxylate to treat diarrhea	3.13	Drowsiness, cognitive impairment and dependence	Nondrug and diet therapy or loperamide	84
Prescription of cyclobenzaprine or methocarbamol to treat muscle spasms	3.06	Drowsiness, agitation and disorientation	Nondrug therapy (physiotherapy application of heat and cold or TENS+)	94

Abbreviations: ASA, acetylsalicylic acid; *COPD*, chronic obstructive pulmonary disease; *NIDDM*, non–insulin-dependent diabetes mellitus; *TENS*, transcutaneous electrical nerve stimulation.
(Reprinted from McLeod PJ, Huang AR, Tamblyn RM, et al: Defining inappropriate practices in prescribing for elderly people: A national consensus panel by permission of the publisher, CMAJ, *Can Med Assoc J* 156:385–391, 1997.)

to examine fully the other 3 tables that cover cardiovascular disease, psychotropics, and analgesics (including nonsteroidal anti-inflammatory drugs). These lists are handy reminders of common errors in prescribing for the elderly patient that can have serious consequences.

A.O. Berg, M.D., M.P.H.

18 Emergencies

Introduction

This short chapter reports and comments on important studies of tissue adhesive in treating minor lacerations, the prevalence of panic disorder in emergency settings (high), and the emergent treatment of arrhythmias.

Randomized controlled trials: Abstracts 18–1, 18–5, and 18–6.

Alfred O. Berg, M.D., M.P.H.

A Randomized Trial Comparing Octylcyanoacrylate Tisssue Adhesive and Sutures in the Management of Lacerations

Quinn J, Wells G, Sutcliffe T, et al (Univ of Michigan, Ann Arbor; Univ of Ottawa, Ont, Canada)

JAMA 277:1527–1530, 1997

18–1

Introduction.—Suture repair of lacerations is a painful and time-consuming procedure. Octylcyanoacrylate (Dermabond) is a new medical-grade tissue adhesive designed to overcome the limitations of previous formulations. It is being studied for use as a medical device for topical skin closure. Octylcyanoacrylate was compared with suture repair for the management of lacerations.

Methods.—The prospective, randomized controlled trial included 136 lacerations treated in 130 patients during a 5-month period. All nonmucosal facial lacerations were eligible for entry into the trial, as were selected extremity and torso lacerations. Each laceration was randomly selected to be closed by octylcyanoacrylate adhesive or monofilament suture. The adhesive was simply painted over the apposed edges of the wound, with care taken not to get any between the wound edges. The wound was held for 30 seconds for complete polymerization, with no dressing applied. The cosmetic results were graded in blinded fashion from photographs of the wounds taken at 3 months' follow-up. Three-month evaluation was available in 98 wounds.

Findings.—On a 100–mm visual analogue scale, mean cosmesis scores were 67 mm in the octylcyanoacrylate group and 68 mm in the suture group. Early and 3-month clinical wound evaluation scores were also similar in the 2 groups. Mean wound repair time was 3.6 minutes with tissue adhesive vs. 12.4 minutes with suture repair. Octylcyanoacrylate repair was also rated as less painful.

Conclusions.—Properly selected lacerations can be effectively closed by octylcyanoacrylate rather than suture repair. Tissue adhesive repair is quicker and less painful, and could avoid the need for suturing in millions of lacerations per year. The clinical and cosmetic results are comparable to those of suture repair.

▶ Does this mark the beginning of the end of simple suturing as we know it? I am especially struck by the use of this new material on small facial lacerations, cause for the most painstaking (and time-consuming) plastic repairs in many emergency departments. This study was funded by the manufacturer of the material; it would be nice to see studies from a variety of centers and researchers demonstrating similar good outcomes. The material is already approved for use in Canada and is in late-stage trials here in the United States. This is a technology to watch carefully and learn about in the next few years.

A.O. Berg, M.D., M.P.H.

Poinsettia Exposures Have Good Outcomes . . . Just As We Thought
Krenzelok EP, Jacobsen TD, Aronis JM (Univ of Pittsburgh, Pa; Carnegie Mellon Univ, Pittsburgh, Pa)
Am J Emerg Med 14:671–674, 1996
18–2

Background.—The poinsettia is reputed to be very poisonous. However, deaths from ingesting poinsettia leaves have never been substantiated. Results of a study demonstrating that the poinsettia is not associated with either significant morbidity or any mortality was presented.

Methods.—A search of the data from the American Association of Poison Control Centers for the years 1985 to 1992 turned up 849,575 plant exposures, of which 22,793 involved the poinsettia. The associated morbidity and mortality were evaluated.

Results.—Exposures were equally divided among males and females, and 93.3% involved children, with 77.3% of them less than 2 years of age. The majority of exposures occurred by ingestion. There were no fatalities. Minor effects were observed in 3.4% of exposures. The majority of patients (96.1%) were not treated in a health care setting. Patients received no therapy in 34.6% of cases, and there was general decontamination or ipecac-induced vomiting in 62.7%. Decontamination procedures had no effect on patient outcome.

Conclusion.—Poinsettia exposure does not carry a significant risk of morbidity or mortality. Most patients do not need to be treated in a medical facility. Decontamination procedures, especially emesis, are not recommended.

▶ The beautiful Christmas plant is safe after all! This large study covering 7 years of national data shows that toxicity from poinsettias is a myth. It is nice to see that scientific research can increase the joy and decrease the anxiety of the holiday season.

J.E. Scherger, M.D., M.P.H.

Panic Disorder in Emergency Department Chest Pain Patients: Prevalence, Comorbidity, Suicidal Ideation, and Physician Recognition
Fleet RP, Dupuis G, Marchand A, et al (Montreal Heart Inst; Université du Québec à Montréal, Montreal; Univ of Missouri-Columbia)
Am J Med 101:371–380, 1996
18–3

Background.—Most patients who come to the emergency department with chest pain are released with a noncardiac chest pain diagnosis. Because psychological factors are suspected and because of research that suggests that approximately 30% of patients with noncardiac chest pain have panic disorder (PD), a study was conducted to establish the prevalence of PD in these patients. The study also compared psychological distress and suicidal ideation in patients with and without PD, evaluated psychiatric and cardiac co-morbidity in patients with PD, and examined physician recognition of this disorder.

Methods.—Self-report psychological and pain questionnaires [Panic-Agoraphobia: Mobility Inventory for Agoraphobia (MIA), Agoraphobia Cognitions Questionnaire (ACQ), Body Sensations Questionnaire (BSQ), Anxiety-State-Trait Anxiety Inventory (STAI), Depression: Beck Depression Inventory (BDI), Pain: the Short Form-McGill Pain Questionnaire (SF-MPQ)] were filled out by 441 consecutive emergency department patients (39% women) with chest pain. Their average age was 56.8 years. Each patient was administered the Anxiety Disorders Interview Schedule–Revised (ADIS-R) by 3 interviewers. Chest pain was classified on the Chest Pain Quality Scale by a cardiologist. Medical tests were performed as appropriate. Data were analyzed statistically.

Results.—There were 108 patients (25%) who met the criteria for PD. They were significantly younger than patients without PD, and 62 (57%) had at least 1 Axis I disorder. Patients with PD scored significantly higher than patients without PD on all psychological and pain measures, except for current pain index. Although a significant number of patients with PD had a history of coronary artery disease, there was no association between PD and a history of coronary artery disease or between PD and cardiac comorbidity. Significantly more patients with PD (25%) than patients without PD (5%) reported suicidal ideation. When depressed patients were excluded from the analysis, the proportion of patients with PD with suicidal ideation remained the same. Significantly more patients with PD (80%) than patients without PD (72%) had atypical or nonanginal chest pain, and 75% of patients with PD were discharged with a noncardiac diagnosis. Patients without PD were significantly more likely to be discharged with a cardiac diagnosis. Cardiologists failed to recognize 98% of patients with PD.

Conclusion.—Panic disorder appears to be responsible for a significant incidence of noncardiac chest pain. Emergency department cardiologists fail to recognize PD in most cases.

▶ Chest pain centers have been established in many emergency departments to facilitate early thrombolytic treatment of patients with an acute myocardial infarction or with severe angina. For such patients, this is great but, unfortunately, many patients with acute chest pain in emergency rooms are not experiencing heart disease. This prospective study of consecutive patients with chest pain seen at a Montreal emergency department revealed that PD and other psychiatric morbidities are very common and are frequently not recognized by emergency department physicians and cardiologists. Interestingly, many of the patients had simultaneous psychiatric and cardiac disease.

This study underscores the importance of taking a comprehensive biopsychosocial approach to patients with chest pain in the emergency room. Not treating the mental health condition may lead to serious consequences, such as suicide.

J.E. Scherger, M.D., M.P.H.

Patients With Acute Hyperventilation Presenting to an Inner-City Emergency Department

Saisch SGN, Wessely S, Gardner WN (Kings College, London)
Chest 110:952–957, 1996   18–4

Introduction.—Little is known about acute and subacute hyperventilation or the clinical characteristics of patients who come to emergency departments with this problem. To prevent misdiagnosis of serious organic disease, such as myocardial infarction, asthma, or diabetic ketoacidosis, and to foster correct treatment, it is important to know more about acute hyperventilation. A consecutive series of patients with hyperventilation who were admitted to an emergency department was studied to learn the cause of hyperventilation.

Methods.—There were 23 patients who were admitted to an inner-city emergency department who had acute hyperventilation diagnosed. Five patients had this confirmed by arterial blood gas values. Tests included chest radiograph, serum biochemistry, blood cell count, and thyroid function. The patients had dyspnea (61%), paresthesia (35%), chest pain or tightness (43%), panic (30%), muscle spasm (9%), dizziness (13%), and palpitations (13%). After they were diagnosed and examined, they were assessed 2 months later.

Results.—In 74%, previous episodes were recorded. In 20 (87%) patients, there was misattribution of the presenting complaints to a cardiac or other life-threatening disorder and was the main reason for the patients coming to the hospital. None of the patients had clinical features of asthma, but 10 (44%) had a history and investigation results suggestive of asthma, and 7 (30%) were known asthmatics receiving treatment. A history of anxiety or depression was found in 2 patients. On the Clinical Interview Schedule interview, 17 (78%) patients exceeded the threshold for anxiety or panic. In 17% of patients, marijuana or alcohol abuse was involved. Past abuse was seen in 26%. At the 2-month follow-up assessment, 13 (57%) were found with resting or stressor-induced hyperventilation having a significant association with asthma but not with a positive Clinical Interview Schedule score.

Conclusion.—Acute hyperventilation has a multifactorial basis, is often misattributed, and the term *hyperventilation syndrome* should be used more carefully in the emergency department. The best therapeutic approach is careful assessment for mild asthma, advice about drug and alcohol abuse, explanation about the possible presenting sequence of events and the symptoms of hypocapnia, and a full organic investigation. In all cases of hyperventilation, arterial blood gas analysis and a chest radiograph are the best tools for detection in the emergency department.

▶ Once a patient is labeled as suffering from acute hyperventilation, a psychosomatic basis is often assumed, and the patient is taken less seriously in the emergency department. This study highlights the complexity of many of these patients and the danger of labeling them as having a mental health condition. With the increasing prevalence of asthma, including asthma mortality, these patients must be evaluated with an open mind and serious concern.

J.E. Scherger, M.D., M.P.H.

Effectiveness of Verapamil–Quinidine Versus Digoxin–Quinidine in the Emergency Department Treatment of Paroxysmal Atrial Fibrillation
Innes GD, Vertesi L, Dillon EC, et al (Royal Columbian Hosp, New Westminster, BC, Canada)
Ann Emerg Med 29:126–134, 1997   18–5

Background.—Patients with paroxysmal atrial fibrillation (PAF) are commonly seen in the emergency department (ED). Prompt, appropriate treatment is essential to avoid potentially life-threatening complications. The evidence suggests that digoxin is inappropriate for acute AF—some treatment that offers quicker and more reliable control of the ventricular response could provide faster conversion of PAF. This would permit faster discharge from the ED and avoid unnecessary hospitalization. The combination of verapamil–quinidine was compared with digoxin–quinidine for the ED treatment of PAF in a double-blind, randomized, controlled trial.

Methods.—The study included 54 adult patients up to 75 years old with new-onset AF. Patients with a ventricular response rate lower than 100 or higher than 200 bpm were excluded, as were those with allergies to the study drugs, hypotension with signs of end-organ hypoperfusion, and conduction abnormalities. Initially, 1 group of patients received digitalis, 1.0 mg over 2 hours, whereas while the other received verapamil, given in sequential 5 mg boluses up to 20 mg. Once the ventricular rate fell below 100 bpm, all patients received oral quinidine, 200 mg. Quinidine administration was repeated every 2 hours until normal sinus rhythm (NRS) was restored, the patient had received a total of 1 g of quinidine, or adverse effects developed.

Results.—After withdrawal, there were 19 patients in the verapamil–quinidine (VER-Q) group and 22 in the digoxin–quinidine (DIG-Q) group. Conversion to NSR occurred within 6 hours in 84% of patients in the VER-Q group vs. 45% in the DIG-Q group. The mean time to conversion was 185 minutes for the VER-Q group and 368 minutes for the DIG-Q group, although the difference was not significant. Sixty-three percent of patients in the VER-Q group were discharged from the ED compared with only 27% of those in the DIG-Q group. Patients receiving VER-Q were more likely to have adverse effects but only minor ones. None of the patients died or experienced significant morbidity.

Conclusions.—At the doses used in this study, the sequential combination of verapamil and quinidine appears to be an effective ED treatment for PAF. It is more effective than the combination of digoxin and quinidine, which should no longer be considered the treatment of choice for uncomplicated PAF. The results may not apply to postcardiac surgery or critical care patients.

Emergency Management of Atrial Fibrillation and Flutter: Intravenous Diltiazem Versus Intravenous Digoxin
Schreck DM, Rivera AR, Tricarico VJ (Muhlenberg Regional Med Ctr, Plainfield, NJ; Robert Wood Johnson Med School, Piscataway, NJ)
Ann Emerg Med 29:135–140, 1997   18–6

Introduction.—Acute atrial fibrillation and flutter (AFF) is the most commonly encountered sustained dysrhythmia. In the emergency department (ED), treatment for acute AFF seeks to gain control of the ventricular rate, preferably through drug treatment in a hemodynamically stable patient. Digoxin is considered the main treatment for AFF, but it has never been directly compared with diltiazem. An open-label, randomized, controlled trial of IV diltiazem vs. digoxin in the ED treatment of acute AFF is reported.

Methods.—The study included 30 consecutive patients seen in an ED with acute AFF during a 1-year period. Patients who had a systolic blood pressure of less than 100 mm Hg or who were being treated with calcium channel blockers other than diltiazem were excluded. One group of patients received IV diltiazem, starting with 0.25 mg/kg given over 2 minutes, then 0.35 mg/kg at 15 minutes, followed by a titratable IV infusion at a rate of 10–20 mg/hr, adjusted to maintain control of heart rate. Another group received IV digoxin, 0.25 mg as a bolus initially and again 30 minutes later. A third group received both treatments at the same dosages. The study definition of heart rate control was a ventricular rate of less than 100 bpm. At specified intervals over 3 hours, the patients' heart rhythms, heart rates, and blood pressures were assessed.

Results.—The mean heart rate at baseline was 150 bpm in the diltiazem group and 144 bpm in the digoxin group. By 5 minutes, the heart rate had decreased to 111 bpm with diltiazem vs. 144 bpm for digoxin. By 15 minutes, there was a significant difference between the combination and digoxin groups; at no time was there a significant difference between the diltiazem and combination groups. Not until 180 minutes after treatment did the digoxin group have a significant reduction in heart rate. At that time, the mean heart rate was 90 bpm in the diltiazem group vs. 117 bpm in the digoxin group.

Conclusions.—For ED patients with acute AFF, treatment with IV diltiazem produces a significant reduction in ventricular heart rate within 5 minutes. Intravenous digoxin, by contrast, requires 3 hours to produce a significant reduction. A combination of diltiazem and digoxin is no more effective than diltiazem alone. Thus, IV diltiazem should be considered to be the drug of choice for emergency treatment of acute AFF. Further study is needed to assess possible adverse effects.

Treatment of Out-of-hospital Supraventricular Tachycardia: Adenosine vs Verapamil
Brady WJ Jr, DeBehnke DJ, Wickman LL, et al (Univ of Virginia, Charlottesville; Med College of Wisconsin, Milwaukee)
Acad Emerg Med 3:574–585, 1996   18–7

Objective.—Adenosine has recently been accepted for use in the acute treatment of supraventricular tachycardia (SVT). It is now the drug of choice for this purpose in the American Heart Association Advanced Cardiac Life Support protocol. Adenosine was compared with verapamil as out-of-hospital therapy for SVT.

Methods.—A 1-year period of prospective adenosine use was compared with a historical 1-year control period of verapamil use in a metropolitan paramedic system. Standard drug protocols were followed during both periods. Patient outcome monitoring included conversion, complication, and recurrence rates. The study included 105 patients with SVT during the adenosine period and 106 during the verapamil period.

Results.—During the adenosine period, 83% of patients with SVT received adenosine. Of these, 69% had conversion to sinus rhythm (SR). In another 8% of patients, vagal maneuvers led to restoration of SR. Although adenosine was sometimes given for rhythms other than SVT, it never produced conversion to SR. Twenty of 25 patients with hemodynamic instability received adenosine; 13 had conversion to SR, whereas 8 required electric cardioversion. Adverse effects related to adenosine were noted in 4 patients.

During the verapamil period, 49% of patients with SVT received verapamil. Eighty-eight percent of them had conversion to SR. Given in 2 patients with wide-complex tachycardia, verapamil produced cardiovascular collapse in both. Eleven percent of patients had SR restored by vagal maneuvers. Five of 16 patients with hemodynamic instability received verapamil, and all 5 had conversion to SR. Electric cardioversion was required by 9 patients. There were 4 patients with verapamil-related adverse effects. Before they arrived at the hospital, 2 patients in each group had recurrent SVT. After arrival in the emergency department (ED), 23 patients in the adenosine group vs. 15 in the verapamil group had recurrences requiring additional treatment. There were no significant differences in hospital diagnoses, patient outcomes, or ED dispositions.

Conclusion.—Both adenosine and verapamil can produce conversion to SR for patients with out-of-hospital SVT of similar origins. There is no significant difference in the SVT recurrence rate. Neither drug affects the future success of therapy in the ED, disposition from the ED, or the need for out-of-hospital electric cardioversion. Rhythm misidentification continues to be a problem in out-of-hospital cardiac care. However, in narrow complex tachycardias, this confusion rarely leads to clinical deterioration after treatment with adenosine or verapamil.

▶ These 3 studies (Abstracts 18–5 to 18–7) provide convincing evidence that the emergency treatment of SVTs has changed. Intravenous calcium channel blockers, verapamil, and diltiazem are more effective in a shorter period of time than IV digoxin. The third article (Abstract 18–7) indicates that verapamil is comparable with adenosine, a drug that is more expensive and possibly more dangerous. Family physicians who regularly treat patients can now use these calcium channel blockers with confidence.

J.E. Scherger, M.D., M.P.H.

19 Issues in Cancer

Introduction

This chapter opens with one of the most provocative articles reviewed this year, showing how cancer treatment has been largely a failure if measured by the ultimate outcome of cancer mortality. Remaining articles in this miscellaneous selection address cancer pain, maternal smoking and childhood cancer, and follow-up for patients with an inherited predisposition to colon cancer.

Randomized controlled trial: Abstract 19–2.

Alfred O. Berg, M.D., M.P.H.

Cancer Undefeated

Bailar JC III, Gornik HL (Univ of Chicago)
N Engl J Med 336:1569–1574, 1997   19–1

Introduction.—Even with intensive clinical and basic science research, cancer continues to be a major cause of morbidity and mortality. Because of advances in diagnosis, the reported incidence of cancer is not a reliable indicator of trends in incidence over time. Age-adjusted mortality is a more useful measure of progress in the fight against cancer. Trends in age-adjusted mortality were analyzed to assess progress against cancer from the 1970s to the 1990s.

Methods.—The analysis used National Center for Health Statistics data on all cancer deaths and on deaths from cancer at specific sites from 1970 through 1994. Cancer deaths were also broken down by age, race, and sex. Age-specific mortality rates were calculated and adjusted to the 1990 age distribution of the U.S. population.

Results.—Age-adjusted cancer mortality increased from 189.6 per 100,000 population in 1970 to 200.9 per 100,000 in 1994. Age-adjusted all-cancer mortality decreased steadily for several decades, then plateaued before undergoing a 1% decrease from 1991 to 1994. Groups achieving the greatest reduction in cancer mortality were African-American males and people younger than 55 years. In recent years, white men aged 55 years or older have had a reduction in mortality (Fig 1). Factors behind these trends include changes in mortality from specific types of cancer, including stomach, cervical, and uterine cancer and leukemia; reductions in cigarette smoking achieved decades ago; and improvements in cancer

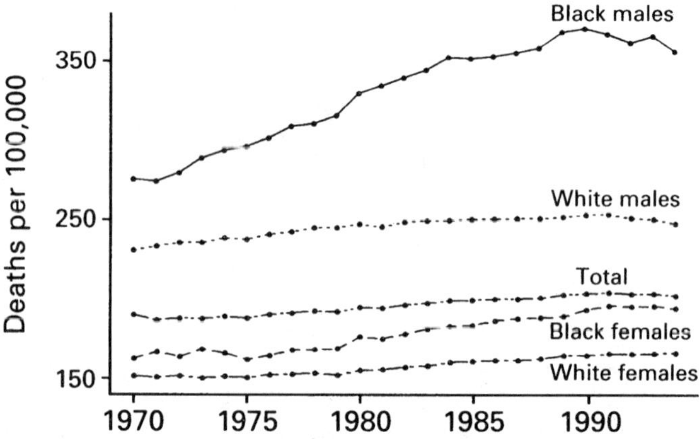

FIGURE 1.—Mortality from all malignant neoplasms, 1970 through 1994, in the total U.S. population and according to race and sex. The rates have been age-adjusted to the U.S. resident population of 1990. (Courtesy of Bailar JC III, Gornik HL: Cancer undefeated. *N Engl J Med* 336:1569–1574, 1997, copyright Massachusetts Medical Society. Reprinted by permission of *The New England Journal of Medicine*. All rights reserved.)

screening. For childhood cancers, mortality rates have dropped by about 50% since the 1970s, with further reductions ongoing.

Conclusions.—Recent years have seen some small reductions in cancer mortality, largely because of changes in cancer incidence or early detection. New cancer treatments have had little impact on mortality. These trends suggest that a focus on prevention—with an attendant shift in the focus and funding of research—is the best approach to reducing cancer mortality.

▶ The first author of this article is one of the leading statisticians in the world with a reputation for clarity and integrity. To those of us in primary care, the main conclusion is not surprising: the future of cancer control lies in prevention and early detection. But among cancer specialists, this article created a furor because it suggests (proves?) that cancer treatment has largely been a failure when measured by the ultimate outcome of mortality (see Fig 1). The suggestion that research dollars might thus more profitably be directed toward prevention (and away from cancer treatment) has made some cancer researchers very angry. This is another example of a changing paradigm in our fast-evolving health system. Interventions of unproven benefit must be moved aside without remorse. Although cancer specialists hope that much will be accomplished with new treatments rooted in molecular medicine, Dr. Bailar takes a more skeptical view, recalling similar arguments over the decades in favor of chemotherapy, virology, and immunology that have not produced benefits as promised. If findings such as these are taken seriously, we could see a dramatic increase in research focused on prevention and early detection. Family medicine researchers are well positioned to contribute if the wind shifts.

A.O. Berg, M.D., M.P.H.

Improving Cancer Pain Management in Communities: Main Results From a Randomized Controlled Trial
Elliott TE, Murray DM, Oken MM, et al (Univ of Minnesota-Duluth; Univ of Minnesota, Minneapolis)
J Pain Symptom Manage 13:191–203, 1997   19–2

Objective.—It is documented that the pain relief cancer patients actually receive is far short of that which is possible to provide. The main barriers to effective analgesia in cancer patients are probably the knowledge, skills, and attitudes of physicians, nurses, patients, and families. There have been no experimental studies evaluating the effects of educational efforts designed to improve cancer pain management (CPM). A community-based educational program designed to improve knowledge, attitudes, and behaviors related to CPM, and to reduce cancer-related pain in patients, was evaluated.

Methods.—The randomized community trial, called the Minnesota Cancer Pain Project, used nested cohort and nested cross-sectional designs. It included 6 medium-sized communities with distinctly defined medical service areas. Three communities were assigned to receive the intervention, while the other 3 served as controls. Numerous approaches were used to educate the intervention communities in modern CPM techniques. Clinical opinion leaders from these communities participated in a minifellowship program, developed community task forces, and interacted with their peers. These interventions were complemented by community outreach programs, clinical practice guidelines, educational materials, and media events. The community-wide interventions were targeted at all practicing physicians and nurses, as well as all cancer patients and their families. The main study end point was the pain intensity scores of cancer patients. A pain management index was developed to assess the responses of health care providers to their patients' pain. Knowledge and attitude scores of professionals, patients, and families were assessed as well.

Results.—The study intervention led to a slight reduction in the prevalence of pain among cancer patients, a slight improvement in pain management index, and a slight increase in pain intensity scores. None of these changes were significant. Neither was there any significant change in the attitude scores of patients and families or in the knowledge and attitude scores of the health care professionals. Physicians and nurses who attended at least 1 interventional program showed a near-significant improvement in their knowledge and attitude scores.

Conclusions.—Community-wide interventions designed to improve CPM are associated with little significant improvement, this randomized trial suggests. Most of the trends are in the right direction, however, so the educational approach used in this trial warrants further study. It could be that a more intensive intervention would be effective. Future attempts at improving CPM should be subject to experimental evaluation, including clinical practice and patient outcome variables.

▶ This is research on a grand scale, randomizing entire communities to intervention or control groups. I include the disappointing results of this trial to highlight the fact that well-conceived and well-executed programs can still fail to show much effect. The intensity of the intervention was about as much as any community is likely to muster, so the finding of little effect should lead to serious rethinking of how to change provider behavior for such a complex problem. Things that seem to be good ideas and make sense still must be proved effective before they can be generally applied.

A.O. Berg, M.D., M.P.H.

Maternal Smoking During Pregnancy and Childhood Cancer
Klebanoff MA, Clemens JD, Read JS (Natl Inst of Child Health and Human Development, Bethesda, Md)
Am J Epidemiol 144:1028–1033, 1996   19–3

Objective.—Although smoking is the causative agent in approximately 30% of cancer deaths in the United States, the role of prenatal smoking in the development of childhood cancers has not been examined. A fourth prospective study on the relation between maternal smoking and childhood cancer was reviewed.

Methods.—There were 54,795 children of 44,621 mothers enrolled in the Collaborative Perinatal Project between 1959 and 1966 who were followed up for 7 or 8 years. Smoking status was reported by the mothers. The incidence of childhood cancers was determined and a survival analysis was done.

Results.—There were 51 children with a diagnosis of cancer, for a lifetime probability of 1.1 per 1,000. Leukemia was the most common cancer found. The cumulative incidence of cancer for children of mothers who were smokers was 0.9 per 1,000 at 96 months. The cumulative incidence of cancer for children of mothers who did not smoke was 1.4 per 1,000.

Conclusion.—Children of women who smoked had no increased risk of cancer during the first 8 years.

▶ Little need be added to these straightforward findings. The length of follow-up and the care with which the cohort was followed up add to the believability of the result. This is a usefully reassuring negative finding.

A.O. Berg, M.D., M.P.H.

Recommendations for Follow-up Care of Individuals With an Inherited Predisposition to Cancer: I. Hereditary Nonpolyposis Colon Cancer
Burke W, for the Cancer Genetics Studies Consortium (Univ of Washington, Seattle; Johns Hopkins Univ, Baltimore, Md; Univ of Texas, Houston; et al)
JAMA 277:915–919, 1997   19–4

Introduction.—Many individuals who are genetically susceptible to hereditary nonpolyposis colorectal cancer can now be identified by genetic testing and need appropriate counseling about cancer surveillance and follow-up options. A task force of experts in medical genetics, oncology, primary care, gastroenterology, and epidemiology was convened by the Cancer Genetics Studies Consortium, organized by the National Human Genome Research Institute. A search of MEDLINE was conducted, and studies of evaluation of cancer risk, surveillance and risk reduction in individuals genetically susceptible to colon cancer were identified. Recommendations were developed during a 14-month period.

Recommendations.—The efficacy of cancer surveillance to lower the risk of cancer in genetically susceptible individuals is unknown. It is recommended that individuals with hereditary nonpolyposis colorectal cancer-associated mutations have a colonoscopy every 1 to 3 years, beginning at age 25 years. Screening for endometrial cancer also is recommended. No recommendations were made regarding prophylactic surgery because of a lack of evidence of clinical benefit. Individuals interested in genetic testing should be advised that the effectiveness of risk reduction measures is unknown. Whenever possible, individuals with cancer-predisposing mutations should receive care within the context of research designed to measure clinical outcome.

Discussion.—Early screening for cancer may reduce access to health insurance and compromise long-term health care. These recommendations are preliminary and controversial, and they do not apply to most individuals with a family history of colon cancer because such families do not have the characteristics of an autosomal dominant inheritance of cancer predisposition. Members of such families have a significantly lower risk of cancer than individuals with hereditary nonpolyposis colorectal cancer-associated mutations.

▶ One of the frustrations in working on the U.S. Preventive Services Task Force was the number of times we ended up with a "C" recommendation, indicating that there was insufficient evidence to recommend for or against providing the intervention. This is especially problematic in groups at higher than average risk. This article is a well-structured attempt to make recommendations in the absence of clear scientific evidence, although the methods used to arrive at the conclusion only partially followed the most rigorous evidence-based standards. For the patient with a familial history of colon cancer (fortunately uncommon), this article represents the state of the art.
                                                            A.O. Berg, M.D., M.P.H.

20 Miscellaneous Clinical Issues

Introduction

This chapter opens with 4 articles giving an overview of the "quality-of-life" debate in measuring outcomes. Two studies follow on end-of-life decisions, with an especially poignant study of physician-assisted suicide in the context of AIDS. The final section contains two articles on alternative medicine, one showing high prevalence of use, and the second reporting a rare randomized trial of treatment (with negative results).

Randomized controlled trial: Abstract 20–8.

Alfred O. Berg, M.D., M.P.H.

Quality of Life and Functional Status

The Problem of Quality of Life in Medicine
Leplège A, Hunt S (Hôpital de Bicêtre, France; Univ of Edinburgh, Scotland)
JAMA 278:47–50, 1997   20–1

Objective.—The concept of quality of life in medicine is subject to a variety of interpretations. Whether the patient's perceptions can be taken into account during evaluations is being debated. A clear conceptual model has not been developed to measure quality of life.

Some Confusions in the Field of Health Status and Quality-of-Life (QOL) Measurement.—Health-related QOL measures fail to consider the interrelatedness of health status and other aspects of life. The limits of the medical model are related to the assumptions that emphasis should be placed on function, which can be broken down into components, and that everyone aspires to an optimum level of functioning. The economic model fails because of the quality-adjusted life years (QALYs) concept that compares different medical interventions and their incremental health improvements for the purpose of formulating health policies. There is debate on the value of including patients' perspectives. In some cases, patient and physician judgments are at odds. Some studies have shown that patients' judgments are highly predictive of outcome. Currently most questionnaires call for patients to address physicians' or policy makers' concerns. Disease processes are not cross-cultural issues, but QOL concerns are.

Cultural factors that influence patient preferences and behaviors are not normally considered as QOL measures.

An Existential Approach.—Measuring QOL status should be individualized. Insight into an individual's preferences and values promotes the emotional and social well-being of the patient as well as the physical well-being. This approach draws attention to the fact that preferences change over a person's life.

Conclusion.—The confusion between health status and QOL underscores the difficulty of trying to develop a single QOL concept. Both medical and economic models fail to describe all aspects of QOL that are important to the patient. Existing health measures need to be combined with individual patient preferences and values in particular circumstances.

▶ "Outcomes research" and "quality of life" are buzzwords one sees everywhere nowadays, as physicians, managed care organizations, and insurers attempt to quantify what it is exactly that medical care accomplishes. This article is required reading for those, like myself, who have been troubled by the vagueness and subjectivity of "quality of life" as currently understood and practiced. This author effectively challenges current received wisdom on the subject, including the central thesis of advocates that physical, emotional, and social well being are its principal components. I share the author's concern of whether quality of life properly belongs in the domains of medical care and health economics at all. He proposes, instead, that perhaps medicine's task should be to optimize those conditions under which a reasonable quality of life might be attainable. This would have the effect of promoting a focus on measurable health outcomes, which I applaud. I also share the authors' concern, however, that more focus on objective health outcomes do not entirely divert attention from patient-centered factors so long ignored by the medical profession.

A.O. Berg, M.D., M.P.H.

Characterizing Quality of Life Among Patients With Chronic Mental Illness: A Critical Examination of the Self-report Methodology

Atkinson M, Zibin S, Chuang H (Univ of Calgary, Alta, Canada)
Am J Psychiatry 154:99–105, 1997   20–2

Purpose.—It is very difficult to demonstrate the effectiveness of treatment programs in psychiatry, as in other specialties dealing with the chronically ill. Such evaluations are made more difficult by the recent emphasis on the use of functional measures, disease-specific outcome indicators, and quality-of-life measures. The quality of life among 3 groups of patients with chronic mental illnesses was examined, and compared self-report and objective measures of quality of life in those groups were compared.

Methods.—Three groups of patients with chronic mental illness were studied: 69 patients with schizophrenia, 37 with bipolar disorder, and 35 with major depression. All were assessed on the Quality of Life Index, which examines health and functioning, socioeconomic factors, psychological and spiritual wellness, and family life. The quality of life of the 3 groups of patients were compared. The results on the Quality of Life Index were compared with other "objective" indicators of life quality, such as medical history, health risk behavior, education and finances, and indicators of social involvement.

Results.—Scores on all domains of the Quality of Life Index were significantly lower for the patients with bipolar disorder and depression than for those with schizophrenia. For the patients with schizophrenia, scores were similar to those of a reference group of patients with chronic physical illness (hemodialysis patients). However, on examination of the objective indicators, the lives of the patients with schizophrenia appeared to be more severely affected than the patients with affective disorders.

Conclusions.—The findings question the use of self-report, quality-of-life measures in patients with chronic mental illness. These measures are likely to be affected by biases related to cognition, periodic affective swings, and recent life events. The findings have important implications for outcome studies in the mental health field. With the development of instruments that are sensitive to change during the course of illness, more attention will be needed to the manner and timing of outcome measurements.

▶ I include this study because it illustrates a problem in the "patient outcome" movement when the outcome is self-reported. These researchers demonstrate the difficulty in correlating self-report with objective measures. Without objective measures, clinicians are entirely at the mercy of the patient in determining whether an intervention is working. Is an objective benefit worth the same regardless of whether one patient reports great improvement and another patient no improvement at all? My view is that we certainly need more studies of patient-oriented outcome, but that too great a focus on patient self-reported outcomes such as quality of life, satisfaction, or happiness could lead us into a scientific swamp. We need to make sure that some objective measures are available to validate the subjective reports.

A.O. Berg, M.D., M.P.H.

Taking Health Status Into Account When Setting Capitation Rates: A Comparison of Risk-adjustment Methods
Fowles JB, Weiner JP, Knutson D, et al (HealthSystem Minnesota, Minneapolis; Johns Hopkins Univ, Baltimore, Md)
JAMA 276:1316–1321, 1996   20–3

Background.—Because health care financing is shifting to a capitation system, physicians are assuming the financial risk that the negotiated lump sum capitation payment will not cover the cost of care. Unless per capita payments are adjusted for health status, physicians with sicker patients will be at a financial disadvantage. The relative strengths and weaknesses of 3 risk-adjusted strategies contrasted with standard demographic adjustment were evaluated.

Methods.—A cross-sectional health status study included results from a mailed 1992 survey and administrative claims data for 3,825 individuals, aged 18–64 years, and 1,955 individuals, aged 65 years or older, enrolled in a network-model HMO in Minnesota. Patient expenditures for survey 1 were analyzed retrospectively and expenditures for the year after the survey were analyzed prospectively. The predictive performance of self-reported functional health status, self-reported chronic diseases, and clinical diagnoses were assessed and compared.

Results.—The demographic model predicted approximately 6% of the prospective results. When chronic disease information was added, the predictive power increased to 11%. Claims-based information increased the predictive power to 12%. The predictive performance of the retrospective model was better than that of the prospective model, increasing the power to 43%. When simulated enrollees were stratified into low-, average-, and high-risk categories, the demographic model predicted rates 7.9% greater than the expenditures of the low-risk group, average predicted expenditures were 8% higher than actual, and the expenditures of the high-risk group were 5.2% lower than actual. According to the demographic model, only 20% of low-risk groups had predicted rates within 5% of actual expenditures. Similar results were seen in the elderly group, although the demographic model tended to perform less well in this age group than in the younger adult group.

Conclusion.—The demographic model predicted higher than actual expenses for the low-risk group and lower than actual expenses for the high-risk group. A risk-adjusted model based on diagnostic information improves predictive performance. Failing that, the use of self-reported measures improves the accuracy of capitation rates.

▶ The variation of disease severity among patients is so great that generalizing about a panel of patients for individual physicians or a small group is inappropriate in setting capitation rates. Inappropriate measures of productivity and compensation will occur unless risk adjustment methods are used. This team of authors reflects the state of the art of risk adjustment methods and reveals that complex functional status measures are not better at this time than self-reported measures of chronic conditions.

J.E. Scherger, M.D., M.P.H.

Health and Functional Status of Long-term Survivors of Bone Marrow Transplantation

Kolb H-J, for the EBMT Working Party on Late Effects and EULEP Study Group on Late Effects (Lawrence Berkeley Natl Lab, Berkeley, Calif)
Ann Intern Med 126:184–192, 1997   20–4

Introduction.—There is relatively little information on the health and functional status of patients who have survived longer than 5 years after bone marrow transplantation for life-threatening hematologic diseases. A retrospective multicenter study reviewed 798 recipients of bone marrow transplants for long-term mortality and performance status.

Methods.—Data were gathered from centers collaborating in the European Group for Blood and Marrow Transplantation. The 798 consecutive transplant recipients, reported from 43 centers in 13 countries, had received the graft before 1986 and had survived at least 5 years. Included in the group were 447 adults and 321 children younger than 18 years. The most common diagnoses were acute myelogenous leukemia (272 cases) and acute lymphoblastic leukemia (208 cases). Most patients (80%) had received total-body radiation and either methotrexate or cyclosporine for prophylaxis of graft-vs.-host disease. Outcomes assessed were survival, clinical performance according to Karnofsky score, and social reintegration.

Results.—The median duration of observation was 8.4 years. Fifty-five patients died more than 5 years after bone marrow transplantation, including 21 who died of recurrent disease and 8 of a secondary cancer. The most important risk factor for survival after more than 5 years is recurrence of leukemia and lymphoma. Other factors statistically significantly associated with late mortality were extended chronic graft-versus-host disease, development of a secondary cancer, female sex of the donor, male sex of the patient, and use of methotrexate. The Karnofsky score was normal or minimally reduced in 93% of patients, indicating a generally high level of clinical status; 89% of patients had returned to full-time work or school. Poorer status was associated with chronic graft-versus-host disease, recurrent leukemia, AIDS, secondary cancer, organ dysfunction, and neurologic or psychological problems. Female sex and older age at transplantation were risk factors for incomplete resumption of social activities.

Conclusions.—Among these long-term (more than 5 years) survivors of bone marrow transplantation, 93% were in good health and 88% had returned to school or work. There remains, however, an increased risk for illness and death, particularly from late recurrence of malignant disease.

▶ These data are a striking reminder of how quickly experimental and risky therapy can become routine and safe. The important caveat here is that the patients were preselected to include only those who survived the first 5 years, and the authors do not disclose the proportion who made it to that important milestone. Still, the excellent function among long-term survivors is quite impressive.

A.O. Berg, M.D., M.P.H.

End-of-Life Issues

Patient Preferences for Communication With Physicians About End-of-Life Decisions
Hofmann JC, for the SUPPORT Investigators (Harvard Med School, Boston; et al)
Ann Intern Med 127:1–12, 1997   20–5

Objective.—The majority of patients and physicians surveyed say they want to discuss end-of-life decisions, but less than 50% of patients have done so. There is no correlation between substituted judgments of physicians or family members and the patients' wishes. To understand the factors influencing patients' end-of-life decisions, barriers to patient-physician communication were identified in a prospective cohort study.

Methods.—The study surveyed characteristics of 1,832 seriously ill patients in 5 tertiary care hospitals and noted their preferences for end-of-life care, perceptions of prognosis, decision-making, quality of life (QOL), and communication with physicians about end-of-life decisions.

Results.—Only 23% of 1,589 responding patients had discussed their cardiopulmonary resuscitation preferences with their physicians. Patients who had discussed preferences with physicians were almost twice as likely to have an advanced directive. Of those who had not discussed preferences, 42% said they wanted to, and 58% said they did not want to. Seventy percent of respondents wanted to be resuscitated, and 30% did not. A quarter of those who did not discuss preferences did not want to be resuscitated. Multivariate analysis showed that factors associated with non-black patients who discussed preferences about resuscitation included not wanting to be resuscitated (adjusted odds ratio [OR], 2.15), having an advanced directive (OR, 2.24), wanting active involvement in medical decisions (OR, 1.48), anticipating a poor prognosis (OR, 1.90), having more limitations in activities of daily living (OR, 1.12), living alone (OR, 1.47), having an income of $11,000 to $25,000 a year (OR, 1.41), and having comorbid conditions (OR, 1.12 per condition). Factors associated with not wanting to discuss preferences included being non-black (OR, 1.48), not having an advanced directive (OR, 1.35), anticipating an excellent prognosis (OR, 1.72), having a fair to excellent QOL (OR, 1.36), and not wanting to be involved in medical decisions (OR, 1.33). Factors associated with wanting to discuss preferences but not doing so were being black (OR, 1.53) and being younger (OR, 1.14 for every decade).

Conclusion.—Most seriously ill hospitalized patients do not discuss resuscitation preferences with their physicians, mainly because they do not want to. Patients who do not discuss preferences, for whatever reason, will probably have interventions that they do not want.

▶ The more I read about end-of-life decisions, the less sure I am that I know what I am doing. Here we have pretty good evidence that patients are independent thinkers on when and how they want end-of-life issues to be addressed. In other words, one cannot assume that certain circumstances or characteristics will make patients more or less willing to talk. I suppose the best advice under these circumstances, as always, is to raise the subject in a supportive and non-threatening way, avoid the times of greatest vulnerability, and let the patient's response guide further discussion and intervention (i.e., use common sense).

A.O. Berg, M.D., M.P.H.

Physician-assisted Suicide and Patients With Human Immunodeficiency Virus Disease
Slome LR, Mitchell TF, Charlebois E, et al (San Francisco; Univ of California, San Francisco; San Francisco Gen Hosp)
N Engl J Med 336:417–421, 1997   20–6

Introduction.—Physician members of the Community Consortium, an association of providers of health care to patients infected with HIV in the San Francisco Bay area, were surveyed about their views on physician-assisted suicide and the frequency with which they actually provided lethal doses of medications to patients with AIDS. Findings were compared with those of a similar survey conducted in 1990.

Methods.—The anonymous, self-administered questionnaire was given to all 228 physician members of the Community Consortium. Included in the survey were sections on demographic characteristics, professional and personal experience with AIDS, beliefs and attitudes regarding physician-assisted suicide, and actual participation in assisted suicide. A case vignette was described, in which a gay man, age 30 years, has requested a prescription for a lethal dose of narcotics. The patient has severe wasting syndrome, is not responding to treatment, and appears to be mentally competent. Physicians were asked what course of action they would take if this patient were determined to obtain assistance in committing suicide.

Results.—Responses were received from 137 (60%) physicians; 19 were no longer in clinical practice and their returns were not analyzed. Compared with respondents to the 1990 survey, physicians completing the 1995 survey were more racially diverse, more likely to be heterosexual, and more likely to have treated a relatively high number of patients with AIDS. Respondents had received a mean of 7.9 direct and 13.7 indirect requests from patients for assistance; 53% said they had granted a request for assistance at least once (mean, 4.2 times). Responding to the case vignette, 48% of physicians said they would be likely or very likely to grant the patient's request for a prescription for a lethal dose of narcotics. Only 28% of respondents to the 1990 survey would have complied with such a request.

Conclusions.—Physicians who regularly care for patients with HIV disease showed a greater acceptance of assisted suicide in 1995 than when surveyed in 1990. Four factors were positively associated with a physician's actual participation in a suicide: having a higher intention-to-assist score (from responses to the case vignette); having a higher number of patients with AIDS who had died; having received a higher number of indirect requests from patients for assistance; and gay, lesbian, or bisexual orientation on the part of the physician.

▶ These are astonishing findings showing that there are substantial "pockets" of physicians who do not follow the party line of most professional groups that stand resolutely against euthanasia and physician-assisted suicide. A recent article from the Netherlands shows that about one quarter of family physicians there assist in suicide or euthanasia at least once in an average year.[1]

The debate rages because the question is rather like the abortion issue: is there a moral absolute, or does it all depend? Is this an issue to be decided by majority vote, by a Supreme Court judgment, or through religious enlightenment? This YEAR BOOK will not answer the question. It is clear, though, that the increasingly visible and vocal minority of physicians who are sympathetic to physician-assisted suicide and euthanasia will leave no place to hide for the current majority who are uncertain, ambivalent, or quietly opposed. The openness of the debate will force more physicians to examine their own views closely, and be prepared to defend them in discussions with colleagues and patients. As with the abortion issue, family physicians will not be allowed to sit quietly on the sidelines.

A.O. Berg, M.D., M.P.H.

Reference

1. Verhoef MJ, van der Wal G: Euthanasia in family practice in the Netherlands. *Can Fam Phys* 43:231–237, 1997.

Alternative Medicine

Use of Alternative Therapies: Estimates From the 1994 Robert Wood Johnson Foundation National Access to Care Survey
Paramore LC (HOPE Ctr for Health Affairs, Bethesda, Md)
J Pain Symptom Manage 13:83–89, 1997   20–7

Background.—The growth of interest in alternative therapies is reflected in the findings of several recent studies that the number of visits to providers of alternative medicine in the United States now exceeds the number of visits to all primary care physicians. Data from the 1994 Robert Wood Johnson Foundation National Access to Care Study (Access Survey) were used to update estimates of the use of alternative therapies among the U.S. population and various population subgroups.

Methods.—Results reported are from the Access Survey's national probability sample of respondents, which consisted of 3,450 individuals and had a response rate of 75%. Included in the general information section of the Access Survey was a series of questions relating to 4 alternative therapies: chiropractic, relaxation techniques, therapeutic massage, and acupuncture. The percentage of those seeing a professional for alternative therapies was estimated for the U.S. population as a whole and for selected subgroups. Other areas of interest included socioeconomic factors such as family income and insurance coverage.

Results.—Nearly 10% of the U.S. population, or almost 25 million individuals, saw a professional for at least 1 of the 4 alternative therapies. The number seeking these therapies was greatest by far for chiropractic (17.6 million), followed by therapeutic massage (8.0 million), relaxation techniques (3.4 million), and acupuncture (1.0 million). Individuals most likely to seek alternative medical treatments were white adults aged 19 to 64 years who had one or more medical conditions. Use of alternative therapies was most extensive in the West and least frequent in the South. Individuals with some post–high school education reported higher use of relaxation techniques and acupuncture; those with less education had more visits to chiropractors. Users and nonusers of alternative therapies did not differ in terms of sex, marital status, or employment status. Those who sought alternative therapies made twice as many visits to traditional medical providers as did nonusers.

Conclusions.—Various forms of alternative medicine are being used by millions of Americans of all ages. Most users seek these therapies for a specific problem such as pain, anxiety, or stress. The higher level of use of chiropractic, compared with other alternative therapies, is probably influenced by insurance coverage. Alternative therapies may have a larger role in a health care system less controlled by the medical establishment.

▶ In the state of Washington we are working with a new law that requires insurance carriers to cover alternative therapies. It's been an interesting ride, forcing those of us in conventional medicine to become realistic about the public demand for more therapeutic options. This well-conducted survey shows that alternative therapies are popular, although the numbers would likely be even higher if the investigators surveyed use of more than the four therapies named (chiropractic, acupuncture, massage, and relaxation are hardly on the "fringe" anymore). The debate between conventional and alternative therapies is increasingly being engaged around which provides better customer service and patient satisfaction. Although these outcomes are undeniably important, they are not necessarily correlated with scientific improvements in physical or mental health. I believe we must develop objective standards of health against which all therapies are measured, conventional and otherwise.

A.O. Berg, M.D., M.P.H.

Homoeopathic Versus Placebo Therapy of Children With Warts on the Hands: A Randomized, Double-blind Clinical Trial
Kainz JT, Kozel G, Haidvogl M, et al (Univ of Graz, Austria; Ludwig-Boltzmann-Institut für Homöopathie, Graz, Austria)
Dermatology 193:318–320, 1996   20–8

Background.—Homeopathy is a system of therapy in which a drug is selected for treatment if it induces symptoms in healthy persons similar to those of the disease to be treated. The agent is made more potent and given in small amounts to the patient. Such treatments have become increasingly popular in recent years. However, scientific proof of its efficacy and mechanisms of action are still lacking. The efficacy of homeopathic therapy was determined in a prospective, double-blind, randomized trial.

Methods.—Sixty children, age 6 to 12 years, were enrolled. All had common warts on the back of the hand. In 30 children, the warts were treated with an individually selected homeopathic preparation of at least a 1:1012 dilution. The other 30 were treated with placebo. The area of the warts was measured before and 8 weeks after treatment by computerized planimetry.

Findings.—Nine children given homeopathic treatment and 7 given placebo responded. A complete cure was documented in 5 patients in the active treatment group and in 1 in the placebo group.

Conclusions.—In these children with common warts, there was no apparent difference in the efficacy of homeopathic preparations and placebos. However, the study design was restricted and did not allow for changes in prescription or the potency of the medication prescribed, as homeopathic physicians would tend to do in practice.

▶ The treatment of warts continues to be a mystery. In many patients warts seem to linger indefinitely; in others they seem to magically disappear. Very often, folk remedies and standard medical treatments are done just before their disappearance. It has been customary to credit the therapies, but trials such as this suggest that there must be a strong placebo (belief) effect on the elimination of warts. My personal opinion is that homeopathy is based in general on strong placebo therapy. This trial supports that homeopathy is effective, but so is placebo.

J.E. Scherger, M.D., M.P.H.

21 Health Policy and Economics

Introduction

This substantial chapter covers many highly topical areas. The 2 opening articles provide a strong defense for the benefits of continuity of care. The section on office strategies outline several useful interventions, including how to deal with walk-in patients, use of the telephone, automated voice messaging, and dealing with the effects of the Clinical Laboratories Improvement Act. Dilemmas in managing patients with chronic conditions are dealt with in the next two articles, followed by a selection of articles presenting a variety of perspectives on large-scale economics, ranging from downsizing the workforce through dealing with uninsured populations. The next section on cost reduction presents two studies on efficient use of radiology consultation and a study of routine presurgical laboratory testing. The concluding section focuses on adverse events and malpractice with further data on the importance of disability (as opposed to actual negligence) and the importance of good physician-patient communication in preventing malpractice claims.

Randomized controlled trial: Abstract 21–17.

Alfred O. Berg, M.D., M.P.H.

Continuity of Care

The Impact of Insurance Type and Forced Discontinuity on the Delivery of Primary Care

Flocke SA, Stange KC, Zyzanski SJ (Case Western Reserve Univ, Cleveland, Ohio)

J Fam Pract 45:129–135, 1997   21–1

Background.—Managed care is coming to dominate the U.S. health care system. Such plans claim primary care as their cornerstone, but effects of managed care on provision of primary care are poorly understood. Annual bidding on managed care contracts may enforce discontinuity of care, with potentially adverse effects. Effects of insurance type on the quality of primary care were studied.

Methods.—In a cross-sectional study, 1,839 patient visits to 138 community-based primary care physicians were studied. A patient questionnaire on physician knowledge of the patient, interpersonal communication, care coordination and continuity, and patients' preference for their regular physician was used to measure primary care quality.

Results.—No significant differences were found between managed care and fee-for-service insurance in any of the 5 indicators. Patients with a forced provider change scored their care significantly lower on all 5 indicators ($P < 0.01$).

Conclusions.—Primary care is the foundation of health care and a generally effective means of providing quality care cost-effectively. It is important in managed care systems. Managed competition incentives are largely economic, and competition on price means that the least expensive plan may change from year to year. Quality appears to depend on continuity of the patient-physician relationship, rather than on specific payment system. Annual bidding on health insurance contracts results in transfer of patients from plan to plan in employers' searches for bargains, disregarding the value of established care relationships. Purchasing and marketing policies should be modified to nurture continuity of primary care rather than impede it. Only thus will primary care's benefits to managed care systems be realized.

▶ This article is important not only because it raises a serious concern about managed care, but also because it reinforces the importance of continuity in the doctor-patient relationship. Hopefully, the frequent changing of primary care physicians is a temporary part of the changing medical marketplace. People in the U.S. move frequently, usually necessitating a change in physicians. It is unfortunate that changing insurance plans causes even greater flux. There is value in the knowledge and experience between patient and personal physician which has been poorly measured. Studies of this type, along with patient discontent, will hopefully cause a renewal in the longer term doctor-patient relationship.

J.E. Scherger, M.D., M.P.H.

Faithful Patients: The Effect of Long-term Physician-Patient Relationships on the Costs and Use of Health Care by Older Americans

Weiss LJ, Blustein J (Columbia College of Physicians and Surgeons, New York)
Am J Public Health 86:1742–1747, 1996

21–2

Objective.—The duration of the physician-patient relationship is believed to have a positive effect on patient well-being and costs, although these positive effects have not been quantitated. With the advent of managed care, many of these relationships have been severed. One survey found that 41% of patients switched physicians when joining an HMO. From publicly available data, the benefits of long-standing physician-patient Medicare fee-for-service relationships were quantitated.

Methods.—Enrollees from 107 sampling units in the United States Medicare program were surveyed. The response rate was 83.3%, or 12,677 patients, of whom 8,068 with specific physician ties were included. Data recorded included provider, duration of tie, health care use, healthy behaviors, cost of care, and sociodemographic and health status measurements. The magnitude and variability effects of the duration of the relationship on each outcome were subjected to multivariate analysis.

Results.—Approximately 55% of the respondents had had relationships of 5 or more years with their physicians, and about 35% had had relationships lasting 10 years or longer. The duration of physician–patient relationships was associated with the receipt of an influenza vaccine the previous winter, hospitalization, Medicare Part A reimbursement, the number of office visits, and Medicare Part B reimbursement. The usual source of care was listed as the physician's office by 78.7% of patients. Of the 251 patients who had been seeing their physician for less than 1 year, 81.1% said they had been seeing another physician previously. Most said they changed because of changes affecting accessibility.

Conclusion.—Relatively healthy older Americans in fee-for-service organizations did not tend to change physicians more frequently. Limitations of this study included that individuals were free to switch providers at any time and the lack of ability to quantify many of the benefits of a long-term physician–patient relationship. Lasting physician–patient relationships are important, even in this era of managed care.

▶ Managed care in the new delivery systems is causing questioning of the value of the physician–patient relationship. Patients are changing health plans and physicians frequently. What impact does this have on the cost of care? How important are long-term physician–patient relationships? This important study addresses 1 part of these questions. Evidence that seniors have a decreased likelihood of hospitalization and lower health care costs as a result of a longer-term physician–patient relationship will, hopefully, influence the design of new delivery systems and avoid frequent disruption of the physician–patient relationship.

J.E. Scherger, M.D., M.P.H.

Office Management Strategies

Meeting Walk-in Patients' Expectations for Testing: Effects on Satisfaction
Froehlich GW, Welch HG (Veterans Affairs Med Ctr, White River Junction, Vt; Dartmouth Med School, Hanover, NH)
J Gen Intern Med 11:470–474, 1996   21–3

Purpose.—Patients often expect to undergo tests during outpatient visits, and physicians may believe that meeting those expectations plays an important role in patient satisfaction. Compared with patients receiving continuity care, those attending walk-in clinics express less satisfaction with care and have more specific expectations. The link between expectations for testing and patient satisfaction was assessed in patients attending a walk-in clinic.

Methods.—The study included 128 patients attending a walk-in medical clinic at a Veterans Affairs medical center. Before the visit, the patients were asked to complete a questionnaire that assessed baseline satisfaction with care and expectations for common tests. Another questionnaire was given after the visit to measure satisfaction with that visit, perceptions of the provider's interpersonal behavior (or "humanism"), and specific tests performed. The effects of met expectations for testing were determined by logistic regression.

Results.—Sixty-two percent of patients expected to undergo some kind of test, almost as many as expected to receive a medication (63%) or to discuss diagnosis or prognosis (70%). According to multivariate analysis of only patients expecting tests, the only predictor of satisfaction at the study visit was provider "humanism." The odds ratio for this predictor was 6.4. No significant association was seen between the proportion of met expectations for testing and patient satisfaction.

Conclusions.—Patient satisfaction at a walk-in clinic does not appear to depend heavily on meeting patients' expectations for testing. Patient perceptions of the physician's interpersonal behavior is a far more important predictor of satisfaction. Thus, ordering tests to meet patient expectations will result in unnecessary testing with no improvement in patient satisfaction.

▶ What a relief! Not testing patients (albeit maybe only male veterans) who expect tests does not affect satisfaction. Actually, this is not counterintuitive; I suspect it is only a few patients who become dissatisfied about the lack of tests. Once again, it is not what the physician knows or what tests are ordered but the personal interaction that counts the most.

M.A. Bowman, M.D., M.P.A.

An Analysis of the Use of the Telephone in the Management of Patients in Skilled Nursing Facilities

Fowkes W, Christenson D, McKay D (Stanford Univ, San Jose, Calif; San Jose Hosp, Calif)
J Am Geriatr Soc 45:67–70, 1997   21–4

Introduction.—Most physician-directed medical care for patients in skilled nursing facilities (SNFs) is provided by telephone communication because of low reimbursement schedules for nursing home visits, time pressures, and practice priorities. Second to poor reimbursement, problems with communication are a great source of frustration for physicians caring for patients in SNFs. The effect of a voice mail system installed to manage the burden of communication between physicians and SNFs was evaluated.

TABLE 1.—Facilities and Calls

Facility	Average Census (%)*	Number of Calls (%)†	Calls/Patient‡
1.	53 (25)	2682 (26)	50.6
2.	38 (18)	1591 (16)	41.9
3.	37 (18)	1169 (11)	31.6
4.	30 (15)	1954 (18)	65.1
5.	11 (5)	759 (7)	69.0
6.	11 (5)	762 (7)	69.3
Total	108 (100%)	8917 (100%)	Average 49.5

Note: Facilities with 10 or more covered patients.

*Average number of patients covered at the facility with the percent of the total to the nearest percentage point.

†Total number of telephone calls received from the facility during a 12-month period, with the percentage of the total to the nearest percentage point.

‡Calls for each facility divided by its average census. The difference in rates between 6 facilities is significant at P 0.001 by chi-square.

(Courtesy of Fowkes W, Christenson D, McKay D: An analysis of the use of the telephone in the management of patients in skilled nursing facilities. *J Am Geriatr Soc* 45:67–70, 1997.)

Methods.—Calls between physicians and SNFs using a standard answering service were evaluated for 1 year. A voice mail system then was installed and patients and staff in SNFs were encouraged to use voice mail rather than the answering service. Medical care providers, the staffs of 13 SNFs, and an average of 207 covered patients were followed up for 1 year. The total number of calls by patients and facilities, reasons for calls, outcome, and timing were evaluated. Comparisons were made between the standard answering service and voice mail.

Results.—The patients and staff of 13 SNFs made a total of 10,264 calls regarding an average of 207 continuously covered patients receiving long-term care. This averaged about 50 calls per year per patient. Most calls were routine; only about 5% of calls were concerning acute illness. A new treatment was started for about one third of calls, but no new orders were issued in response to 23% of calls. About 1 in 200 calls resulted in hospitalization. About 1 in 5 calls did not require a return call. Some facilities had significantly higher numbers of calls per patient per month, reflecting either a higher level of care provided or less frequent contact with providers on site (Table 1). A recent follow-up indicated that of 692 calls received in 1 month, 93% were received through voice mail.

Conclusions.—Communication between SNFs and physicians is driven by patient need and the Omnibus Reconciliation Act of 1987, which requires that any significant condition change be reported to the resident's physician. The voice mail system described can help relieve some of the significant communication burden of caring for patients in SNFs.

► I think we all know that nursing home patients generate a lot of telephone calls, but this puts objective numbers to our feelings of burden—nearly 50 calls per patient per year, many based on regulatory requirements. At 2¼ minutes apiece, this is 112 minutes a year. The only good news was that most occurred during the day. Using voice mail, about one fifth did not even need to be returned (but someone probably had to pull a chart to record the call). This may not be fully generalizable because the study was done in California and no standing orders were permitted by law. My bottom line: state and federal governments should reduce the regulatory burden and/or pay for telephone calls!

M.A. Bowman, M.D., M.P.A.

The Feasibility of Automated Voice Messaging as an Adjunct to Diabetes Outpatient Care

Piette JD, Mah CA (Veterans Affairs Palo Alto Health Care System, Calif)
Diabetes Care 20:15–21, 1997
21–5

Background.—The treatment of many diabetic patients continues to fall short of recommended standards of care. The value of automated voice messaging (AVM) systems as an adjunct to primary care for diabetic patients was investigated.

Methods.—Sixty-five diabetic patients were included. An AVM monitoring protocol was developed to inquire about patients' symptoms, glucose monitoring, foot care, diet, and medication adherence. The system used included specialized computer technology to telephone patients, communicate messages, and collect information.

Findings.—A total of 216 AVM calls were completed successfully; they averaged 3.3 or 4 calls per patient. A variety of problems were reported, signaling the need for follow-up. Many patients said they had not checked their blood glucose or feet. One in 4 patients reported problems with medication and diet adherence. The AVM reports were judged to be reliable and valid. Ninety-eight percent of all patients said that the calls were helpful, 98% reported that they had no difficulty responding to the calls, and 77% said that receiving AVM calls would increase their satisfaction with their health care.

Conclusion.—Diabetic patients respond to AVM queries and believe that such calls are helpful. This strategy is feasible for identifying health and self-care problems that would otherwise go unnoticed.

▶ The actual answers of diabetics to the questions posed through the AVM system are less interesting than the ability to make the system work and the high acceptance by the patients. I have not yet tried one of these systems, but I see great potential. These diabetic patients were often given prevention reminders included with the AVM. For example, instead of mailing cards to remind patients about immunizations, telephone reminders with patient responses could be used, thus identifying individuals who may have received flu shots elsewhere and did not need further follow-up. Between office visits, we could get more home-recorded blood sugar or peak flow information, thus encouraging patients to obtain such data, and also to determine whether action needs to be taken.

Unfortunately, the authors did not report on the cost, which I suspect is still higher than postage, particularly if telephone companies charge for local use. Also, this system requires patients to be able to understand the spoken message and reply to a series of queries with the correct digit entry, which will obviously exclude even some with touch-tone phones.

M.A. Bowman, M.D., M.P.A.

Should Doctors See Patients in Group Sessions?
Terry K
Med Economics 74:70–75, 1997   21–6

Introduction.—About 30 primary care doctors run group sessions for about 400 seniors at Kaiser Colorado, and other Kaiser divisions are experimenting with the idea. In group appointments, a doctor or nurse can take care of up to 25 patients in a 90-minute session. Patients have a better perspective on their disease process and situations because they see other people with similar or worse problems and they learn how others cope with their difficulties.

Patients' Perspective.—At Kaiser Colorado, some group members attend 1 or 2 meetings, whereas others come to about 8 of the 12 annual meetings. It works better when the patient's own doctor is running the session. Older patients receive much-needed social support. For patients, the biggest benefit is that these sessions bring people together. Patients learn from each other how to manage their own health better, and they receive valuable tips from one another. Group patients believe they are getting more attention from the doctor than those who make office visits because they spend more time with the doctor. Some patients believe they also gain in self-confidence.

Cutting Overutilization.—Kaiser has measured the impact of group sessions in controlled, randomized trials, which showed that seniors who attended groups made 1½ fewer visits to their primary care doctors than the control subjects. Among the group patients, there were also fewer nursing home admissions, hospitalizations, and emergency department visits. Little is known about cost savings, however, and it is still difficult to predict whether money will be saved in the long run.

Disadvantages.—Doctors who do not lead group sessions cite insufficient time allotted for care, inadequate patient education, excessive callbacks, redundancy of care, and inability to meet each patient's needs. There's still no proof that group patients have better outcomes and no hard evidence that group members manage their own conditions better than other patients.

▶ I will have to try this. Although I have been involved in group patient education, I have not tried group visits. It does not seem that these can replace all individual appointments, but I can see a potential value. The article emphasizes that it probably works best with individuals who have chronic illnesses and usually see the physician frequently, and that the group should be led by their personal physician. Although there seemed to be some benefits (fewer hospitalizations, nursing home admissions and emergency department visits), more study of cost-effectiveness is clearly needed.

M.A. Bowman, M.D., M.P.A.

What Do Patients Think About During Their Consultations: A Qualitative Study

Cromarty I (RAF Brampton, Cambridgeshire, England)
Br J Gen Pract 46:525–528, 1996   21–7

Introduction.—The consultation has been the object of considerable research, but most studies and consultation models focus on the physician's viewpoint. Eighteen patients took part in semistructured interviews designed to elicit information about the range and types of thoughts that patients have during their consultations.

Methods.—Study participants were drawn from a group of 121 patients of general practitioners who had agreed to have a video recording made of their consultation. Eighteen of 30 patients randomly selected from this group were willing to take part in unstructured interviews. The patients were asked for their recollections of the consultation in 3 stages: unprompted, prompted by video playback, and prompted by a transcript of the consultation. They were encouraged to comment freely throughout the interview. Interviews took place at a mean of 2.8 days after the consultation and lasted between 80 and 130 minutes. The interviews were then analyzed and data grouped around several dominant themes.

Results.—Although patients thought most about the problems that had led them to seek medical care, they also considered the available time and the behavior of the physician. Matters that the physician introduced were given less attention. The patients' primary goal was to gain understanding, information, and a solution. Professional ability of the physician was not doubted, and patients placed great value on long-term, open, and friendly relationships. All but 2 patients complained about shortage of time, but most were concerned about taking more than their fair share of the physician's time. In only half of the consultations did the physician appear to have an overt agenda. The main source of dissatisfaction was a failure of understanding.

Discussion.—In this white, middle-class study population, patients were found to have a central desire for understanding during their consultations. Even those who did not feel rushed also felt that their consultation time was too brief. Consultation models should be developed to include patient perspectives and to address the complexity of the event.

▶ This was a time-intensive and in-depth look at what patients are thinking about during a medical visit. Reading the comments made by patients indicates that they have a silent script running full-time, with a search for meaning at the center. The complexity of the interaction is striking: both patient and physician communicate with verbal and nonverbal cues, all the while with a parallel set of evaluative insights and perceptions going on silently in each participant.

These findings emphasize once again that the physician's view of what is going on during a visit is a poor predictor of the patient's perspective. Research like this also reassures that the physician-patient relationship can never be replaced by protocols, guidelines, or computer-assisted patient education. At the center of a visit to the physician is a fundamentally human relationship that transcends the objective facts describing it.

A.O. Berg, M.D., M.P.H.

Impact of CLIA on Physician Office Laboratories in Rural Washington State

Roussel PL (Tacoma Family Medicine, Washington)
J Fam Pract 43:249–254, 1996

21–8

Background.—Regulations implementing the Clinical Laboratory Improvements Act (CLIA) of 1988, published by the Health Care Financing Administration (HCFA) in 1992, imposed a licensing scheme on all clinical laboratories, including physician office laboratories (POLs). Many physicians worried that the regulations' costs and complexity would force many POLs to close or downsize, especially in rural areas, resulting in increased patient costs and decreased access to health care. The impact of CLIA on POLs in rural Washington state was studied.

Methods.—A survey eliciting data on tests done before and after the implementation of CLIA was mailed to all members of the rural practice section of the Washington Academy of Family Physicians. Usable responses were received from 76% of the 414 family physicians contacted.

Findings.—Significant changes in the complexity of laboratory tests done before and after implementation of CLIA were noted. Among the POLs of independent family physicians, waived-status laboratories, which perform only the simplest and lowest risk tests, increased from 1% to 34%; laboratories performing tests of moderate complexity decreased from 76% to 53%; and laboratories doing high-complexity tests declined from 23% to 13%. The shift to waived-status laboratories was more marked among solo and small-group physicians in smaller communities.

Conclusion.—In rural Washington, there has been a significant shift to waived-status laboratories from moderate- and high-complexity testing laboratories among POLs run by independent family physicians. The HCFA has seriously underestimated the effect of CLIA on rural POLs.

▶ Ah, just as we suspected. I just wish this had created more of a political brouhaha and that the HCFA had reversed itself. Our only hope seems to be that many of the tests are becoming simpler and simpler. If this simplicity is recognized by the HCFA, perhaps our repertoire can re-expand.

M.A. Bowman, M.D., M.P.A.

Care of the Chronically Ill

Persons With Chronic Conditions: Their Prevalence and Costs

Hoffman C, Rice D, Sung H-Y (Univ of California, San Francisco)
JAMA 276:1473–1479, 1996

21–9

Background.—Beginning in the 1920s, public health officials and statisticians noted that chronic illnesses were becoming more prevalent than infectious diseases in the United States. And although this trend has continued through the century, the nation's health care system is centered on episodic and acute care. Data from the 1987 National Medical Expenditure Survey (NMES) were used to determine the number and proportion of Americans living with chronic conditions and the direct and indirect costs associated with these conditions.

Methods.—Members of the NMES Household Survey database were 34,459 individuals who were representative of the civilian noninstitutionalized United States population in 1987. Survey respondents provided information about health conditions, including medical services and supplies used in 1987 and periods of disability. United States Census data for 1987 were used for estimation to the full population and total expenditures. Estimates of indirect costs were based on the 1990 National Health Interview Survey and *Vital Statistics of the United States.*

Results.—In 1987, 90 million Americans were living with at least 1 chronic condition; 39 million of these individuals had more than 1 chronic condition. Overall, more than 45% of noninstitutionalized Americans have 1 or more chronic conditions. The resulting direct costs account for 75% of health care expenditures in the United States. Total costs projected to 1990 for individuals with chronic conditions amounted to $659 billion, of which $425 billion were associated with direct health care costs and $234 billion with indirect costs. Direct care costs do not include the costs of institutionalized patients in nursing homes. The disproportionate health care expenditures for chronic conditions is consistent across all age groups. Deaths caused by chronic conditions in 1990 represented more than three fourths of all deaths in the United States that year.

Discussion.—The total prevalence of chronic conditions may be minimized because most reports are limited to individuals with disabilities resulting from such conditions. Although the majority of those with chronic conditions are not disabled, they are subject to recurrent exacerbations, the risk of long-term limitations, and increased direct and indirect health care costs. The health care delivery system needs to understand the magnitude of the problem of chronic illness and its associated costs.

▶ This article supplies hard numbers to support the general impression all physicians must feel that more and more of practice is devoted to care rather than cure. The size of the imbalance between acute and chronic care still surprises, though. There is not much of a new message here, only a reminder that as the population ages, improving patient function with a chronic condition will more and more dominate practice. The authors provide some provocative speculation on the implications of this for health care providers, policymakers, and managed care organizations.

A.O. Berg, M.D., M.P.H.

Differences in 4-Year Health Outcomes for Elderly and Poor, Chronically Ill Patients Treated in HMO and Fee-for-Service Systems
Ware JE Jr, Bayliss MS, Rogers WH, et al (New England Med Ctr, Boston; Tufts Univ, Boston; Harvard School of Public Health, Boston)
JAMA 276:1039–1047, 1996   21–10

Background.—Enrollment in HMOs has increased 10–fold since 1976, and government policies now seek to shift publicly insured patients to HMOs. The Medical Outcomes Study compared 4-year health outcomes for chronically ill patients treated in well-established HMOs and fee-for-service (FFS) plans serving the same medical marketplaces in Boston, Chicago, and Los Angeles. Only those with hypertension, non–insulin-dependent diabetes mellitus, recent acute myocardial infarction, congestive heart failure, and depressive disorder were monitored. This study focused on patients aged at least 65 years who were covered by Medicare and those near or below the poverty line.

Methods.—The study group consisted of 2,235 adult patients with 1 of the 5 index conditions who were sampled in 1986 and monitored through 1990. Medicare and low-income patients were analyzed separately. The 36-item Short-Form Health Survey was used to determine differences in physical and mental health over the 4-year study period.

Results.—Overall, physical health declined and mental health remained stable over the 4-year follow-up period of this study. These physical declines were significantly larger for the elderly than for the nonelderly in the study group. For the average patient, physical and mental health outcomes were not different between the HMO or FFS systems. For elderly Medicare patients, physical health declines were significantly more common in HMO than FFS plans. For patients near or below the poverty line, outcomes were more favorable in the FFS system than in HMOs.

Conclusions.—The Medical Outcomes Study observed adult patients treated in HMO and FFS systems for 4 years to determine changes in medical status. Although no difference in medical outcome between these two systems was noted for the average patient, health outcomes were worse in HMOs than in FFS systems for poor and elderly patients. These results indicate that vulnerable subgroups need to be separately monitored by health care plans to ensure that their needs are being adequately met.

▶ This was an extremely important and troubling study that since its publication has generated quite a debate. It is not difficult to pick the study apart methodologically because it was nonrandomized and only studied patients in

3 geographic areas, but expecting a randomized trial on this scale replicated in more localities is not a credible goal. Further, the findings resisted all attempts by the authors (and others) to make the findings disappear through the usual statistical sleight of hand. In short, the message to policymakers is *deal with it.* The authors' conclusions are modest enough and ethically the only ones that are defensible: carefully monitor the outcomes of vulnerable elderly and poor subgroups at risk in any system of care.

A.O. Berg, M.D., M.P.H.

System Economics

Downsizing the Physician Workforce

McClendon BJ, Politzer RM, Christian E, et al (Bureau of Health Professions, Health Resources and Services Administration, Rockville, Md)
Public Health Rep 112:231–239, 1997   21–11

Background.—An oversupply of physicians, and particularly specialists, is a contributing factor to rising health care costs. Several reports have suggested changes in the size and composition of the physician work force. However, the response to these recommendations has been slow. A Bureau of Health Professions study of the need for downsizing of the physician work force, with specialty-specific recommendations, is reported.

Methods.—The study was based on the conservative assumption that the 1993 physician-to-population rates would be maintained, with no further increases in any of the specialties. The growth in the supply of specialists needed to maintain these figures was calculated by adding losses from death and retirement to the increases needed to keep pace with population growth. These figures were compared with the number of new physicians currently being produced, as estimated from the average annual number of board certificates issued from 1990 to 1994. The necessary downsizing for a system increasingly dominated by managed care was then estimated, using several different sources of data.

Results.—The 1993 ratio of active physicians to population was 199.6 physicians per 100,000 individuals. The number of new physicians needed each year to maintain this ratio would be 14,644. However, the average number of new physicians certified during the 1990s was 20,655, which means there is an excess of more than 6,000 physicians per year. The 1993 ratio of active non–primary care physicians to the population was 132.2 per 100,000. The number of new non–primary care physicians needed per year to maintain this ratio would be 9,698. However, the average number of new non–primary care physicians produced per year was 14,527, which suggests the need for a 33% reduction.

The 1993 ratio of active primary care physicians was 66.8 per 100,000 individuals. A total of 4,946 new primary care physicians per year would be needed to maintain this ratio compared with an average of 6,128 new certifications per year. This suggested the need to produce about 1,200 fewer primary care physicians per year, which indicates a downsizing of 20%. The only specialties that did not need to be downsized were family practice, neurosurgery, otolaryngology, and urology. The study identified 17 hospital- and medical-based specialties, including 7 of the 10 internal medicine subspecialties, that were in need of downsizing by 40% or more. The need for downsizing was generally less in the surgical specialties and in psychiatry.

Conclusions.—The findings suggest the need for reductions in the numbers of new physicians produced in most specialties. The need for downsizing is particularly great among the internal medicine subspecialties and hospital support specialties, and is less so among surgeons and primary care physicians. With the expansion of managed care in the health care system, further reductions in the non–primary care specialties will probably be needed.

► Studies of physician requirements by specialty are always controversial. Concerns about an oversupply of some specialists have been expressed since 1980. This analysis uses 1993 as a benchmark and shows that many subspecialists are being overtrained. An increase in managed care will make this situation much worse. Regulatory policy regarding the training of physician specialties is seriously needed in the United States. Until recently, most physicians in training, regardless of specialty, assumed that there would be 1 or more positions available to them. The absence of jobs after long and hard years of training is a tragedy that we must try to avoid.

J.E. Scherger, M.D., M.P.H.

The Impact of Managed Care on the Physician Marketplace
Simon CJ, Dranove D, White WD (Univ of Illinois, Chicago; Northwestern Univ, Chicago)
Public Health Rep 112:222–230, 1997   21–12

Background.—The rise of managed care has major implications for the health care system and for public policies affecting the physician work force. One possible effect is to reduce the income of specialists and to discourage the training of new specialists, which would bring into question the need for regulatory initiatives. National data were used to assess the effects of managed care on the supply of and demand for primary care and specialist physicians, including physician incomes, practice locations, and the specialty choices of new physicians.

Methods.—The analysis used data from the Socioeconomic Monitoring System of the American Medical Association (AMA), which comprises a nationally representative, 1% random sample of postresidency physicians providing patient care. The growth of managed care from 1985 to 1993 was assessed for its impact on inflation-adjusted physician incomes and the physician-to-population ratios for primary care physicians and specialists. Trends in specialty choices among new physicians were analyzed using data from the National Residency Matching Program.

TABLE 1.—Growth in Managed Care Penetration, 50 U.S. States and District of Columbia, 1985–1993

Quartile	Percentage increase in physician revenues from managed care
Lowest Alabama, Alaska, Arkansas, Delaware, Kentucky, Maine, Mississippi, Montana, Pennsylvania, South Carolina, South Dakota, West Virginia, Wyoming	1.6–10.1
Second Georgia, Hawaii, Idaho, Indiana, Iowa, New Hampshire, Nevada, New York, North Carolina, North Dakota, Ohio, Oregon, Utah, Wisconsin	12.6–15.8
Third Arizona, Florida, Illinois, Louisiana, Nebraska, New Mexico, Oklahoma, Rhode Island, Tennessee, Texas, Virginia, Washington DC	17.0–20.9
Highest California, Colorado, Connecticut, Kansas, New Jersey, Maryland, Massachusetts, Michigan, Minnesota, Missouri, Vermont, Washington state	21.4–30.7

(Courtesy of Simon CJ, Dranove D, White WD: The impact of managed care on the physician marketplace. *Public Health Rep* 112:222–230, 1997.)

Results.—During the study period, the incomes of primary care physicians grew by 4.78% per year in states with the highest rates of managed care growth compared with 1.20% in states with the lowest managed care growth rates (Table 1). This translated into a cumulative increase of $33,526 for physicians in states with the highest rates of managed care growth and $7,448 for physicians in states with the lowest rate. In contrast, income for medical and surgical subspecialists increased at a similar rate, regardless of managed care growth (2.5% to 4% per year) (Table 2). Managed care also affected the incomes of radiologists, anesthesiologists, and pathologists (RAPs): their annual increase was 0.14% ($1,700) in the highest quartile of managed care growth vs. 4.14% ($58,558) in the lowest quartile.

Managed care growth had no impact on the number of subspecialists per capita. However, the number of RAPs per capita grew fastest in states in the lowest quartile of managed care growth. The 1990s saw a 32% increase in the number of family practice and pediatric residency positions filled, no change in the number of medical and surgical subspecialty positions filled, and a 14% decrease in the number of RAP positions filled.

Conclusions.—As managed care spreads, income growth is greatest for primary care physicians and least for RAP physicians. Areas with the least managed care growth are seeing an increasing number of RAP physicians.

TABLE 2.—Growth in Physician Income by Quartile, 1985–1993

Increase in median real physician income

Quartile	Primary care			Subspecialists			Radiologists, anesthesiologists, and pathologists		
	Annual growth rate*	Real dollar change†	P	Annual growth rate	Real dollar change	P	Annual growth rate	Real dollar change	P
Lowest	1.20	7,448	0.04‡	3.15	39,417	0.03‡	4.14	58,558	0.01‡
Second	3.27	21,705	… ‖	3.62	46,109	… ‖	3.30	45,450	… ‖
Third	3.63	24,489	0.03§	4.08	52,743	… ‖	3.27	44,802	… ‖
Highest	4.78	33,526	0.05§	2.55	31,260	… ‖	0.14	1,701	0.03§
P-value, all quartiles equal			0.01¶			… **			0.01¶

*Annualized percentage rate of growth in median real physician income.
†Cumulative real dollar growth in median physician income.
‡Significantly different from 0.
§Significantly different from the lowest quartile.
‖Not significantly different from the lowest quartile.
¶Significantly different from each other.
**Not significantly different from each other.
(Courtesy of Simon CJ, Dranove D, White WD: The impact of managed care on the physician marketplace. *Public Health Rep* 112:222–230, 1997.)

Managed care appears to have had little impact on the income and practice location of medical and surgical subspecialists. The number of primary care residency positions filled is increasing as the number of RAP positions filled decreases.

▶ Managed care has had an equalizing effect on physician incomes and has provided an incentive to enter primary care careers. This article nicely documents these changes over approximately 10 years. Despite all of the negative rhetoric about managed care from practicing primary care physicians, these effects must be seen as positive.

J.E. Scherger, M.D., M.P.H.

The Two Cultures and the Health Care Revolution: Commerce and Professionalism in Medical Care

McArthur JH, Moore FD (Harvard Business School, Boston; Harvard Med School, Boston; Partners HealthCare Inc, Boston)
JAMA 277:985–989, 1997

21–13

Introduction.—Two distinct cultural traditions, the commercial and the professional, have shared a central role in the evolution of U.S. society and its institutions. The quality and scope of medical care is now threatened by the invasion of commerce into the profession of medicine. There is conflict between these cultures, and there are hazards in commercial medicine. A national agency in the private sector should set standards for medical care.

The Two Cultures.—The essential image of a medical professional is that of a practitioner who values the patient's welfare above his or her own. In contrast, the goal of commerce in providing medical care is to achieve an excess of revenue over costs. Reductions in volume or quality of services are central to reduction of costs and increase of profit. Physician-employees of a corporation cease to act as free agents and owe their primary loyalty to the for-profit employer. Some physicians and administrators in commercial health systems receive earnings beyond the reasonable and customary rewards for such services.

Potential Hazards of Commercial Medicine.—Specific dangers include diversion of funds from care of the sick to corporate objectives, price increases to ensure profitability, denial of care to those most in need (and potentially most expensive to treat), and shifting of the burden of caring for patients at high risk to public providers. Personnel who are most highly qualified may be discharged in an attempt to save money by using employees with less experience and fewer credentials. Gag rules, which prevent criticism of quality of care, constitute loss of free speech. Compromises of clinical care place the physician in an ethical dilemma, torn between patient needs and business practices. Physicians are increasingly becoming entrepreneurs, and hospitals are turning away from community responsibility, teaching, and research.

The Need for Standards.—A new national agency is proposed, one that would establish standards applicable to all prepaid health plans, corporate providers, HMOs, and managed care plans, whether for profit or non-profit. This National Council on Medical Care would also provide an approval mechanism that would be the basis for state enforcement through licensing. Two models are outlined, one growing out of the National Academy of Sciences and the other with a consortium of national charitable foundations as the initiating force. It is hoped that the health care industry's cooperation with such an agency would provide a public standard of acceptance and uniformly high quality of service, merging medical professionalism with the constraints of commercial enterprise.

▶ It is becoming increasingly clear that the United States will not have a government-run health care system, but rather a combination of systems that operate in a commercial market. Because of the importance of health care to society, a national agency is necessary to ensure quality and regulate against abuse. This article provides an important perspective on how such a national agency might be formed, and on the important issues that it must address.

J.E. Scherger, M.D., M.P.H.

Extending Health Maintenance Organization Insurance to the Uninsured: A Controlled Measure of Health Care Utilization
Bograd H, Ritzwoller DP; Calonge N, et al (Kaiser Permanente of Colorado, Denver)
JAMA 277:1067–1072, 1997   21–14

Introduction.—The more than 42 million Americans who are now without health insurance may eventually become insured by an HMO. Previous studies have found that the uninsured, who have less access to health services, also use fewer health services than the insured. To determine whether the previously uninsured would exhibit high rates of utilization once they received HMO coverage, perhaps because of a large pent-up demand, a group of previously uninsured, low-income patients were compared with a control group of newly enrolled patients drawn from a commercially insured HMO population.

Methods.—The study setting was Kaiser Permanente of Colorado, a prepaid group-model, non-profit HMO, which began a dues-subsidy program for the medically uninsured in late 1991. Financial eligibility was established at or below an income of 200% of the federal poverty level. Patients eligible for Medicaid were not accepted, and coverage was limited to a once-in-a-lifetime 24-month period. Utilization data were collected for the period from January 1992 through December 31, 1993. The study group included 346 previously uninsured patients and 382 controls with a similar age and sex distribution and the same benefits package.

Results.—The study group had a significantly higher total of outpatient visits per enrollee per year, but stratification by type of visit showed that differences existed only for specialty care visits. No differences were observed between study and control groups in number of visits for mental health or for emergent or urgent care. The 2 groups were also similar in hospital admissions and hospital days and in prescriptions, laboratory tests, and number of radiographic tests. When participants were surveyed on health status measures, the study group reported a significantly lower self-perceived health status. As noted in other studies of low-income populations, children in the study group spent significantly more days in bed and missed significantly more days of school because of illness than control children. Both study and control groups used fewer services with increasing distance from the time of HMO enrollment.

Conclusion.—Previously uninsured, low-income patients used no more costly services, such as hospital admissions and radiology services, than control subjects with similar HMO coverage. Although outpatient visits were 30% higher during any month of the 2-year study period for study patients, about half of this increase was related to their worse self-perception of health status.

▶ There is a common belief that low-income, uninsured patients generate higher health care costs than the general population. In addition, it is believed that a previously uninsured population, given comprehensive insurance coverage, would result in a wave of utilization of services. This study suggests that both of these beliefs are myths. Those working in the health care system, especially in emergency rooms, get exposed to a skewed segment of the low-income, uninsured population. Many such persons stay at home without health care and will not seek health care more than the normal population, even if given the chance. Negative attitudes regarding the uninsured should not get in the way of expanding health care coverage to this population.

J.E. Scherger, M.D., M.P.H.

Costs of Care and Administration at For-Profit and Other Hospitals in the United States
Woolhandler S, Himmelstein DU (Cambridge Hosp, Mass; Harvard Med School, Boston)
N Engl J Med 336:769–774, 1997   21–15

Background.—Studies performed in 1990 showed that administrative costs account for one fourth of total U.S. hospital costs, a proportion nearly double that found in Canada. Studies from the 1970s and 1980s have documented high costs—particularly administrative costs—at for-profit hospitals. Medicare data were used to compare administrative costs of for-profit and not-for-profit hospitals.

Methods.—The analysis included fiscal-year 1994 data on administrative costs for 6,227 nonfederal hospitals and on total inpatient care costs at 5,201 acute care hospitals. Data for 1990 were considered as well. Administrative costs were compared for private not-for-profit, and public hospitals. The findings were adjusted for type and size of hospital, geographic area, and proportion of revenues for outpatient care. The data on inpatient costs were adjusted for local wages, reporting periods, and case mix.

Results.—Administrative costs as a percentage of total hospital costs rose in 1990 to 26.0% in 1994. For-profit hospitals saw a greater rise, 2.2%, to a total of 34.0%. The increase was 1.2%, to a total of 24.5%, for private not-for-profit hospitals, and by 0.6%, to 22.9%, for public hospitals. At psychiatric hospitals, administrative costs were 44.4% at for-profit hospitals. At rehabilitation hospitals, the figures were 33.0%. On multivariate analysis, for-profit status raised the administrative proportion of total spending by 7.9% compared with public hospitals and by 5.7% compared with private not-for-profit hospitals. Adjusted cost per discharge was $8,115 at acute care for-profit hospitals vs. $7,490 at private not-for-profit and $6,507 at public hospitals. The administrative component of these costs per discharge was $2,289, $1,809, and $1,432, respectively.

The findings were little affected when alternative methods of allocating care maintenance costs were considered. Neither were they attributable to a small number of high-cost hospitals. For-profit hospitals had higher costs across geographic ranges and in 75 hospitals that switched to for-profit ownership between 1990 and 1994, administrative costs increased by an average of 2.5%, compared with a 0.4% increase at 105 hospitals with not-for-profit or public status during that period. Wage and salary costs were lower for short-term general hospitals. Almost all of this difference was related to lower costs for clinical personnel.

Conclusions.—For-profit hospitals have higher administrative costs and higher costs per inpatient day and per discharge than do private not-for-profit hospitals. The cost figures may underestimate total overhead. It is uncertain why administrative costs are rising in for-profit hospitals—the shortened lengths of stay at these institutions have not resulted in lower costs per admission. Market forces appear to be "upsizing," rather than downsizing, administrative costs. The findings raise question about whether our recent reliance on market forces to lower health care costs is having the desired effect.

▶ One of the great problems of health care, if not a scandal, is the large amount of health care dollars that go into administration. Health care has become a big business in the United States, now consuming 15% of all expenditures (gross national product). Running hospitals as profit-centered businesses results in extensive administration. Hopefully, the 21st century will produce greater efficiency, with more health care dollars going into actual health care.

J.E. Scherger, M.D., M.P.H.

Racial and Ethnic Disparities in the Use of Cardiovascular Procedures: Associations With Type of Health Insurance

Carlisle DM, Leake BD, Shapiro MF (Univ of California, Los Angeles)
Am J Public Health 87:263–267, 1997   21–16

Background.—Coronary heart disease is the leading cause of death among African Americans, Latinos, and Asian Americans. Possible disparities in the use of cardiovascular procedures in these populations compared with whites, within health insurance categories, were investigated.

Methods.—Data were obtained from the hospital discharge records of Los Angeles County residents with possible coronary artery disease. A total of 104,952 charts were reviewed.

Findings.—The odds of procedure use were found to be lower for African American and Latino patients for most types of insurance, after adjustment for confounding variables. The odds of procedure use among Asians and Pacific Islanders were comparable to those of white patients. There were no such disparities among the privately insured.

Conclusion.—Race- and ethnicity-related disparities in the use of cardiovascular procedures were evident for all insurance types except private insurance. Of particular concern is the finding that HMO enrollment does not reduce disparities for African American and Latino patients.

▶ This is an interesting and disturbing study of differences in aggressiveness in diagnosing and treating cardiovascular disease by ethnicity. The authors did a retrospective study of patients discharged from Los Angeles County hospitals with diagnoses related to coronary artery disease. They abstracted over 100,000 charts. Although it was a retrospective study, the large number of study subjects adds to the power of the findings. The authors were able to compare numbers and types of procedures by ethnicity and type of insurance payment. Their findings were consistent across all insurance types except private fee-for-service insurance.

Does this study show racism in our approach to our patients? I don't know. I cannot see any other reason for the significantly lower rates of cardiac catheterization and subsequent intervention between black and Latino patients on the one hand, and white and Asian patients on the other. My purpose in including this study is simply to raise our collective awareness that this may be an issue and that we must try as hard as possible to make decisions based on medical criteria, which are blind to gender or ethnicity.

R.C. Davidson, M.D., M.P.H.

Cost Reduction Strategies

Effect of Mandatory Radiology Consultation on Inpatient Imaging Use: A Randomized Controlled Trial

Bree RL, Kazerooni EA, Katz SJ (Univ of Michigan, Ann Arbor)
JAMA 276:1595–1598, 1996

21–17

Background.—Utilization review for diagnostic imaging has been widely adopted because of the belief that these tests are used excessively, but there is no consensus on the best technique for controlling utilization. A randomized, controlled trial examined the effect of mandatory consultation service on radiology resource use in inpatient internal medicine services. The authors hypothesized that radiology resource use would be lowered by at least 20% through the mechanism of request denials or changes.

Methods.—The study setting was 4 internal medicine services at a university hospital. Six radiologists performed the intervention on 2 of the services over a 12-month period; the other 2 services served as controls. A total of 1,022 patients were admitted to intervention services and 1,178 to control services. All radiology studies except emergencies required approval by the attending radiologist. Consultants were urged to substitute lower-cost, but equally effective, tests for higher-cost tests. Four classes of radiology tests were examined: x-ray, MRI, CT, and ultrasonography.

Results.—Outcome was determined on the basis of relative resource costs, number of examinations per patient, proportion of patients with 1 or more tests, and mean length of stay. Relative resource costs were measured in relative value units (RVUs). The intervention and control groups were similar in age, sex, and distribution of diagnosis-related groups (DRGs). Mean RVUs did not differ significantly for intervention (356.1) and control (336.0) groups, even after adjustment for differences in DRGs. The mean quantity of examinations per admission, the percentage of patients having radiology examinations, and the length of stay were all similar or identical for the mandatory consultation and control services.

Discussion.—Radiology resource use was not reduced in these internal medicine services by the implementation of a mandatory precertification program for inpatients. The consultation was time consuming, and only a few requests were denied. Managed care organizations might achieve cost savings, however, if outpatient radiology resource use was targeted.

▶ I loved this one: an experiment that failed. Journal editors often forego publishing "negative" studies: most research that makes it into print demonstrates that whatever it is "works." Why publish this one? The results are surprising, for one thing. One might have expected an intervention of this intensity to produce the intended outcome. The message in this study importantly points out that untested interventions are just that: untested. The findings should have a cautionary effect on those who may be implementing utilization review schemes merely because they "make sense."

I was puzzled by the authors' concluding comments that outpatient resource use might be a better target. I would guess that the variety of outpatient problems and the subtleties of use of x-ray studies in the outpatient setting would confound attempts at intervention just as surely as in the hospital. Also, I would think the cost of the intervention would be higher because of the inherently lower efficiency of the consulting process in the ambulatory setting.

A.O. Berg, M.D., M.P.H.

Assessment of Joint Review of Radiologic Studies by a Primary Care Physician and a Radiologist

Knollmann BC, Corson AP, Twigg HL, et al (Univ Med Ctr, Washington, DC; George Washington Univ, Washington, DC)
J Gen Intern Med 11:608–612, 1996   21–18

Background.—Data supporting the practice of reviewing radiologic studies by primary care physicians in hospital settings are limited. The error rate of initial radiologic diagnosis is 20% to 30%, but this improves after further clinical information is obtained. A joint review of radiographs by a radiologist and a primary care physician may improve diagnostic accuracy.

Methods.—All radiologic studies ordered during a 1-year period at a college health clinic were reviewed by both the clinic physician and radiologist. The net cost of this review process was calculated. The outcome measures were (1) a change of radiologic diagnosis and patient management and (2) cost of the review process.

Results.—There were 323 films ordered, of which 305 were reviewed. Revision of the initial reading occurred in 23 films. Of these revisions, 16 resulted in a change in patient management; the other revisions were clinically insignificant. Revision of the 16 readings simplified or eliminated further workup and resulted in a savings of nearly $2,000. The cost of the extra physician time was $5,500. The net cost of the review process was just over $3,500. For the patients, fewer diagnostic studies were needed, but there was no other therapeutic benefit. The positive predictive value of the readings was 85%, and the negative predictive value was 99.7%.

Discussion.—This population was young and in good health, and the review process had little effect on patient management or outcome. The process may have been more cost-effective if only abnormal films had been reviewed. Routine review of all radiographs may be more beneficial in populations with a higher rate of disease.

▶ This study is the health services research equivalent of a clinical study on patient outcomes because it tests a health services intervention in a typical clinical setting, determining the real effect in a real setting. The authors provide powerful evidence that radiologist overread of all films is unnecessary and costly in a typical low-prevalence primary care setting. As the authors point out, the findings are especially relevant for settings in which a radiology "carve out" is being considered, removing the radiologist from the immediate clinical setting and making the readings harder to link to the clinical circumstances. This article is an important bit of information if you are in a position to influence the provision of radiology services to primary care physicians.

A.O. Berg, M.D., M.P.H.

Outcomes of Patients With No Laboratory Assessment Before Anesthesia and a Surgical Procedure

Narr BJ, Warner ME, Schroeder DR, et al (Mayo Clinic, Rochester, Minn)
Mayo Clin Proc 72:505–509, 1997   21–19

Purpose.—Previous studies have found that preoperative tests have little or no impact on the outcomes of anesthesia and surgery. The authors' center has therefore stopped performing routine preoperative screening tests on healthy surgical patients younger than 40 years. The impact of this policy change on perioperative morbidity was assessed.

Methods.—The retrospective study included 56,119 patients undergoing surgical or diagnostic procedures with anesthesia during 1 calendar year. Of these, 5,120 patients had no laboratory tests performed within 90 days before their elective surgical procedure. A random sample of 1,044 such patients was analyzed to demonstrate the absence of preoperative tests, the presence of pre-existing disease, the type of anesthetic used, and the intraoperative and postoperative test outcomes. The patients' median age was 21 years, with a range from 0 to 95 years. The study was designed to demonstrate, with a 95% confidence level, that true morbidity was less than 0.4%.

Results.—None of the patients died or experienced major morbidity. Although blood typing and screening were performed in 10 patients, none required blood transfusion. During surgery, 17 laboratory tests and 1 ECG were performed; the results were abnormal in 3 of these. Of 42 blood tests performed postoperatively, 5 showed abnormal results, most often the hemoglobin level. One of the 2 ECGs performed postoperatively showed premature ventricular contractions; otherwise, both were normal. None of the intraoperative or postoperative tests altered the patients' medical or surgical management. One patient undergoing outpatient surgery had unexpected blood loss and was hospitalized for observation.

Conclusions.—This study demonstrates the absence of perioperative morbidity in patients undergoing no laboratory tests before anesthesia and surgery. As long as the history and physical examination show no preoperative indications for laboratory tests, anesthesia and surgery can be safely performed without routine testing. Intraoperative and postoperative tests can be ordered as indicated.

▶ Findings from this study are less than completely satisfying because the design was a simple case series, although quite a large one. Still, it provides some of the first outcome data showing that the academic surmise of little benefit of testing in low-risk patients is likely correct. The authors do not provide specific criteria for what "relatively healthy" means, but given the likelihood that Mayo physicians are more aggressive than most in ordering possibly useful laboratory testing, a common-sense approach regarding whether a young person is healthy is not likely to get you into trouble if you choose not to obtain "routine" preoperative tests.

A.O. Berg, M.D., M.P.H.

Adverse Events and Medical Malpractice

Adverse Drug Events in Hospitalized Patients: Excess Length of Stay, Extra Costs, and Attributable Mortality

Classen DC, Pestotnik SL, Evans RS, et al (LDS Hosp, Salt Lake City, Utah)
JAMA 277:301–306, 1997
21–20

Introduction.—Adverse drug events (ADEs) account for a major proportion of drug-related morbidity and mortality, and may be responsible for up to 140,000 deaths in the United States each year. About 30% of hospitalized patients have an adverse event attributable to drugs during their stay. There are no specific data on the effects of ADEs on mortality, length of hospital stay, or resource utilization. The impact of ADEs during hospitalization on length of stay, costs, and mortality was analyzed.

Methods.—The case-control study included 1,580 patients with ADEs occurring during their stay at a tertiary care hospital. They were matched to 20,197 control subjects for primary discharge diagnosis-related group, age, sex, acuity, and year of admission. The 2 groups were compared for mortality and length of stay, both crude and attributable to ADEs. Hospital costs also were compared.

Results.—The rate of ADEs during the 4-year period studied was 2.43 per 100 hospital admissions. The crude mortality rate was 3.5% for the patients with ADEs vs. 1.05% for the control subjects. The mean length of stay was 7.69 days for patients vs. 4.46 days for control subjects, with an extra 1.74 days attributable to ADEs. Mean hospital costs were $10,010 vs. $5,355, with an extra cost of $2,013 attributable to ADEs. On linear regression analysis, an ADE increased the length of stay by 1.91 days and hospital costs by $2,262. In a logistic regression analysis, patients with an ADE were at a 1.88 times higher risk of death.

Conclusions.—Adverse drug events carry a significant impact for hospitalized patients. These events are associated with increased lengths of stay, higher hospital costs, and a nearly doubled risk of death. Adverse drug events have major potential costs to the hospital and to the nation as a whole. A system-wide approach to improving the processes of drug use, including monitoring for ADEs, is recommended.

▶ It takes courage to publish an article like this, in which one raises a quality of care issue in one's home institution. Most physicians would not be surprised to find similar results at their own hospitals. This article appeared in an issue of *JAMA* containing 3 other articles or editorials on the subject, all tending to raise the level of concern about adverse drug events. If these results are typical, and I can think of few reasons to doubt it, the increases in length of stay, costs, and mortality become enormous when multiplied by the number of hospitalizations occurring nationwide each year. Of course, hospitals have been aware of the problem for a long time, although perhaps not its dimensions. There is even an emerging research base to suggest the educational and management structures that stand a chance of addressing the problem. This is an issue to bring to your hospital quality improvement team.

A.O. Berg, M.D., M.P.H.

Relation Between Negligent Adverse Events and the Outcomes of Medical-malpractice Litigation
Brennan TA, Sox CM, Burstin HR (Harvard School of Public Health, Boston)
N Engl J Med 335:1963–1967, 1996   21–21

Introduction.—Malpractice research indicates that many medical injuries caused by physician negligence do not lead to claims, whereas many of the claims that are brought do not involve any medical injury or demonstrable physician negligence. However, the litigation system can still be accurate if compensation is awarded only for the cases in which it is merited. Factors predicting payment to plaintiffs were studied to assess the relation between negligent adverse events and the outcomes of malpractice litigation.

Methods.—Fifty-one litigated medical malpractice claims were followed up for 10 years to see whether the malpractice insurer had closed the case. The outcome of each case was predicted on the basis of detailed case summaries obtained from the insurers. The litigation files were reviewed when the actual outcome differed from the predicted outcome.

Results.—Forty-six of the 51 cases were closed at the time of the review. Twenty-four cases were classified as involving no adverse event; of these, 10 were settled for the plaintiff, with a mean payment of nearly $29,000. Also settled for the plaintiff were 6 of 13 cases involving adverse events but no negligence, with a mean payment of about $98,000, and 5 of 9 cases involving adverse events caused by negligence, with a mean payment of $67,000. These included 7 of 8 claims involving permanent disability, with a mean payment of $201,250. Permanent disability was the only factor significantly associated with payment on multivariate analysis. Payment was unrelated to adverse events of any type, including those caused by negligence.

Conclusions.—In malpractice cases, the size of the payment is related to the severity of the patient's disability, not to the occurrence of an adverse event or an adverse event caused by negligence. The results question the reliance on determinations of negligence when considering compensation for medical injury. No-fault compensation and other malpractice litigation reforms may be more effective in compensating injured patients and avoiding preventable medical injuries.

▶ This is an important article that, in the end, supports the idea of no-fault medical malpractice insurance. The size of malpractice awards is related to the severity of the patient's disability, not the "magnitude" of the negligence. Here is the direct quote from the article that says it all: "If the permanence of a disability, not the fact of negligence, is the reason for compensation, the determination of negligence may be an expensive sideshow." In the medical malpractice environment of the future, a no-fault system surely makes more sense than what we have.

A.O. Berg, M.D., M.P.H.

Physician-Patient Communication: The Relationship With Malpractice Claims Among Primary Care Physicians and Surgeons
Levinson W, Roter DL, Mullooly JP, et al (Oregon Health Sciences Univ, Portland; Johns Hopkins Univ, Baltimore, Md; Kaiser Found Hosps Ctrs for Health Research, Portland, Ore; et al)
JAMA 277:553–559, 1997

21–22

Background.—Malpractice litigation tends to occur at the conjunction of bad outcome and patient dissatisfaction. Patient dissatisfaction may occur as a result of problems with communication. To evaluate the association between communication behaviors and malpractice litigation history, routine communications between physicians and patients were taped and analyzed.

Study Design.—This study was designed to compare the routine communication style of physicians with and without a history of malpractice litigation and stratified by years of practice and specialty. The study was conducted in 1993 in Oregon and Colorado and included primary care physicians and surgeons. Communication style was evaluated through audiotapes of 10 sequential office visits for each of the 124 physicians who participated in this study. The participating physicians were 94% male and 92% white. Patients were eligible if they were at least 18 years of age, spoke English, were not in acute distress, and were not on their initial visit to the physician. Eighty-five percent of the participating patients were white, 63% were college-educated, and 45% were male. The 1,265 audiotapes were coded for content by 3 trained, blinded coders using the Roter Interaction Analysis System (RIAS).

Results.—Compared to primary care physicians with previous malpractice claims, those without claims spent more time on patient education and orientation, used more humor, and tended to use more facilitation. The physicians without prior claims spent more time with each patient than those with prior claims. Although these differences in communication style were relevant for primary care physicians, they could not be used to distinguish between surgeons who had prior malpractice claims and those with no history of malpractice claims.

Conclusions.—This study of physician-patient communication behavior identified differences in the communication style between primary care physicians with no history of malpractice claims and those with a history of malpractice claims. Physicians and insurers can use these findings to improve communication and decrease the risk of malpractice litigation for primary care physicians. These communication behaviors did not explain the difference between surgeons with no history of malpractice claims and those with a history of claims. It cannot be assumed that these communication behaviors are equally appropriate or important for all specialty groups.

▶ Communication is considered important for risk management in the prevention of malpractice claims. This is the most elaborate study I have seen on this issue, and includes large insurance plans from Colorado and Oregon. It is interesting to note that communication is an important factor in avoiding claims for primary care physicians, but not for surgeons. Spending more time educating patients certainly pays off with respect to avoiding the high expenses of malpractice claims. I found it interesting that laughing and using humor was also a significant factor, suggesting that a personable and enjoyable relationship between the doctor and patient is important.

J.E. Scherger, M.D., M.P.H.

22 Miscellaneous

Introduction

This selection of abstracts contains studies that are nonetheless important if defying usual clinical categories. I found especially interesting the articles on the effects of obtaining consultation on various hospital outcomes, the growing prevalence of latex allergy, and the (once again) discouraging evidence of the appropriateness of information distributed by drug companies.

Alfred O. Berg, M.D., M.P.H.

Infectious Diseases Consultation: Impact on Outcomes for Hospitalized Patients and Results of a Preliminary Study

Classen DC, Burke JP, Wenzel RP (LDS Hosp, Salt Lake City, Utah; Med College of Virginia, Richmond; Virginia Commonwealth Univ, Richmond)
Clin Infect Dis 24:468–470, 1997   22–1

Background.—Ongoing changes in the health care system will substantially reduce the need for many highly specialized physicians in the United States. With more attention focused on cost containment, some research studies suggest that resource use is higher with medical specialists than with generalists. Infectious diseases physicians, who provide services beyond direct patient care and consultation, may be shielded from such changes if the value of their contributions can be demonstrated. A preliminary study was conducted to examine the crude impact of an inpatient infectious disease consultation on use of resources and length of hospital stay.

Methods.—The study site was the LDS Hospital, a tertiary care facility in Salt Lake City. Data were obtained from HELP (health evaluation through logical processing), an information system used at the hospital for more than 15 years. Costs were calculated with a microcomputer software system (Standard Cost Manager) electronically linked to the HELP system. After the crude economic impact of an inpatient infectious diseases consultation was determined, important matching variables were identified for more refined analysis.

Results.—A total of 496 patients who were seen by an infectious diseases consultant (cases) were matched with 3,117 patients who were not seen by an infectious diseases consultant (controls). The 2 groups were matched on the basis of age, sex, exact discharge diagnosis–related group, length of hospital stay, and 2 measures of severity of illness (nursing acuity score and number of secondary diagnoses). No attempt was made to match for the exact site of infection. Compared with controls, cases had a longer mean hospital stay (14.7 vs. 8.97 days), a longer, mean ICU stay (4.59 vs. 2.6 days), used a higher number of different antibiotics (mean, 2.7 vs. 1.26) and had higher antibiotic costs (mean, $1,448 vs. $446). An opposite trend appeared, however, when consultations performed during the last one third of hospitalization were analyzed. In this setting, cases had a shorter length of hospital stay and lower antibiotic costs.

Conclusion.—Infectious disease practitioners contribute most of their effort to direct patient care, and the crude impact of inpatient infectious disease consultations is to increase hospital and ICU stay, antibiotic use, and antibiotic costs. But such consultations may indicate a more severely ill patient, and severity of illness was not adequately controlled for in the design of this study.

▶ I selected this preliminary study to use as a touchstone, and perhaps as a cautionary tale. A disturbing trend in medicine was illustrated to me recently in a most uncomfortable way. While signing my son in for his allergy shots, there, next to the sign-in list, was the face sheet of an article, highlighted by the allergist, claiming generalists should not/could not provide adequate care for asthma and allergy. This certainly raised my ire but also got me thinking, and talking with some of my specialist colleagues. Although this article, at first blush, seemed to point to more cost-effective care without involving an infectious disease specialist, the data really provided no firm basis for any conclusions on the matter.

I fully understand the economic pressures on specialists in the current climate of managed care. I also enjoy what has been tagged the "gatekeeper" role (though not the paperwork). However, it seems that this has created an unhealthy competition between specialists and primary care physicians, evidenced by the recent spate of articles — typically by specialists — arguing for recapturing their "market share." Money, or — more to the point — real or perceived loss of income is what seems to be the force behind these articles, despite the stated intention of evaluating outcomes.

The authors of the article abstracted here, at least, freely state that the impetus for this article was "financial risk." Should outcomes truly differ (read these articles carefully!), then, by all means, let's all (primary care physicians, specialists, administrators, patients) come to the table and figure out the best scheme for achieving desired outcomes. Frankly, even were the system to train many more allergists, we could not possibly supply enough to care for the number of people (15% of the population) with asthma. There needs to continue to be dialogue and collegiality. I would like to think the sniping will stop. It will not. I suspect this is just the beginning. Open the dialogue now.

W.W. Dexter, M.D.

Sudden Death in Young Competitive Athletes: Clinical, Demographic, and Pathological Profiles
Maron BJ, Shirani J, Poliac LC, et al (Minneapolis Heart Inst Found, Minn; Albert Einstein College of Medicine, Bronx, NY, et al)
JAMA 276:199–204, 1996   22–2

Objective.—There is no general agreement on characteristics of cardiovascular malformations that contribute to the sudden death of young competitive athletes nor on the value of preparticipation examination in identifying those athletes at risk. A clinical and pathologic profile of young athletes who died suddenly was developed.

Methods.—A prospective analysis of autopsy reports and information gleaned from interviews with family, witnesses, and coaches was performed for 158 U.S. athletes with no evidence of drug use who died suddenly from 1985 through 1995. Diagnostic cardiovascular evaluations were conducted.

Results.—In 24 patients, death was the result of noncardiovascular causes. The remaining 134 athletes (90% male), aged 12–40 years, were 52% white, 44% black, 2% Asian, 0.5% Hispanic, and 0.5% Native American. Most of the athletes (62%) were in high school, 30% were in college, 9% were professional, and 9% were in junior high school. Most (62%) played basketball or football. Most (90%) collapsed during or immediately after playing or practicing and died instantaneously, 63% between 3 and 9 PM. Hypertrophic cardiomyopathy was the most common cause of death (36%) and was significantly more prevalent in black athletes (all male) (48%) than in white athletes (26%). Coronary anomalies were responsible for 13% of deaths; 6 of 14 female athletes who died suddenly had coronary anomalies. Only 4 of 115 athletes who had preparticipation evaluations had suspected cardiac disease, and only 1, with Marfan's syndrome, received a correct diagnosis.

Conclusion.—Sudden death of young athletes commonly occurs during or after playing or practicing and is most often the result of hypertrophic cardiomyopathy. In few at-risk athletes was the condition diagnosed at preparticipation evaluations.

▶ The tragedy of a young, apparently healthy athlete collapsing and dying during sports has captured public attention. Sports physicians, trainers, and coaches have come under fire to anticipate and avoid these situations. Although we all share this public health goal, this study confirms the great variation of conditions that can cause sudden death in athletes. Reasonable and optimal screening criteria have yet to be established to prevent all these conditions. Exercising at maximum capacity, something which is necessary for success in many sports, is risky behavior. Athletes and their families need to be aware that not all of this risk can be predicted and controlled.

J.E. Scherger, M.D., M.P.H.

Normal Oxyhemoglobin Saturation During Sleep: How Low Does It Go?

Gries RE, Brooks LJ (Case Western Reserve Univ, Cleveland, Ohio)
Chest 110:1489–1492, 1996
22–3

Objective.—Measurement of arterial oxyhemoglobin saturation (O_2 Sat) is useful in the diagnosis and follow-up of various respiratory disorders, including sleep apnea and chronic obstructive pulmonary disease. Reported normal nadir values for O_2 Sat vary significantly, from a low of 84% to a high of 91%. The O_2 Sat in normal subjects was determined and compared with the findings in those patients with uncomplicated obstructive sleep apnea (OSA) and asthma.

Methods.—The study included 350 subjects with no history of lung or heart disease and normal findings on overnight polysomnography. One hundred eighty-four were male, and 166 were female, and the age range was 1 month to 85 years. All underwent all-night pulse oximetry, the results of which were carefully analyzed to exclude periods of motion artifact. The analysis determined the lowest saturation point recorded during the night (Low Sat), the median saturation point (Sat 50), and the saturation point below which the patient spent 10% of the time (Sat 10).

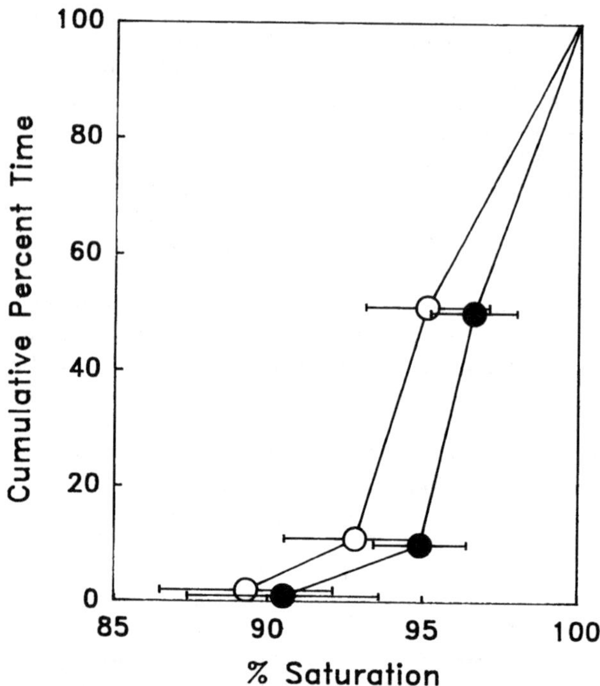

FIGURE 2.—Range of normal (mean ± 2 SDs) of O_2 saturation (Sat) for healthy research subjects younger than 60 years of age (*solid circle*) and 60 years or older (*open circle*). Points represent Low Sat, Sat 10, and Sat 50. (Courtesy of Gries RE, Brooks LJ: Normal oxyhemoglobin saturation during sleep: How low does it go? *Chest* 110:1489–1492, 1996.)

TABLE 3.—O₂ Sat in Patients with Asthma, OSA, and Healthy Control Research Subjects

	Healthy	Asthma	OSA
No. of subjects	350	21	25
Sat 50*	96.5±1.5	96.0±1.9	93.5±3.8†
Sat 10*	94.7±1.6	94.2±2.5	87.1±10.9†
Low Sat*	90.4±3.1	89.0±5.3	65.9±22.6†

*Values are means plus or minus standard deviations.
†$P < 0.005$ compared with healthy research subjects and patients with asthma.
Abbreviations: Sat, saturation; *OSA,* obstructive sleep apnea.
(Courtesy of Gries RE, Brooks LJ: Normal oxyhemoglobin saturation during sleep: How low does it go? *Chest* 110:1489–1492, 1996.)

The findings were compared with those of 25 patients with OSA and 21 patients with stable asthma.

Results.—The normal research subjects had a mean Low Sat of 90.4%, a mean Sat 50 of 96.5%, and a mean Sat 10 of 94.7%. None of these values were significantly related to sex, race, or body mass index. In research subjects older than 60 years, the mean Sat 10 was 92.8% and the mean Sat 50 was 95.1% (Fig 2). There was no difference in O₂ Sat between patients with asthma and healthy research subjects. However, all 3 values were significantly lower than normal in the patients with OSA (Table 3).

Conclusions.—This study defines the normal O₂ Sat values of healthy individuals. Values for Sat 50 and Sat 10 are reduced in older adults, perhaps because of accumulated occupational exposures and aging-related alveolar changes. Oxyhemoglobin saturation values are lower than normal in patients with OSA, especially in terms of Low Sat.

▶ With the increasing use of continuous monitoring of O₂ Sat by pulse oximetry, we are frequently left with the dilemma of what is adequate. In our own practice, we have used a relatively artificial cutoff of 90% as acceptable. This is the first study that I have found looking at a population of healthy individuals and what happens to their O₂ Sat during sleep.

This was a retrospective study of 350 people evaluated in a sleep laboratory. They excluded individuals with known problems. They divided the patients into 3 subsets: those that were healthy, those with asthma, and those with OSA.

The authors found no significant difference in O₂ Sat in healthy individuals and in patients with asthma. As expected, they found a significantly lower O₂ Sat in patients with OSA. The mean minimum level of O₂ Sat in the 350 healthy patients was 90.4%.

For me, this study gives credibility to the efficacy of using a cutoff O₂ Sat of 90% as low normal. My only hesitancy is that this is not a representative sample of patients because they were all referred to a sleep laboratory. However, it does give baseline data on what happens to the O₂ Sat in healthy patients during sleep.

R.C. Davidson, M.D., M.P.H.

Latex Allergy: Epidemiological Study of 1351 Hospital Workers

Liss GM, Sussman GL, Deal K, et al (Ontario Ministry of Labour, Canada; Univ of Toronto; McMaster Univ, Hamilton, Ont, Canada; et al)
Occup Environ Med 54:335–342, 1997

22–4

Introduction.—Allergy to natural rubber latex is an important occupational concern in recent years, especially for health care workers. A large cohort of health care workers was evaluated to determine the prevalence of latex sensitization, to assess the occupational and nonoccupational factors associated with latex allergy, and to characterize exposure from wearing gloves or airborne exposure.

Methods.—All 2,062 employees of a general hospital in Hamilton, Ontario, Canada who routinely used latex gloves were invited to take part in baseline screening consisting of a questionnaire, latex skin testing, and serum samples. Glove extracts were assayed for antigenic protein, and exposure to airborne latex protein was estimated once during summer and once during winter. The skin sensitivity to 3 latex reagents, 3 common inhalants, and 6 foods was assessed by skin prick test.

Results.—The mean (SD) latex protein concentrations were 324 (227) μg/g and 198 (104) μg/g, respectively, for powdered surgical gloves and powdered examination gloves. Of 1,326 employees who underwent testing at baseline, 160 (12.1%) tested positive to latex. Participants who were sensitive to latex were significantly more likely than their nonsensitive cohorts to be atopic, and were significantly more likely to have positive skin tests to 1 or more foods. Employees who were sensitive to latex were more likely to have work-related symptoms that included hives, eye symptoms, and wheezy or whistling chest. Laboratory workers (16.9%) and nurses and physicians (13.3%) had the highest prevalence of latex sensitivity among exposed employees. Glove consumption per health care worker for each hospital department was grouped into tertiles. The prevalence of latex skin positivity was most prominent in the higher tertiles of glove use for sterile surgical gloves, but not examination gloves.

Conclusions.—The prevalence of positive skin prick tests to latex was about 12% in this cohort of health care workers. There were positive associations between latex positivity and atopy, positive skin tests to foods, work-related symptoms, and departmental use of gloves per health care worker. Participants will be retested in 1 year to determine the incidence of development of latex sensitivity.

▶ I have become a believer. I must admit to initial skepticism about this entity, but as a result of accumulating evidence and professional experiences, I have become convinced. The authors in this study went to great lengths to prove the existence and extent of latex sensitivity in this admittedly focused population. With the explosion of the use of latex gloves over the past 2 decades, it is not surprising that the prevalence of latex sensitivity is so high. The ubiquitous nature of latex in the medical profession magnifies the problem — for the affected workers and for the employers. What will I do with this information? Be on the lookout for this entity (it's common), and look forward to the follow-up study.

W.W. Dexter, M.D.

Sleep History Is Neglected Diagnostic Information

Haponik EF, Frye AW, Richards B, et al (Bowman Gray School of Medicine, Winston Salem, NC)

J Gen Intern Med 11:759–761, 1996   22–5

Background.—Despite the prevalence and impact of sleep problems, most physicians are not formally trained in detecting or managing such problems. Little is known regarding how often physicians obtain the history needed to diagnose sleep disorders.

Methods.—The frequency of sleep histories obtained during encounters with simulated patients was determined. Twenty experienced primary care physicians, 23 uninstructed medical interns, and 22 interns who had had instruction regarding sleep disorders participated in the study.

Findings.—None of the experienced practitioners and only 13% of the uninstructed interns obtained sleep histories. However, 81.8% of the interns who had received instruction in sleep disorders asked the patients about sleep.

Conclusion.—These findings suggest a general lack of knowledge of the importance of sleep history or low prioritization of sleep among the many important issues that need to be discussed with a patient in a limited time. Focused instruction regarding sleep problems can positively affect physician behavior.

▶ Because of the type of simulated patient used, there was no cuing to the primary care physician, and, obviously, these physicians did not view a sleep history as a part of a history taken to "promote the patient's cardiovascular health." This is probably true in practice also, in spite of the association of obstructive sleep apnea with hypertension, congestive heart failure, myocardial infarction, and stroke. Are sleep questions a routine part of your written or oral review of symptoms?

M.A. Bowman, M.D., M.P.A.

The GP-Hospital Interface: Attitudes of General Practitioners to Tertiary Teaching Hospitals

Isaac DR, Gijsbers AJ, Wyman KT, et al (St Vincent's Hosp, Melbourne, Australia)

Med J Aust 166:9–12, 1997   22–6

Introduction.—During the past 30 years, general practitioners (GPs) in Australia have ceased to be involved in the public hospital care of most of their patients. Recent developments in health care, however, may serve to strengthen linkages between GPs and hospitals and other health services. A questionnaire-based survey of GPs assessed their perceptions of liaison with hospitals in their practice areas.

Methods.—The study setting was 2 tertiary teaching hospitals in inner-city Melbourne, Australia. All GPs practicing in the Melbourne and North West Melbourne Divisions of General Practice were surveyed for the study. These divisions include diverse populations, with both socioeconomic disadvantage and high socioeconomic status. The survey included questions about GPs' experiences of hospital referrals, interactions with hospitals, and responses to new initiatives.

Results.—The questionnaire was returned by 350 (60%) of the 587 GPs identified from a database. Most respondents were men (70%) in private (87%), full-time (68%) practice. In cases involving uninsured patients without urgent clinical problems or a need for immediate hospital admission, most GPs telephoned a private specialist (49%) or a GP colleague (42%). The GPs had no clear strategy for obtaining public hospitalization in semiurgent cases. When urgent admission was required, almost one third sent patients to the emergency department without first telephoning. Hospitals usually failed to notify GPs of patient admission (84%) or discharge (75%), and GPs were not told of major changes in patient condition (87%), including death. Factors regarded by GPs as important to facilitate hospital visits included adequate parking (91%), the opportunity to discuss patients with hospital staff (76%), and reimbursement (62%). Three fourths of respondents favored having GPs involved in the workup of their patients before elective admission for studies or treatment. Although shared care was generally considered desirable, many GPs voiced concerns about scarce time and about communication difficulties with the hospital.

Conclusion.—Many factors serve to prevent the development of professional relationships between GPs and hospitals. Hospitals need to develop procedures and allocate resources to improve the effectiveness of the hospital-GP liaison.

▶ In the United States, an increasing trend is for family physicians to give hospital work to hospital-based specialists. In other parts of the western world, GPs do not provide hospital care. One might assume that in such countries, well-established methods of communication provide important patient data from the hospital to the GP. This article from Australia suggests that, at least in that country, many problems occur. If the patient's personal family physician is not involved with hospital care, communication of such care to the primary care physician is critical. This article should serve as a warning to new health systems in the United States, which are increasingly separating the family physician from the hospital.

J.E. Scherger, M.D, M.P.H.

Characteristics of Materials Distributed by Drug Companies: An Evaluation of Appropriateness
Stryer D, Bero LA (Univ of California, San Francisco)
J Gen Intern Med 11:575–583, 1996   22–7

Purpose.—Drug companies provide large amounts of informational material about their products to physicians. Although the industry and many physicians find this information to be educational, others maintain that it is promotional in nature. There is little scientific knowledge about the information provided by this material, or about whether it complies with United States Food and Drug Administration (FDA) labeling regulations. The appropriateness of materials distributed by pharmaceutical companies to physicians in 3 different settings was analyzed.

Methods.—Over a 7-month period, 486 consecutive items distributed by pharmaceutical companies were collected. The materials were distributed to physicians in an internal medicine residency program, a private internist's office, and an HMO. The nature of these materials was analyzed, including the characteristics of the drugs described. The material was examined for promotional vs. educational characteristics, and its compliance with FDA regulations was assessed.

Findings.—The materials included 207 reprints, 196 advertisements, 51 general informational materials, and 32 other types of materials. Residents were more likely to receive reprints than were physicians at the private internist's office or the HMO, whereas the internist's office was more likely to receive personal correspondence. Only 10% of the drugs covered in the materials were real improvements over the other choices. Forty-two percent of the materials were non-compliant with at least 1 of 3 FDA regulations: the requirements for fair balance, instructions for use, or discussion of approved uses only. Three percent discussed unapproved uses for the drugs promoted. Promotional characteristics were seen in many materials that were not obviously promotional in nature. Scientific data to support the claims made were found in only 39% of the materials analyzed. Only 20% of the materials included new data or listed references newer than 3 years old.

Conclusions.—Some of the materials provided to physicians by drug companies contain useful information for making prescribing decisions, but many do not. These materials rarely provide any information about real treatment breakthroughs, and may fail to comply with FDA labeling regulations. The materials show both educational and promotional characteristics. Measures to reduce physicians' reliance on materials put out by the pharmaceutical companies are recommended.

▶ These findings will come as no surprise to the thoughtful physician who thinks back over the week's harvest of drug company "stuff." Of course, most of it is promotional. We deceive ourselves, however, in imagining that we can ignore the promotional and only pay attention to the "real" information. Published research (and unpublished market research) proves otherwise. It would be interesting to see what would happen if a larger proportion of the enormous investment that drug companies put into promotion could be directed in more educationally useful ways. Would drug sales increase, decrease, or stay the same? Would physicians learn to value and trust the information?

A.O. Berg, M.D., M.P.H.

Subject Index

A

Author Index

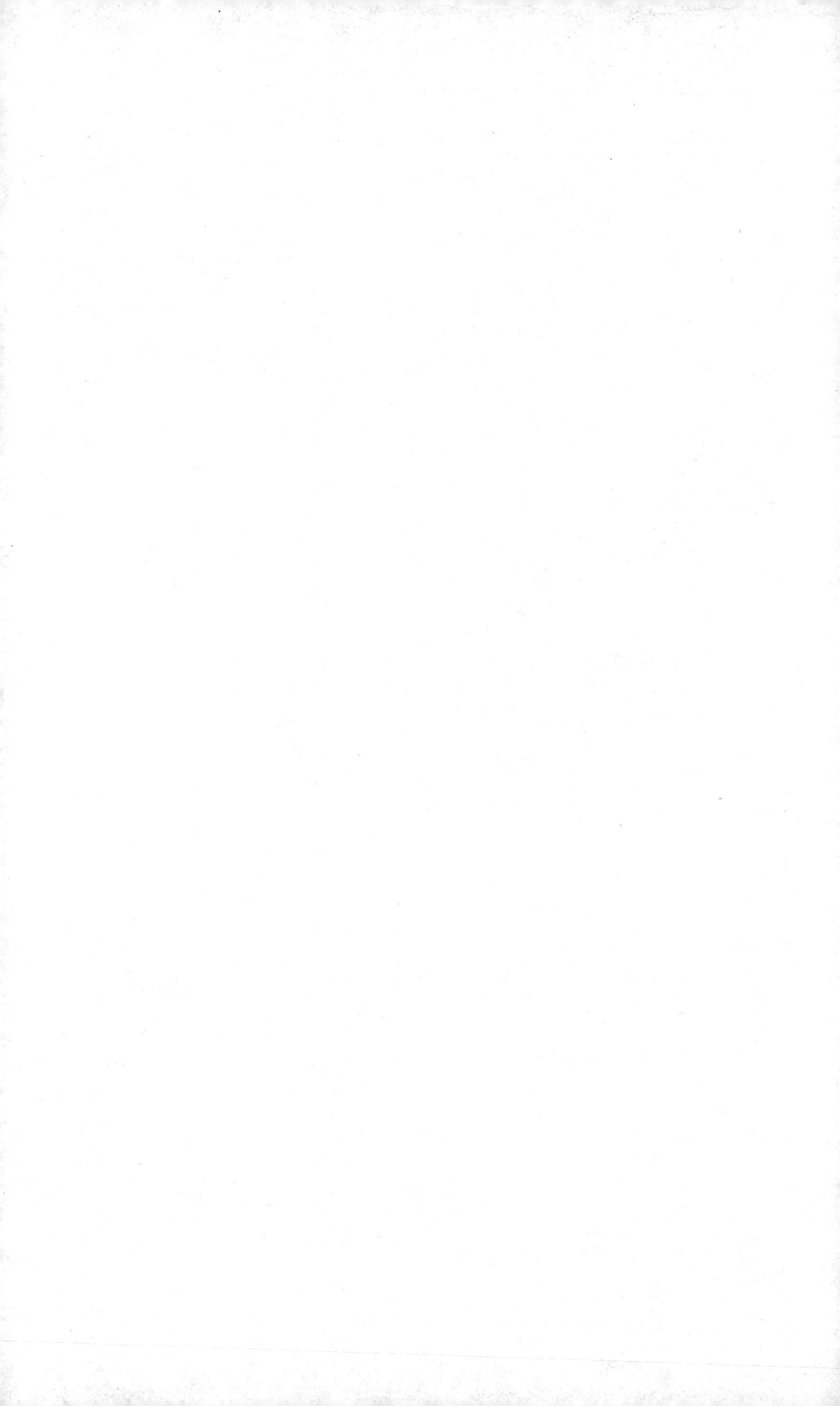